The Living Dance

An Anthology of Essays on Movement and Culture

Second Edition

Judith Chazin-Bennahum

University of New Mexico

KENDALL/HUNT PUBLISHING COMPANY
4050 Westmark Drive   Dubuque, Iowa 52002

Cover photo credit: Eva Encinias Sandoval
Photographed by Ann Bromberg in her studio, Albuquerque, New Mexico

Copyright © 2003, 2007 by Kendall/Hunt Publishing Company

ISBN 13: 978-0-7575-3924-4
ISBN 10: 0-7575-3924-6

Printed in the United States of America
10   9   8   7   6   5   4   3   2   1

Contents

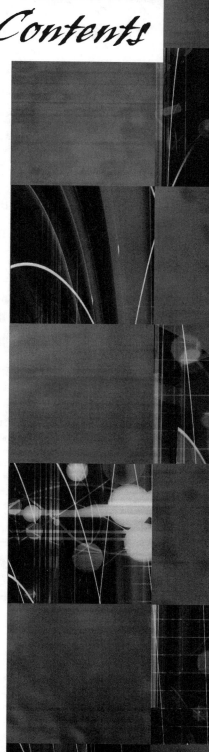

Acknowledgments

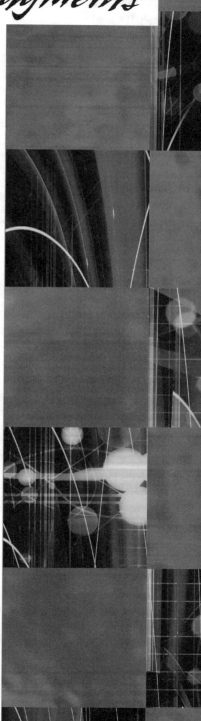

Many people have been very helpful in this endeavor to write a collection of essays on dance that is both relevant to the world of dance and to the dance in New Mexico. First I must thank my husband David for his continuing support of my work and especially for his computer worldliness. The team in my department was extremely forthcoming including Sarah Waff, our graduate student coordinator, Linda Skye, Melinda Jordan, Patricia Morris and Marvin Archuleta who encouraged me to finish this project. Interviews with Lola Lestrich and Edna McIver on African-American dance in New Mexico, Kay Brooks on Ballet in New Mexico, and Aline Chavez on the Matachines in New Mexico brought new and valuable advice to the text. Kathleen Howe led me to the wonderful Catherine Baudoin from the Maxwell Museum who aided my efforts in retrieving photos of Native-American dance. I am grateful to Lynn Garafola for astutely commenting on the introduction as did Larry Lavender and Jennifer Linnell. I thank Jill Sweet and Sally Sommer for immediately offering their articles to this project. I especially want to acknowledge Noah Carroll's early epistolary support for the chapter on modern dance. Almost the last minute, Marcia Siegel provided her usual pristine writing. We received counseling from Monica Moseley on photographs when we sought help from Phil Karg and Paul Kolnik. Eva Encinias and Maria Benitez generously gave a great deal of time to the essay on Flamenco. Finally I am deeply thankful to all the authors in this book, to Jay Hays for his charming and strong support and to Kendall/Hunt for publishing the book.

In this exciting go round of the second edition of this anthology, I am especially indebted to Melinda Jordan who took on the whole responsibility of working with the authors and the publishers, and keeping all of us on a reasonable time line with her graceful and competent nudgings. I am indebted to the authors who wished to revise and update their work, and especially to Katita Milazzo who with vim and verve agreed to create an entirely new chapter on tap and jazz. Mary Anne Newhall tastefully and perceptively offered advice on various topics that needed to be addressed. I also appreciate Brad Rahmlow's upbeat comments on hip hop and popular dance forms in New Mexico.

About the Authors

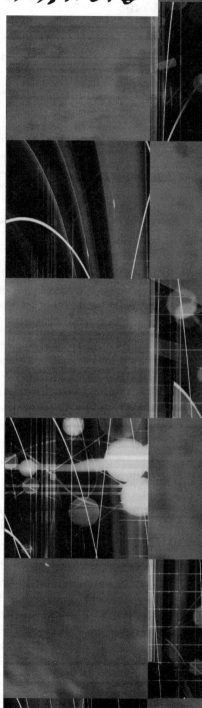

Tom Bahti is the author of the books *Southwestern Indian Ceremonials, Southwestern Indian Tribes, Southwestern Indians: Arts and Crafts, Tribes, Ceremonials,* and *An Introduction to Southwestern Indian Arts and Crafts.* He has illustrated the books *Before You Came This Way* and *When Clay Sings.*

Ninotchka Bennahum is currently an Associate Professor at Long Island University's Brooklyn Campus where she directs an M.F.A. in New Media Art & Performance and, "LIU @ ABT," a Bachelor's program for American Ballet Theatre dancers. She holds a Ph.D. in Performance Studies from New York University's Tisch School of the Arts and a B.A. in History & Art History from Swarthmore College. In 2000, she published *"Antonia Mercé, 'La Argentina:; Flamenco & the Spanish Avant-Garde"* (Wesleyan University Press) and is currently working on a second manuscript that traces the Gypsy migration from the Middle East to Spain. She has written widely on ballet, modern and flamenco for *Dance Magazine, Pointe Magazine, The New York Times, The Denver Post, The Village Voice, the Albuquerque Journal* and currently serves as the Editor for the *Congress on Research in Dance Published Proceedings.* She has taught dance history for American Ballet Theatre's pre-professional summer intensive program since its inception in 1996 and loves working with ABT's staff and students.

Ananya Chatterjea is Assistant Professor in the Department of Theater Arts and Dance in the University of Minnesota, Minneapolis. She is also the Artistic Director of her company, *Women in Motion,* a contemporary South Asian dance company, dancing to push for social change. Ananya believes in the integral interconnectedness of her creative and scholarly research and in the identity of her art and activism. Her book, *Butting out! Reading cultural politics in the work of Chandralekha and Jawole Willa Jo Zollar,* is currently in publication with Wesleyan University Press. Ananya has recently performed in Delhi (India International

Center, Habitat Center), Bombay (National Center for Performing Arts), Kuala Lumpur (Sutra Dance Theater), and London (Nehru Center).

Judith Chazin-Bennahum was Principal Soloist with the Metropolitan Opera Ballet Company when Antony Tudor was Artistic Director. She is the author of *Dance in the Shadow of the Guillotine* (1988), *The Ballets of Antony Tudor: Studies in Psyche and Satire* (1994); *The Lure of Perfection: The Culture of Fashion and Ballet 1780-1830* (2004) and *Teaching Dance Studies* (2005), both published by Routledge Press. She became Distinguished Professor Emerita in the Department of Theatre and Dance in 2006. Currently she is working on a biography of René Blum.

Lynn Garafola is a Professor of Dance at Barnard College. She is the author of *Diaghilev's Ballet Russes* and *Legacies of Twentieth-Century Dance*, and the editor of several books including *The Diaries of Marius Petipa, Rethinking the Sylph: New Perspectives on the Romantic Ballet*, and *José Limón: An Unfinished Memoir*. Curator of the New-York Historical Society's exhibition "Dance for a City: Fifty Years of the New York Ballet and several smaller shows," she is a former Getty Scholar and editor of the book series "Studies in Dance History." A *Dance Magazine* senior critic, she has written for *Ballet Review, The Nation, Times Literary Supplement*, and many other publications. She holds a Ph.D. in Comparative Literature.

Beth Genné is Associate Professor of Dance Studies and History of Art, University of Michigan. She has written the book *The Making of a Choreographer: Ninette de Valois vii and Bar aux Folies-Bergére* and she has published chapters on film in dance in the books *Envisioning Dance on Film and Video* (2002) and *Re-thinking Dance History* (forthcoming from Routledge). Her articles have appeared in *Dance Research, Dance Chronicle, Dancing Times, Art Journal* and others.

JoMarie Griego-Lubarsky is 30 years old and received her Bachelor of Fine Arts degree in December of 2003. She recently married the love of her life and plans to devote her time to her family full time. She currently owns an internet business. This is her first publication on dance.

Larry Lavender is Head of the Dance Department at the University of North Carolina at Greensboro. He earned his MFA in Choreography at University of California Irvine and his Ph.D. in Dance Education at New York University. Larry has published numerous articles on dance criticism and dance making. His book, *Dancers Talking Dance: Critical Evaluation in the Choreography Class* (1996), is widely used in college and university dance programs worldwide.

Bridgit Luján is a native New Mexican born in an artistic and agrarian family where she was immersed in the rich culture and traditions of New Mexico. Bridgit began studying Mexican Folkloric and Spanish dance at age two. Bridgit is the Artistic Director of Dulce Flamenco Internacional and is on the dance faculty at the Santa Fe Community College. She has an M.A. in Dance History and Criticism and an M.B.A. in International Business in Latin America both from the University of New Mexico. Bridgit has furthered her understanding of the Latin cultures and their dance while living abroad in Mexico and Spain.

Katita Milazzo, a member of the Society of Dance History Scholars, has completed two Masters degrees, a MA in Dance History/Criticism from the University of New Mexico and a MALS in Spanish Dance and Culture from Empire State College. Her inquiries into Spanish Dance in North America earned a research fellowship at Jacob's Pillow. Presently she is working on her Ph.D. in dance studies at the University of Surrey in Great Britain and is residing in Germany where she is enjoying the accessibility of doing research in Europe.

Barbejoy Ponzio is a dance educator, choreographer, and dance writer, who holds an M.A. in Sports Medicine from San Francisco State University and another M.A. in Dance History and Criticism from the University of New Mexico. She currently directs the dance program at John F. Kennedy High School, in Denver, Colorado, and has had extensive experience teaching and establishing dance programs at all levels of education across the United States and overseas in Kinshasa, Zaire and Cairo, Egypt. In 1996, she was awarded the Selma Jean Cohen Award for Dance Scholarship, by the Society of Dance History Scholars. In addition to scholarly articles, she was the dance writer for *The Austin Chronicle* and created *Speaking of Dance*, a theatrical-based lecture series on dance, history and culture.

Jennifer Predock-Linnell, Ph.D., is a Professor of Dance in the Department of Theatre and Dance at the University of New Mexico. She holds a B.F.A. in Art Studio, and an MA and Ph.D. in Psychological Foundations of Education. She is a past recipient of an NEA Choreographer's Fellowship. Her dance/video works have been performed in the United States, Australia, France, Portugal, Israel and New Zealand. Recipient of a Rockefeller Foundation Grant for Cultural Exchange USA-Mexico. ROSTROS/FACES, Collaborative Choreographic project between UNM, and UNAM, Mexico City Utopia Danza Theatro. Her articles have been published in *Siences*, Mexico, *Psychological Reports: Perceptual and Motor Skills, Impulse*, 16th & 17th Volume of the *Institute of Psychoanalytic Studies of the Arts, 50 Contemporary Choreographers, Dance: Current Selected Research*, AMS Press, *The International Dictionary of Modern Dance, Research in Dance Education*.

Marcela J. Sandoval taught in the Albuquerque Public School System for twenty-five years. She started a Ballet Folklorico dance class and performing group at Albuquerque High School. Marcela danced professionally with Miguel Caro's Fiesta Mexicana for twenty years.

Marcia B. Siegel, dance critic, teacher and historian, is the author of *The Shapes of Change—Images of American Dance; Days on Earth—The Dance of Doris Humphrey*; and *Howling Near Heaven—Twyla Tharp and the Reinvention of Modern Dance*, as well as three collections of reviews and commentary. Her work is a subject of *First We Take Manhattan—Four American Women and the New York School of Dance Criticism* by Diana Theodores. From 1983 to 1999 she was a member of the resident faculty of the Department of Performance Studies, Tisch School of the Arts, New York University. Siegel is the dance critic of the *Boston Phoenix* and the *Hudson Review*.

Sally Sommer, historian, is a Professor in the MA program in American Dance Studies at Florida State University. She has published numerous articles on dance and popular culture for *Village Voice, The New York Times, Dance Magazine, The Drama Review, Dance Ink, Dance Research Journal* and various encyclopedias, and wrote *Ballroom* (1987). She worked on three PBS television documentaries on tap dance, social dance and the Peabody Award-winning *Everybody Dance Now!* and produced a documentary on club dancers and dances, *Check Your Body at the Door*.

Jill D. Sweet is Professor of Anthropology at Skidmore College. She received her BA and MFA in Dance from the University of California, Irvine, and her MA and Ph.D. in Anthropology from the University of New Mexico in 1981. Since then she has published extensively on the effects of tourism on Tewa Indian ritual dance events.

Introduction

Dancing the Southwest

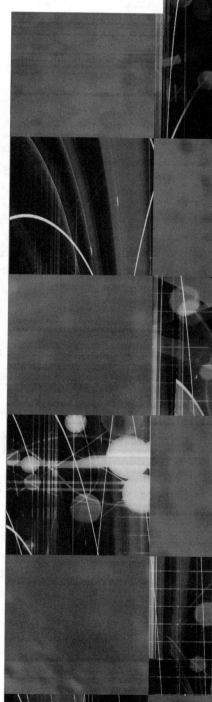

When I first came to New Mexico, I was struck by the diversity of dance experiences that could be found here, not only by the native dances of the Southwest, but the Mexican, Flamenco, country western and all the imported stage and social styles, from tap to Southeast Asian to ballet. Watching these dances has been deeply satisfying; they mirror the complexity of this region and certainly seem necessary to any text I was to write. A marvelous congruence of transmigrations have come and stayed in New Mexico, attracted by its desert mountains, open spaces, and huge sky. With their different traditions they live side-by-side, practicing their own ceremonies, speaking their own languages, telling their stories while sharing the parched land.

Since this text was created in the Southwest, initially for students here at the University of New Mexico, we have located the dances as they exist and flourish here, as well as in their places of origin, such as New York, Paris or Northern India. *The Living Dance* attempts to demonstrate how important the local knowledge of movement styles informs our essential understanding of how dance functions on many levels. Throughout the book, we witness the way dance responds to conquest, fusion, the advancement of subcultures, the studious attention given to gender roles, to the fashions of clothing the body wears while dancing, and to the survival of communities. New Mexico is in many ways a microcosm of the world of dance and so we describe those dance forms that prevail here and also hold currency in the scholarly narratives written about dance. It is important to acknowledge that dances that were brought here by settlers and citizens began in a very modest manner, since New Mexico's populations have been extremely small.

The beginning chapters of this book reveal that indigenous dances born in this environment cannot be viewed apart from this culture and geography. Ideally someone writing about movement and dance should study all the activities and artistic forms of the people that produced them and also should have a deep understanding of the social processes and aesthetic precepts that lay behind them. Movement and dance are "systems of knowledge," and as such, they belong to a larger description of the culture. They also help us to understand questions such as the roles of men and women in a given community and its sociopolitical discourses. Many do not view their dances as "art," but may see the dances as having religious or recreational value. This ritualistic approach to vital activities that magically transform our lives, parallel to some extent, the power of art in the western world.

New Mexico is an integral part of the American West of rodeos, cattle drives, cowboys, and rough weather-scored mountain ranges; it retains a frontier flavor. Rectangular in shape, New Mexico is the fifth largest American state, with Colorado to the north, Oklahoma and Texas to the east, Texas and the Mexican state of Chihuahua to the south and Arizona, which, from 1850 to 1863, was part of the Territory of New Mexico to the west.

Living in this sun-drenched country, one experiences extraordinary landscapes and senses the presence of mystery. At twilight, driving north to Santa Fe from Albuquerque, the imposing Sandia Mountains loom boldly to the east. Further north lie the foothills of the Rockies—pink-hued, studded with piñon and juniper trees. Thunderhead clouds thrust up over the rim of the Sangre de Cristo Mountains, warning of a torrential downpour. Flanked on the west by the Rio Grande River, and on the east, by the High Plains, the Rockies rise to 13,161 feet at Wheeler Peak. This area of mountain range embraces three of the seven life zones found in western North America, (from the ponderosa pine of the transition zone to the tundra of the arctic-alpine.) Sudden weather changes are the norm in New Mexico, and between day and night there is often a forty-degree drop in temperature.

The Conquistadores, in search of the fabled seven cities of gold, brought Spain's sixteenth-century culture, elements of which still survive in the Northern part of the state and the Sangre de Cristo Mountains. Some still speak a dialect that is more than 300 years old. The region became part of the Mexican Republic in 1821, and its inhabitants considered themselves Mexican. But in 1850, New Mexico became an American territory by conquest and in 1912, became the forty-seventh state. To some extent, New Mexicans felt themselves very isolated from the busy cross-roads of Mexico and America, although the Santa Fe Trail maintained a constant flow of trade with the United States. The remoteness of the Sangre de Cristo plateaus insulated villages from outside influence, freezing customs and language in a time frame long eclipsed in other parts of the Southwest. It was a forgotten world, but one rich in history. In 1598, nine years before the English settled Jamestown, in the village of Chimayo, soldiers of the conquistador Juan de Onate staged los moros y los cristianos, The Moors and the Christians—probably the first European drama performed in what is now the United States. With wild cries, the opposing forces charged and clashed in a melée of furious horses, sword against scimitar and shield against buckler. When it ended, a Christian victory had been won and the sultan was converted from Islam. The play has survived in New Mexican villages for four centuries.

Driving North from Albuquerque, one passes many pueblos or reservation villages that are Native American. Different Indian cultures have farmed and hunted on the land for at least 20,000 years before European explorers appeared. The more peaceful agriculturists, including the later Anasazi whose pueblo ruins dot the state, held sway longer and had well-developed irrigation systems by the time the wandering, invading Navajos arrived from the north, perhaps in the thirteenth century. Violent confrontations took place between the original indigenous populations and the invading Spanish Conquistadores. Even later, the Mexicans were conquered by the "Anglo" or American pioneers.

Anthropologist, Jill Sweet and author Tom Bahti both describe the profound influence of Native American ritual on this cultural geography. Bahti details the action of the Zuni Shalako dance, so that we live this event in its profound complexity for all 49 days. Sweet writes about the meanings associated with the space and time in which the Tewa dances occur. She acknowledges the importance of structure in their lives—the structure of their space, their homes and their performance of ritual. Native American or Indian religious ceremonials have survived despite massive efforts to obliterate them. In the name of "civilizing" and "christianizing" the Indians, masks and other religious objects were destroyed. The anti-Indian forces endured from the time of the Spanish conquest. Finally, in 1889, The Code of Religious Offenses in an effort to totally crush Pueblo religious dances and ceremonies, banned virtually all their activities. In 1934, the repressive code was abolished, and Native American religious rights were reinstated.

After the chapter on Native American dance, writers Bridgit Lujan and Marcela Sandoval discuss the Mexican and New Mexican folk dances that accompany many popular festivals and incorporate both European and Mexican elements. Mexican folk dances continue to be performed at various celebrations, often along with concerts by mariachi bands. Lujan and Sandoval paint a rich panorama of dances whose costumes and customs have the élan and vitality of peoples who continue to love their history.

When people live side by side, they borrow goods and habits from one another. Even enemies adapt one another's practices. An example of this occurrence is the Matachines dance, a unique and passionate dance drama described here in detail by JoMarie Griego Lubarsky, a young woman whose grandparents faithfully participated in the dance every year. Spanish and Indian, Mexican and Anglo traces are manifested in this colorful ceremony. No one really knows how long the dance has been practiced but one has found it in the calendars of both Native American pueblos and Spanish towns in New Mexico for hundreds of years.

Another example of a dance that represents a mingling of different movement styles is country western; we've included it here because so many New Mexicans find their way to clubs in Albuquerque to do line dancing and country western dances. In her essay on country western dance, Barbejoy Ponzio explains that New Mexico's country western roots lay in square dancing, with African-American, Spanish, and Mexican influences. She recalls the words of commentators from the nineteenth century who describe the fairly raucous and wild events when women were few and poorly understood.

Ninotchka Bennahum begins her Flamenco essay by traversing the road from Albuquerque to Santa Fe in her description of the history of Flamenco in New Mexico. She expands her narrative with the long voyage of gypsies from India to southern Spain. Bennahum explores the tricultural environment of Islamic Spain in which Flamenco was born and evolved. She draws connections between the multi-culturalism of New Mexico and its unique Flamenco festivals and the rich environment of Andalucia, Spain. In particular, she studies the world-renowned Flamenca, Maria Benitez, a thirty-year veteran of the stage, and discusses her contribution to New Mexican dance along with that of Eva Encinias-Sandoval's, producer of Festival Flamenco Intenacional de Alburquerque, the largest American Flamenco festival which has taken place at the University of New Mexico for 20 years. The famed Maria Benitez, whose roots originate in this region, developed Flamenco in Santa Fe and travels widely with her company.

European Legacies and Dances in the Diaspora

Many dance styles have their roots in Western European traditions, including the enduring theatrical forms of modern dance and ballet. In her essay Marcia Siegel tells the rich and variegated history of modern dance. She concentrates her attention on the movements and figures that are closer to us, evoking the momentum and fury of late twentieth-century choreographic heroes and heroines. They became the existential moderators in fierce arguments about what is art, what is gender and what is performance.

Initially modern dance was called aesthetic, barefoot or interpretive dancing. Both ballet and modern dance took root relatively late in New Mexico. Many factors accounted for this—the lack of concert theatres, the large distances between populated areas, and a general disinterest in what was not Mexican, New Mexican, or American popular fare such as minstrelsy, vaudeville and musicals. Touring companies played in downtown Albuquerque in the early twentieth century. The Atchison, Topeka, and Santa Fe Railroad ran through New Mexico and facilitated connections to the outside world.

Modern dance made its way here with the Denishawn dancers in 1926. They were followed by Jane McLean, a Martha Graham exponent, Trudi Schoop, and the Miriam Winslow Dancers who performed in the 1930s. Martha Graham herself came to Santa Fe in 1930 to visit friends. She was deeply stirred by the Native American dances she saw and by an Easter festival of the Penitentes that she witnessed in Northern New

Mexico. Her dances, *Primitive Mysteries* and *El Penitente* reflected her encounter with this New Mexican material.

In the early 1940s, modern dance was taught at the University of New Mexico by Mela Sedillo who also instructed Mexican dance classes. She was later replaced by Elizabeth Waters who danced with Hanya Holm. One of Waters' precocious students was Tim Wengerd who became a leading performer in the Martha Graham Dance Company. As Albuquerque grew, more modern dance touring companies visited and excited interest. In 1972, Jennifer Predock-Linnell was hired by the university to build their dance program. She, in turn, recruited Lee Connor and Lorn MacDougal for the modern area, Judith Chazin-Bennahum for the ballet area and Eva Encinias for the Flamenco area. In recent years, Bill Evans has taught at the university and performed regularly with his talented and dynamic company. When Larry Lavender became Head of Dance, he expanded the program to include other dance styles, such as African, Mexican Folk and Hip Hop. Important recent additions to the dance faculty are the Head of Dance, Donna Jewel who values the landscape and creates site-specific works, and Mary Anne Newhall who digs into the legacies of modern dance, recreating some of its most powerful works, such as Mary Wigman's *Hexentanz* and Daniel McKayle's *Rainbow Round my Shoulder*.

Contemporary dance in Albuquerque thrives with the Keshet Dance Company, a downtown dance studio that caters to all of society including the poor and the homeless. Shira Greenberg founded the company ten years ago with the goal of providing an arts organization that works conscientiously with its community.

Years ago, other modern dancers settled in Santa Fe, including Eleanor King, a former dancer with Doris Humphrey who created original pieces based on her interest in Native American ritual and Eve Gentry who left New York and became very interested in injury prevention. Both King and Gentry affected many students and young dancers.

Recently, the charm of Santa Fe attracted the famous ballet dancer Jacques D'Amboise to locate a branch of his National Dance Institute in 1995. NDI continues to grow and spread popular dance among school children. Its Director, Catherine Oppenheimer, spearheaded a successful drive to create a spacious building with four studios and a theatre. Another unique dance company and school in Santa Fe recently founded by Ronn Stewart is the Moving People Dance Theatre that brings together, as a consortium, many different dance forms for periodic performances.

The first ballet dancers who toured Albuquerque on their way to the west coast, also known as the "Death Circuit," had appropriately elegant French names and came with a revue in 1918. It was also touted that the great Russian ballerina Anna Pavlova passed through town in the late 1920s with her own train and 100 company members including an orchestra. By the 1940s and 1950s, a number of American and European ballet teachers had settled in Albuquerque and opened studios and developed a taste and inclination for classical ballet. Nadia and Sulin Krasnoff initiated a very professional approach to teaching ballet in New Mexico, soon thereafter Dr. Charles and

Katherine Fishback (1945), Kay Windsor Brooks, Bill and Lucy Hayden, Karen Alwin, Linda Kennedy and Suzanne Johnston settled in Albuquerque to open studios. Johnston created the New Mexico Ballet Company in 1969. From 1980 to 1990 Edward Androse's Southwest Ballet Company performed full seasons with professional dancers and a repertoire that included both nineteenth and twentieth century works. Today there are several local studio ballet companies producing classical and contemporary ballet, notably Patricia Dickinson's Southwest Ballet Theatre and Ballet Theatre of New Mexico directed by Katherine Geise. Celia Dale from the Hayden School, mounts student ballet productions and runs the Contemporary Dance Ensemble as well.

Ballet in Santa Fe fares well with the establishment of the Aspen Santa Fe Ballet Company in the year 2000, the only truly professional ballet company in New Mexico. Its directors, Tom Mossbrucker and Jean-Philippe Malaty brought the company of eleven classically-trained dancers to perform an eclectic and robust repertoire. The associated school is run by Gisela Genschow, formerly of the Hamburg Ballet and other European dance companies.

Lynn Garafola synthesizes the complex 500-year-old history of ballet in her chapter on the Ballet. Garafola points to the Renaissance origins of ballet in Italy, and how it moved to France, heralding the beginning of its long voyage through Europe to Russia where it became a quintessential, classical art form. It then traveled around the world, to Asia, South Africa, Australia etc. There is no question that ballet travels well and continues to beautifully represent Western European aristocratic values.

Katita Milazzo and Sally Sommer write about the definitive role that African-Americans have played in the development of American dance. Sommer concentrates on the richness of black participation in social dance during the twentieth century, while Milazzo unravels the connections between Irish and African-American dancing in her narrative that discloses how tap became a valued American dance form. In addition, she describes the vibrant development of jazz as an art form with its origins in tap dancing and its growth influenced by modern, ballet and other dance forms.

A rather small population of African-Americans has lived in New Mexico since the Buffalo soldiers and homesteading in the late nineteenth century. With the railroads and ranching, more African-Americans settled in this racially diverse country. Initially, most of the African-American population was located in cities such as Clovis and Hobbes in the southern part of the state. The 1940s brought African-American soldiers to Kirtland Air Force Base and other military compounds near Albuquerque. Although living in relative isolation due to segregation, African-Americans made a strong contribution to the cultural sensibility of New Mexico. They inspired the dancing that took place in the juke joints and dancing halls along Route 66, such as Club 66 and the Old Town Dance Hall. The Flame was a popular juke joint situated on South Broadway. Such celebrated jazz artists as Louis Armstrong, Lionel Hampton, Count Basie and Duke Ellington played in the white night clubs, but went to African-American nightspots late in the evening in order to connect with the black community. They stayed in black rooming houses, as Albuquerque did not have hotels for blacks; before the 50s there was one hotel with a restaurant, Ruby's café. Interestingly enough, in 1952, Albuquerque was the first city in America to pass a bill prohibiting discrimination in public places because of race, creed or color. In the late 40s and 50s, young African-Americans might earn a little money doing jitterbug acts at white clubs and at clubs at the local air force base. (Lola Lestrich interview Sept. 2, 2002).

Today, one of the most vigorous dance communities continues the tradition of breaking and popping, with its hip hop competitions and performances. Originally from Philadelphia, Karen Price choreographs and teaches hip-hop at the University of New Mexico, stimulating great interest in the dance form, as she participates in national arenas. Several groups of "B-boys" and "B-girls" fuse popping and locking with house styles in various opportunities to perform around New Mexico. Some of the most current are PFR, PHO, 505 crew and KYS (Killin' your Style).

As ideas for this text began to materialize, it seemed important to include dance forms from South Asia, far from New Mexico. The reason for this was twofold. First, there is a significant East Indian population in New Mexico. The India Association has played a central role in promoting lively dance performances. They sponsored Angela Singh who was one of the first to teach Bharata Natyam. Second, Indian dance poses questions about nationalism and colonialism that bear thinking about in connection with the history of New Mexico. In her engaging essay on East Indian Dance, Ananya Chatterjea writes about the prejudicial history of the dancing body, its submission in various conquests, and about the women whose "bodies" are dancing.

One of the most important aspects of American dance experience is to be found in the movies and television and no less so in New Mexico. In her essay on dance in film, Beth Genné traces the remarkable history of dance on film during the twentieth century. For New Mexicans, movies and video may be the most significant way that they encounter theatrical dance and learn about dancing in its many guises. During the 1920s and 1930s, there were at least five movie palaces in downtown Albuquerque, and people thronged to them, especially the musicals. The television screen succeeded the silver screen. It was a window to the world as well as entertainment.

In recent years film and video technology have fascinated experimental artists, including many non-dancers who are experts in motion-based computer graphics. One of the results of this experimentation is that the living body may be superseded and blurred by digitized screen effects. In her essay, Jennifer Predock-Linnell asks hard questions about the performance of "screen" or "video" dance. Where will it go now that choreographers have begun to incorporate technology such as motion-capture and figure animation? How do we conceptualize this new kind of dance? Do we want to live in places where the world of technology and dance dictate the images of our unconscious?

Finally, Larry Lavender asks us to look at dance as a living activity, as something that grows and changes, and breathes with every person who performs the dance. He takes us through the steps we need to make in order to write clearly about dance. Lavender emphasizes the richness of writing and how it helps us to understand the power of dance in the present.

This book is about the world of dance. It begins with dance as seen from the region of the Southwest and takes us through a number of geographies in our quest for mutual understandings. While seemingly remote, New Mexico has a vision of life that includes many cultures. In the Pueblo and Navajo ethos, the world is near the "Sipapu" or the birthplace of all human kind. It is also where Trinity site in 1945 witnessed the first explosion of the Atomic Bomb. The past and the future merge in this high desert and mountain space.

Judith Chazin-Bennahum
Albuquerque, New Mexico
September 2006

Chapter 1

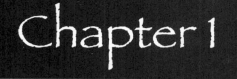

Native American Dances of New Mexico

Zuni Ceremonial

Tom Bahti

The Zuni have probably the most complex of all native religions in the Southwest. Every aspect of traditional Zuni life is completely integrated with their religion. Numerous religious organizations, through an intricate system of interlocking ceremonials, interrelate the whole of Zuni culture.

Six esoteric cults (in addition to the ancestor cult to which all Zuni belong) form the basis of Zuni ceremonialism. These are the cults of the Sun, Rainmakers (which is in charge of 12 priesthoods), *Koko* (or katsinas), Priests of the Koko, War Gods, and Prey Gods (representing the animal patrons of 12 related curing societies). Each cult has its own priests, fetishes, rituals, and ceremonial calendar.

Basic to the religious philosophy of the Zuni is the recognition of man's oneness with the universe and the absolute necessity of maintaining this harmony through the correct execution of prescribed rituals. If the ceremonies are properly performed, the rains *will* fall, the harvests *will be* bountiful, the life of the people *will* be long and happy, and the fertility of the plant and animal worlds will continue.

Creation Myth

In the beginning there was only fog and mists. "Above" existed three deities: *Awonawilona*—a bisexual supreme being (Creator of All); Sun, the giver of light, warmth, and life; and Moon, the deity responsible for dividing the year into 12 months and delineating the life span of man. "Below" existed two superhuman beings, *Shiwanni* and his wife *Shiwanokia*.

Awonawilona created clouds and water with the breath of his heart. Shiwanni formed the constellations from bubbles of his saliva. Shiwanokia, using her saliva, created Mother Earth. The *Ahshiwi* (Zuni) are the children of Shiwanni and Shiwanokia—they were born in the innermost of the underworlds.

From *Southwestern Indian Ceremonials* by Tom Bahti and Mark Bahti. Copyright 1997 by KC Publications. Reprinted by permission.

Emergence and Migration Myth

The Underworld which the Ahshiwi inhabited was totally dark—the people lived in holes and subsisted on wild grass seeds. They are said to have been peculiar creatures with tails, gigantic ears, webbed hands and feet, moss-covered bodies, and a foul odor.

Sun Father created two sons, *Kowituma and Wahtsusi,* out of bits of foam and sent them to the Underworld to bring the Ahshiwi into the Upperworld. The sons, known as the Divine Ones, made light for the people by kindling fire. Following a path marked with sacred meal, they led the Ahshiwi to the North where they planted a ponderosa pine. They climbed the tree to make their way into the Third or Water Moss World. The next trail led to the West—here a Douglas fir was grown to allow the Ahshiwi to enter the Second or Mud World. The third trail went South to an aspen which was used to reach the First World of Wings (Sun's Rays). The last journey was to the East, and the Ahshiwi climbed a silver spruce to emerge into the Upperworld. The actual entry was made through a spring or small lake whose waters parted to allow passage.

At the time of emergence the Divine Ones used their stone knives to transform the animal-like Ahshiwi into human form. They also taught the Zuni how to make fire and to cook their food. Corn was acquired from *Paiyatemu,* assistant to the Sun.

The Zuni then began their wanderings to seek the Middle Place (the middle of the world) where they were to settle. Many years were spent in the search and numerous villages were built only to be later abandoned. At one stage in the wanderings Shiwanni of the North sent his son and daughter to seek a village site. During their search the brother suddenly became enamored of his sister's beauty and possessed her. The same night ten offspring were born to them—the first was normal and became the ancestor of *the Kokokshi,* the Rainmakers. The other nine became the *Koyemshi* (Mudheads), the idiot offspring of this incestuous union.

The brother created the Zuni and Little Colorado rivers by marking the sands with his foot, and at their junction a lake (Listening Spring) was formed. Within the waters of this lake he created a village, *Kothluwalawa* (sometimes called *Wenima*), the home of the Council of the Gods.

The Council of the Gods came into being as the result of a river crossing by the Ahshiwi during their migration. The children of the Wood Fraternity were being carried across, but became panicky and fell into the rushing water. Immediately they were transformed into various water creatures—turtles, tadpoles, frogs, and snakes—which made their way to Kothluwalawa. Here they matured instantly and became the Council of the Gods.

In their migration to the Middle Place the Ahshiwi were stopped by a tribe known as *Kianakwe,* which was led by *Chakwena,* the Keeper of the Game. The Divine Ones grew weary of leading the Ahshiwi in fighting the Kianakwe, so they petitioned their Sun Father to send them two War Gods as replacements. The Sun impregnated a waterfall and the *Ahayuda* (as they are known in time of peace) or *Uyuyewi* and *Masailema* (as they are known in time of war) were created.

With the help of the War Gods the Ahshiwi defeated the Kianakwe in a four-day battle. They captured the village and released the wild game held captive by Chakwena. The ruins of the village are said to be some 50 miles south of the present town of Zuni.

The Ahshiwi continued to wander and live in several villages (the ruins of which may still be seen) before they finally settled in the Middle *Place*, *Itiwanna*, the Zuni name for their pueblo.

Afterworld

At death the corpse is bathed in yucca suds and rubbed with cornmeal before burial. The spirit of the dead lingers for four days, during which time the door of its former home is left ajar to permit its entry. On the morning of the fifth day the spirit goes to the Council of the Gods in the village of Kothluwalawa beneath the water of Listening Spring. Here the spirit becomes a member of the *Uwannami*—a Rainmaker. If the deceased was member of the Bow Priesthood, he becomes a lightning maker who brings water from the "six great waters of the world." The water, in the form of rain, is poured through the clouds which are the masks worn by the Uwannami.

Shalako

The *Shalako*, a winter ceremony held in late November or early December, is the major ritual performed at the pueblo of Zuni. Usually referred to as a house-blessing ceremonial, it is a 49-day re-enactment of the Zuni emergence and migration myths. In addition, it is a prayer for rain, for the health and well-being of the people, and for the propagation of plants and animals. During the Shalako the spirits of the dead return to be honored and fed. As the final element of this lengthy ceremonial, a hunting rite is performed. The description that follows can do little more than touch the surface of this highly complex ceremonial.

Participants in the Shalako (both impersonators and the sponsors of the Shalako houses) are chosen during the previous Winter Solstice ceremony. Preparations for the numerous and varied rites begin immediately afterward and occupy much of the participants' time for the intervening ten months. Long and complicated chants must be learned, prayer sticks must be placed each month at certain shrines that mark the migrations of the Zuni in ancient times, and minor rituals must be performed each month.

In addition to this, the houses that will honor the Shalakos must be built or extensively remodeled. (The floor is left unfinished and dug deep enough to accommodate the tall Shalakos.) Ideally, eight houses are used—six for the Shalakos, one for *Sayatasha* and the Council of the Gods (usually called the Long Horn House), and one for the *Koyemshi*. To sponsor a Shalako house is a tremendously expensive undertaking—added to the cost of construction is the expense of providing food for the participants and a myriad of visitors.

The principal masked figures that appear during the ceremony are:

Shalakos—the Giant Messengers of the Rainmakers—one to represent each of the six kivas. The masks and bodies of these ten-foot figures are carried on pole frames by the impersonators. Each Shalako has two impersonators who take turns dancing.

Sayatasha—the Rain God of the North—often called "Long Horn" for the projection from the right side of his mask which is said to symbolize long life for the people. Sayatasha oversees all the activities preceding the actual appearance of the Shalakos.

Hututu—the Rain God of the South—is the deputy of Sayatasha. Both carry rattles of deer scapulae, bows and arrows, and numerous prayer plumes.

Shulawitsi—the Fire God—is a representative of the sun. The part is always played by a young boy from the Badger Clan. Shulawitsi carries a fawn skin filled with seeds.

Yamuhakto—Spirits of the Forest—these two figures are also called Warriors of the West and East. They have sticks of cottonwood tied to the tops of their masks that represent their authority over forests and trees. The antlers that they carry are symbolic of the deer that live in the forests.

Salimopya—are the warriors who carry yucca whips to guard the performers and keep spectators from coming too close. There are six—one for each of the six directions, with masks painted accordingly—but only two appear during the Shalako.

Koyemshi—the Mudheads—are led by *Awan Tachu*, Great Father. The others are called Deputy to the Great Father, Warrior, Bat, Small Horns, Old Grandfather, Old Youth, Water Drinker, Game Maker, and Small Mouth.

Members of the Council of the Gods taking part in this ceremony include Sayatasha, Hututu, two Yamuhakto, and Shulawitsi.

Eight days before the arrival of the Shalakos, Koyemshi appear in the village to exhort the people to complete their preparations for the coming of the gods.

Four days later Shulawitsi and Sayatasha arrive from the west, having retraced the migration of the Ahshiwi. The Fire God lights fires on the way to guide the Council of the Gods to the Middle Place.

Forty-Eighth Day

Shulawitsi and Sayatasha appear in the village to inspect the six holes—-one for each kiva—that have been dug to receive prayer plumes. Later in the day the Fire God and his ceremonial father deposit their prayer sticks. They are followed by Sayatasha, Hututu, and the two Yamuhakto who bless the shrines in brief ceremonies and also leave prayer plumes. They then retreat to their Shalako house to perform blessing ceremonies for the building and the altar that has been installed, and to place special prayer sticks near the roof beams. After this they smoke cigarettes of native tobacco. The smoke, symbolic of clouds, will bring rain to the land.

At dark the giant Shalakos arrive at the south side of the river where they use a narrow footbridge to cross over into the village. Upon reaching the north side the impersonators briefly leave their masks and go to the Shalako houses. They return shortly and the birdlike creatures rise and approach the houses with much clacking of beaks and strange whistling sounds. Before they enter, the houses must be properly blessed in ceremonies similar to those conducted at the Long Horn House.

After bringing the Shalako inside, the impersonator leaves his mask and enters into a lengthy dialogue with the sponsor of the houses. This recitation of the emergence and migration myth consumes a great part of the evening. Food is then taken by the Shalako impersonators to the river where it is offered to the spirits of the dead who live at Kothluwalawa.

General feasting follows and the kitchens of the Shalako houses bring forth unbelievable quantities of food for performers, townspeople, and visitors.

Dancing by the Shakalos begins after midnight. The Salimopyas and Koyemshi also make the rounds to all of the Shalako houses to perform. A Zuni version of the Navajo Yeibichai is also staged—to the great delight of the Navajos who are present. It is said that this dance commemorates a time when the Navajos performed this ceremony at Zuni to cure the people of an epidemic that caused swellings.

Forty-Ninth Day

The dancing continues until sunrise, at which time Sayatasha climbs to a rooftop to offer prayers on behalf of the Zuni people. The dancers are purified with a hair-washing rite.

About noon on the final day, the Shalakos and their attendants leave the pueblo, crossing the river to an open field south of the old village. Here the Shalakos race, placing prayer plumes in six specially dug sites before returning to Kothluwalawa. The race depicts the manner in which the Shalakos, as couriers of the gods, deliver messages and prayers for rain throughout the year.

As the Shalakos disappear in the distance, the young men run to catch them. Those who succeed in "capturing" a Shalako believe they will have future success in hunting deer.

Tewa Village Rituals

Jill Sweet

Tewa village rituals bombard the senses. Through crowds of spectators, the visitor sees masses of rhythmically moving bodies arrayed in colorful costumes and paraphernalia. Excited children run through the village, their laughter mingling with the voices of singers and the repetitive sounds of bells, rattles, and drums. The smells of freshly baked bread, burning piñon, and steaming stews permeate the air. Together, the careful ritual preparations, the group movement sequences, the closely interrelated dance and music, the costumes, and the audience itself create a performance that communicates important images and messages to performer and observer alike.

Some Tewas agree to dance and sing in the village rituals more often than others. Women may be needed at home to care for youngsters or cook food for feasting. Some people may be unable to take time off from their jobs. Though participating is seen as a community responsibility, no one individual is expected to dance in every ritual event. Those who choose not to sing or dance are still considered important participants in the ritual performance. There is no "audience" in the Western theatrical sense of the word because the Tewas do not passively watch the action but instead consider the role of dance watching to be one of active listening. Tewa audiences contribute their thoughts to the communal prayer that is dramatized by the singers and dancers.

The Performance

Each ritual event is part of an annual cycle of village performances, a cycle that reflects seasonal changes and the traditional subsistence activities associated with each season. Only certain dances can be performed in the spring and others in the summer, winter, or fall. The village council, often referred to by the Tewas as the tribal council, usually selects the dances and dance dates, although a few specific dances must be requested by special groups. For example, at the village of San Juan, the unmarried men request the deer dance each year, and the women's society, the cloud or basket dance.

Once the dance and date are chosen, the war captains and their assistants ask the village composers to prepare the songs. The composers must recall traditional songs for some dances, such as the deer, yellow corn, Comanche, butterfly, and harvest dances, while for others, such as the turtle, cloud, and basket dances, they compose new songs each year. The war captains' group then requests the lead male singers—those considered most musically gifted—to meet and practice with the composers in the kiva. Later, the other male participants join this group for practice and the dance steps are set. Again, for some dances, traditional movement patterns are recalled, and for others new choreographic combinations are created.

Finally, the war captains' group invites the women participants to attend the practice sessions in the kiva. Assistant war captains go to the women's homes and make formal requests: "We have chosen you to enlighten us and to help us gain life" (Garcia and Garcia 1968:239). If the woman is married, they must speak to her in front of her

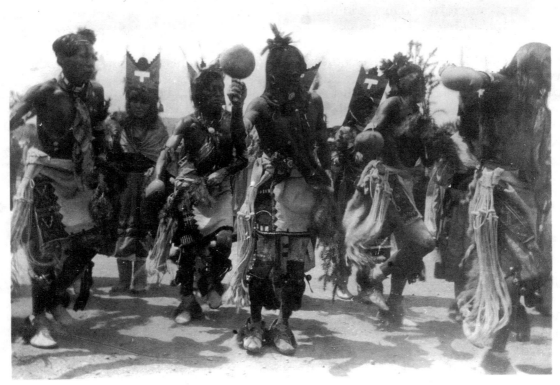

Santa Clara Pueblo Corn Dance, c. 1911.

Photographer Matilda Coxe Stevenson. Courtesy of National Anthropological Archives, Smithsonian Institution (Neg. No. 1982-B).

husband, but the decision to take part is hers alone. If she is not married, the request must be made in front of her father, who usually gives his permission.

On the fifth night before the dance, an expedition of young men gathers the evergreens that will be worn or carried by the dancers. Traditionally, they walked many miles to the mountains, collected evergreen branches with prayers, and carried them back to the village, all in one night. Today, pick-up trucks may take the gatherers into the mountains, but the evergreens are still collected with reverence because they remain powerful symbols of life.

The length of the practice period varies, but four evenings in the kiva is commonest. Throughout the practice period, costumes and paraphernalia are prepared. On the evening of the performance, the participants may present a short prelude dance in the plaza. The next day, a final practice session may be held before emergence from the kiva.

Tewa dance style is formal, controlled, and repetitive, with relatively simple steps. The dancers move in unison with torsos held erect and limbs close to the center of the body. Tewa dancers usually contract their elbows to about a ninety-degree angle and hold them four or five inches from the body. Most gestures are made through space in a flat arc, rather than in a straight line projecting out from the dancer's body.

For most steps, the dancers contract their knees only slightly, so their feet remain close to the ground. The men usually lift their feet a bit higher than do the women. The *ântegeh* (from the Tewa "foot," ân, and "to lift," *tegeh*) is the most basic step in Tewa dance. Kurath and Garcia (1970:82) described it as "foot lifting with emphasis on right foot: upbeat of raising right knee while supporting weight on left foot; accented lowering of right foot, while raising left heel and slightly flexing knees; unaccented raising of right knee while lowering left heel" This step may be done in place or traveling forwards, sidewards, or diagonally.

Other common Tewa steps include a stylized deer walk and a buffalo walk. The deer dancer holds a canelike stick in each hand and leans forward, bearing his weight on the sticks while bending his legs. He meanders slowly, creating the illusion of a four-legged animal. The buffalo walks upright in a gait that shifts the body weight from side to side, the knees bending deeply in a heavy, lumbering walk. Occasionally the choreography calls for small jumps (springing from and landing on both feet), hops (springing from one foot and landing on the same foot), and small, low leaps (springing from one foot and landing on the other). Knee bends in place with weight on both feet are sometimes used, in addition to a shuffle step (see Kurath and Garcia [1970] for notation of these steps).

In the most sacred Tewa dances, a single file of men ântegeh in place, occasionally pivoting to change their facing direction. This choreographic pattern is considered to be the most sacred and is primarily associated with males because it is the same pattern found in the private kachina dances performed by men in the kivas. Other dances may take a double file formation, especially when a large number of women participate. The lines usually alternate men and women, or a line of men faces one of women.

Less frequently, the dance formation takes the form of a circle that typically rotates counterclockwise.

The performers usually follow a prescribed spatial circuit repeating a five-verse dance set in each designated area. Sometimes they perform the final set of the circuit within the kiva, then after a short rest, return for another circuit through the village. There rarely are fewer than four, and sometimes as many as ten, circuits completed during the day, and some Tewa dances include extra prelude and postlude sections. A day of dancing often begins at dawn and lasts until sunset.

In any Tewa performance, music and dance are tightly interwoven. Each song is a prayer. More than mere accompaniment for the dancers, the songs are an integral part of the event, helping to communicate the meanings of the ritual. Ethnomusicologists have noted this interdependence in their work with Tewa song composers, who find it difficult to perform a song without also dancing or to comment on silent films of Tewa dance. Tewa women caring for infants or preparing food indoors can often describe the section of the dance in progress, simply by hearing the music. Although most Tewa villages permit photography and even silent filming of their public performances, permission to make sound recordings is typically more difficult to obtain; songs are powerful and must be protected.

Only after the singers have learned the songs can the dancers begin their practice using the music to guide them through the choreography. The tempo of the music, of course, sets the dancers' speed. Usually the tempo is constant, but in some cases, such as that of the San Juan cloud dance, a slow beat accelerates until it is very fast, then suddenly drops back once again, the dancers following suit. The tremolo, or rolling of drum or rattle, musical phrasing, and changes in the beat are techniques that cue the dancers to a change in facing direction or formation. A switch from the usual double beat to triple beat—called a *t'an*—often signals a slight hesitation in the ântegeh step.

Self-accompanied dances such as the San Juan turtle dance most dramatically express the relationship between music and movement. Here, the dancers are simultaneously the musicians as they ântegeh in place, each with a tortoise shell rattle tied behind the right knee. The rattle sounds with each step, and the dancers sing as they move. Other percussion instruments used by male dancers include painted gourd hand rattles and commercially made sleigh bells sewn onto a leather belt. In addition, men who take the role of the buffalo in the buffalo dance wear kilts edged with rows of cone-shaped tin tinklers.

The Tewas purchase or trade for drums which are made from hollowed cottonwood tree trunks. Pueblo drum makers cover the ends with horse or bull hide and sometimes paint the body with bright colors. Drumsticks are carved from soft pine, and a stuffed hide ball is tied to one end. The best known Pueblo drum makers are from the Keresan Pueblo village of Cochiti, where many Tewa drums originate.

Performers treat their drums with respect and sometimes give them names. After using a drum, the performers may ritually "feed" it with a sprinkle of cornmeal. The pitch of a drum can be altered by changing drumsticks or by turning it over and

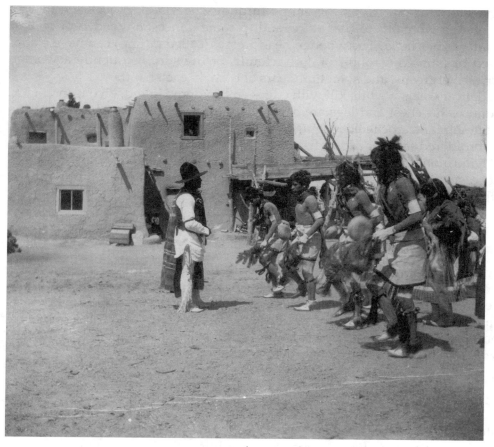

Santa Clara Pueblo, c. 1913.

Photographer Barbara Freire-Marreco. Courtesy of School of American Research,
W. W. Hill Collection Maxwell, Museum Photo Archives.

beating on the opposite end, changes that a good drummer can accomplish without
losing a beat. The number of drummers varies with the dances from one to as many as
four or five, and drummers often alternate during a long ritual performance.

Tewa performance costumes vary according to village, dance, and time of year, but
there are some common elements in all costume designs (see Roediger 1961). The
woman dancer generally wears a *manta*-dress, made of black or white wool or heavy
cotton fabric and bordered with geometric patterns in green, black, and white embroidery. Under this heavier garment, she may wear a cotton shirt or dress trimmed in lace.
A brightly colored, lace-trimmed shawl may be pinned at her right shoulder, and a red
woven sash tied at her waist. For some dances, she will be asked to dance barefooted,

and for others to wear moccasins. Silver and turquoise necklaces, bracelets, and pins always decorate a woman's festive attire, and in some dances, a wooden or feather headdress adorns her head. The wooden headdresses, called *tablitas*, can have elaborately carved or painted symbols of corn, clouds, or the sun. Frequently a woman dancer carries evergreens, and sometimes ears of corn, in each hand.

A male dancer wears a white kilt with edges embroidered in red, green, and black. For some dances his chest and legs are bare except for body paint, and for others he wears a white shirt and crocheted leggings. At his waist, the male dancer usually wears bells, an embroidered sash, or a long-fringed white rain sash. He carries a gourd rattle in his right hand along with evergreen sprigs, while in the left hand he holds only evergreens. Moccasins on the feet and usually a few feathers tied at the top of the head complete the man's costume.

Some Meanings and Messages

Tewa village ritual performances are rich with layers of symbolic meaning and messages encoded in songs, gestures, actions, costumes, and paraphernalia. Along with the central theme of new life, other important Tewa concepts find expression in ritual, including those of subsistence, society, beauty, space, time, and humor. Communication of these concepts is directed toward the performers themselves, toward fellow Tewas, and toward the supernaturals.

Subsistence, Society, and Beauty

Subsistence themes ensure, celebrate, and give thanks for plant and animal life and for the rainfall essential to it. Because the Tewas traditionally depended upon agriculture and hunting, the importance of these messages cannot be overemphasized. Through performances the people communicate statements about the abundance and fertility of plants and animals in their environment.

A key subsistence symbol is corn. For centuries a crucial and versatile food source, corn plays an important role in Tewa mythology, and all aspects of the plant are considered to be symbolically powerful. Its life cycle is seen as a paradigm of all other natural life cycles. Corn designs may be embroidered on a dancer's manta or carved in her wooden tablita headdress, and she often carries ears of corn in her hands. Tewas sprinkle cornmeal as they stand watching the village ritual performances, a sacred offering to the supernatural world. Corn and the related need for rain are central themes in many Tewa songs (Spinden 1933:95):

Ready we stand in San Juan town,
Oh, our Corn Maidens and our Corn Youths!
Oh, our Corn Mothers and our Corn Fathers!

Now we bring you misty water
And throw it different ways

To the north, the west, the south, the east
To heaven above and the drinking earth below!

Then likewise throw your misty water
Toward San Juan!
Oh, many that you are, pour water
Over our Corn Maidens' ears!
On our Wheat Maidens
Thence throw you misty water,
All round about us here!

On Green Earth Woman's back
Now thrives our flesh and breath,
Now grows our strength of arm and leg,
Now takes form our children's food!

A second group of symbolic meanings expresses the social dimensions of the world. The performances make explicit and implicit statements about Tewa society, not only reflecting social roles, relationships, and responsibilities but also helping to establish, shape, and reinforce them. The village performances are arenas for demonstrating how the Tewas interact socially and what it means to be a member of Tewa society. During a performance, for example, an aunt might help a nephew prepare for his first deer dance. The women of a household will work together preparing a feast for dancers and visitors. A clown may ridicule a man because he neglects his family. Each of these acts makes public the Tewas' notions of social roles and responsibilities.

One of the more obvious statements of social responsibility that is expressed during many village rituals is the "throw," "giveaway," or "throwaway." People from the community bring out large baskets filled with fruit, packaged snack foods, candy, cigarettes, money, and even small household items such as towels, brooms, pots, and pans. These they throw out to the dancers and singers as a statement of community sharing. The performers catch or pick up the gifts as they continue to dance and sing. Relatives of the performers quickly take the gifts home so that the dance is not disrupted. Throws may also be directed toward the observers, both Indian and non-Indian. When this happens, there is often more laughter and scrambling for the goods. Non-Tewa visitors who catch items are expected to accept them as gifts.

The most fundamental social statement is communicated simply by the act of participating in a village ritual performance. When a Tewa decides to sing or dance in, or attend, a ritual performance, he or she demonstrates a commitment to being Tewa and contributes to the cohesiveness of the social group, which is distinguished from all "outsiders." Some Tewa Indians claim that to remain a Tewa, one must, in some capacity, participate in village performances (Ortiz 1979b:287–98). As the Tewas participate, they make commitments of time, effort, and money to traditions and to the community. They may forfeit a few days wages to spend the required time at practice. Their costumes may need costly and time-consuming repairs, and they must purchase and cook large quantities of food for feasting. Through participation they are reminded of their cultural heritage and renew their strength to continue as members of Tewa society.

In addition to subsistence and society, Tewa conceptions of beauty are expressed during a village ritual performance. For the Tewas, beauty is found in the power of group movement, in repetitive and understated choreography and song composition, and in a serious, respectful, and dedicated performance. The motion of the entire group together is more important and more beautiful than the performance of any individual; there are no stars. Those who do stand out are criticized for being "too showy" or for dancing "too hard." A single dancer must not destroy the illusion of the group moving as one.

Group unity is facilitated, in part, by the repetitive or redundant nature of the dances and songs. Redundancy not only makes aesthetic expression predictable and familiar, producing a sense of pleasurable security, but it also simplifies execution. By keeping the movement and song vocabulary relatively simple, and by recombining and repeating this vocabulary, a large group of non-specialists is more likely to dance and sing successfully in unison. Performance in unison is not only an aesthetic imperative, but it also reinforces a Tewa concern for the needs of the whole community over those of specific individuals.

Tewas see beauty in the subtle understatement of the dance performance. Gestures are typically close to the body, and steps are usually small progressions with little elevation. The women keep their eyes cast down and their manner demure and contained. This understated performance style also helps to keep any one individual from standing out from the group.

The Tewas also find beauty in songs. They admire their composers for their skill at creating new songs or remembering the traditional ones. The beauty of repetition and understatement are important aspects of Tewa songs. Singers also bring beauty to the ritual when they sing with strong clear voices. Note the simple yet elegant use of metaphor in the following section of a Tewa song (Spinden 1933:94):

Oh our Mother the Earth, oh our Father the Sky,
Your children are we, and with tired backs
We bring you the gifts that you love.
Then weave for us a garment of brightness;
May the warp be the white light of morning,
May the weft be the red light of evening,

May the fringes be the falling rain,
May the border be the standing rainbow.
Thus weave for us a garment of brightness
That we may walk fittingly where birds sing,
That we may walk fittingly where grass is green,
Oh our Mother the Earth, oh our Father the Sky!

The beauty of the performance results from the concentration and commitment of the participants. Tewas speak of this as dancing and singing with respect, or "from the heart," which, as one Tewa man said, "makes the meaning straight." Another said, "You've got to concentrate a lot. Dance with your whole heart in it. Nothing else in your mind—just what is taking place there. Give it all you've got. Singing is the same way. When I sing, I sing from my heart up."

An example of the communication of all three themes—subsistence, society, and beauty—is the cloud dance, also called the corn maiden dance or the three times dance. It is unique among Tewa dances because each time the long line of male dancers appears, only two women participate with them. Eight women are selected for these roles, a different pair for each of the four appearances. They wear elaborate eagle feather headdresses and brightly colored shawls and carry an ear of corn in each hand. They travel with small steps in front of the line of men, who sing and step in place.

The cloud dance communicates many messages, but those about subsistence, society, and beauty are most obvious. Usually held in February, the dance is a reminder that the cold winter months are nearly over, and spring, with its promise of new life, is near. The prominence of the women dancers expresses this message because Tewas associate femaleness with agriculture and warmth (Ortiz 1965:390). The ears of corn carried by the women underscore the theme of agriculture. The women's headdresses symbolize rainbows and clouds, both harbingers of the rain needed for crops, and cloud designs embroidered on the women's dresses also invoke rain.

The men's costumes reinforce the message of seasonal change and a new agricultural cycle. The long fringes on white sashes represent falling rain; tortoise shell knee rattles promote fertility; and evergreen branches symbolize life. One Tewa man described the sound of gourd rattles as "like the sound of summer showers."

The social messages communicated during the cloud dance refer to the structure of Tewa society, carefully classifying the people who make up the village. Cloud dance songs typically mention all the leaders and social groups in the village, such as the women's societies, clown societies, moieties, and native priests. Ties between families and friends find public expression as, for example, an aunt pins a one, five, or twenty dollar bill on her niece's costume, a gesture of appreciation that can take place while the dancer is performing or between dance sets. In either case, the dancer maintains a serious expression and does not overtly acknowledge the gift. Pinning money becomes a public statement about personal relationships. While the cloud dance defines social

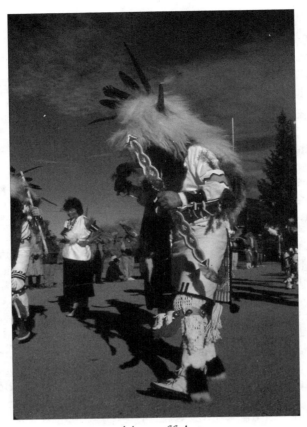

Pojoaque Pueblo Buffalo Dance, 1989.

Photographer Jaqueline Dunnington. Courtesy of School of American Research, W.W. Hill Collection, Maxwell Museum Photo Archives.

groups and personal ties, a concomitant "throw" expresses community cohesiveness and social responsibility. As dancers, singers, and observers catch the tossed gifts, the notion of community support is made public.

The choreographic structure of the cloud dance epitomizes notions of beauty. The dancers begin each dance set by forming a long line, shoulder to shoulder; two women take positions near the ends of the line, and the lead singers stand in the middle. The whole line ântegeh in place, the movements of individuals subordinate to the powerful totality of the group. Slowly and unobtrusively the two women move out from the line, face each other, and begin to move toward each other with small diagonal steps. They meet, pass, and continue traveling to the opposite ends of the line, then turn and travel back to their starting positions. They repeat this pattern again and again. Near the end of the dance set, each woman must be near her starting position so she may slip back into her place in the line as a music cue directs her. Although the cloud dance highlights women, their movements remain small and eyes cast down because those judged most beautiful are the women who contain their movements, appear demure, and dance "from the heart" with deep concentration and quiet dedication. Dancing "from the heart" also helps to unite participants with the supernaturals. The entire performance is a prayer to the supernatural world, the women dancers symbolizing the two corn mothers, central figures in the Tewa origin myth.

Space, Time and Humor

The Tewa Indians give great importance to spatial definitions of their world. In ritual performances, this concern with space appears in frequent and persistent references to the four cardinal directions and their intersection. Through gesture and song, space is symbolically ordered and the Tewa world is spatially defined.

Each direction is designated by a color, an animal, a bird, a mountain, and other natural phenomena. Tewas associate the north with the color blue, the mountain lion, the oriole, and *Tse Shu P'in* (Hazy or Shimmering Mountain), while the west they associate with the color yellow, the bear, the bluebird, and *Tsikumu* P'in (Obsidian Covered Mountain). To the south is assigned the color red, the wildcat, the parrot, and *Oekuu P'in* (Turtle Mountain), and to the east belongs white, the wolf, the magpie, and *K'use' P'in* (Stone Man Mountain) (Harrington 1916:41–45; Parsons 1939:365–366; Ortiz 1969:19). Tewas view the directional mountains as sacred because they define the boundaries of the Tewa world. These mountains border an area approximately 140 miles by 35 miles, and each contains a lake or pond and a sacred stone shrine. Each Tewa village also holds sacred certain neighboring hills with additional stone shrines. These nearby features both designate the directions and mark the boundaries of the land immediately surrounding each village.

In Tewa ritual performances, gestures and songs refer to the cardinal directions in the sequence north, west, south, and east. Dancers, singers, and religious leaders may gesture in this sequence during rituals, and dancers often change their facing direction, performing first toward the west, then suddenly pivoting to repeat the movements facing east. Most Tewa dance movements, sequences of movements, or entire dance appearances are repeated four times or in multiples of four, indicating a close connection with the four directions.

When asked about the content of Tewa songs, one composer replied:

> The words we mention in the songs are the directions. We start from the north, we go to the west, south, and east. And when we mention the colors we start with the blue, yellow, red, and white. And of course we do mention the sacred mountains that are the mountain to the north, the mountain to the west, the mountain to the south, and the one to the east. And then there are some sacred lakes that we have names for there in the north, west, south and east. And then sometimes we mention the rain clouds, the

rain, the thunder, the lightning, the rain gods, and sometimes we mention the rattle we use, and the turtle, and the feathers.

A segment of the San Juan turtle dance song of 1974 illustrates the references to the directions in Tewa songs (Ortiz 1979a):

Away over there, at the dawning place,
Dawn Youths are heard, singing beautifully!
Away over there, at the dawning place,
Dawn Maidens are heard, beautifully making their calls!

Away to the north, holy people are gathering from every direction!
They come, with their corn-growing powers,
And still they come!
Until here they have arrived! (loud rattling)

Away to the west, holy people are gathering from every direction!
They come, with their wheat-growing powers,

And still they come!
Until here they have arrived! (loud rattling)
Away to the south, holy people are gathering from every direction!
They come, with their squash-growing powers,
And still they come!
Until here they have arrived! (loud rattling)

Away to the east, holy people are gathering from every direction!
They come, with their power to raise all cultigens,
And still they come!
Until here they have arrived! (loud rattling)

The intersection of the four directions marks the center of the Tewa world. Each Tewa Indian, however, also sees his or her village as a center because it is the reference point for the cardinal mountains and lakes (Dozier 1970:209). Within each village, the plazas and kivas are additional centers. How can there be more than one center? In cultural groups like the Tewas, where space is regarded as a most important factor in defining the world, the center is often so significant that it is considered spiritually powerful and sacred. Because of its sacredness, the center of the world can be symbolically represented by several actual places. That is, the center, as sacred space, is forever renewable and can symbolically exist in several places at once (Eliade 1954:20–21; Ortiz 1972:142).

By defining the spatial dimensions of their world through ritual, the Tewas reinforce and strengthen their relationship to the physical environment. Tewa history and culture is intimately connected with the land because unlike many Native American groups, the Tewas managed to remain in the territory settled by their ancestors. Indeed, Tewa cultural survival stems partly from their not having been forced from their ancestral lands. A deep relationship with the land, symbolically stated and restated in ritual, helps the Tewas maintain their distinctive culture.

Time, like space, is perceived differently by different cultural groups. Some think of time as exact measurements along a linear progression. Others, like the Tewas, see time as a never-ending cyclical rhythm connected with solar and lunar movements. This view suggests repeated renewal of life as seasons alternate endlessly and all forms of life begin, grow, die, and begin once more (Ortiz 1972:137, 143). The dance circuit patterns of

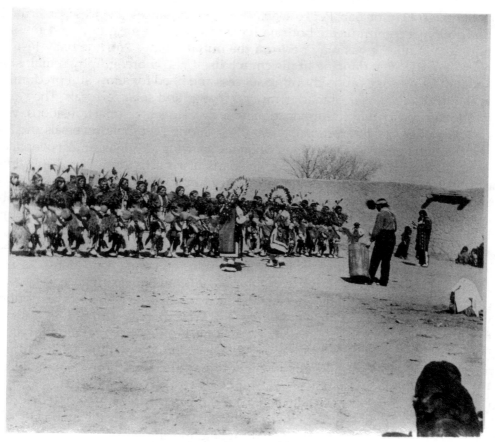

Santa Clara Pueblo, 1911.
Photographer Barbara Freire-Marreco. Courtesy of School of American Research, W.W. Hill Collection, Maxwell Museum Photo Archives.

village ritual performances reflect this cyclical concept of time. Throughout the day, the dancers and singers perform in several designated areas, following the same prescribed circuit with each appearance. At times, the entire performance seems to be a continual cycle of repeated movement patterns with only subtle choreographic variations.

The structure of their ritual calendar, in which each event is associated with traditional seasonal tasks, also reflects the Tewas' view of time. The native calendar, however, is not the only one that dictates when a village ritual will be held: since contact with Europeans, the Tewa people have also observed certain Catholic holy days. The Catholic and native calendars coexist, with the result that some traditional winter dances are regularly held on or near Christmas and some spring dances are held at Easter. In addition, all the Tewa villages have patron saints who are commemorated by native dances on feast days each year. Santa Clara Tewas, for example, celebrate their feast day every August 12, Saint Clare's Day. Some villages celebrate other saints' days, such as Santiago Day or San Pedro Day, with native dances. Dances performed on Christian holidays communicate both native and Christian meanings and messages. Although the Nambe Tewas may perform the buffalo dance "for the baby Jesus" on December 24 or 25, even dancing in the church itself, the choreography remains unaltered and native messages about hunting success and need for snow still predominate.

The equinoxes and solstices mark temporal change and solar reversals. They are important times for Tewa ritual performance because they signal seasonal transitions. Village events acknowledge these transitional times, often through symbolic reversals and inversions and through humor. In September, when the growing season is almost over and the hours of sunlight decrease, the clowns become particularly active, publicly displaying behavior that is backwards, improper, and often very funny. Their performances temporarily turn the social world topsy-turvy. Dancers and singers may also take part in symbolic reversals during the equinoxes and solstices. In some events, men impersonate women, and vice versa. Symbolic reversals may include the imitation of outsiders, as performers dress and act like Anglos, Hispanics, or other Indians such as Kiowas, Comanches, or Navajos. Just as the natural world is in a state of transition and "confusion" during the equinoxes and solstices, so the Tewa world mirrors it through performance.

In order to better understand Tewa symbolic reversals, as well as Tewa notions of humor, consider the antics of the clowns. Tewa clowns are powerful figures associated with fertility, health, and the sun. As masters of burlesque, they make fun of dancers and singers in solemn public performance, village residents and officials including the governor, and even the sacred kachinas. Clowns may also tease non-Tewa people: perhaps the local Catholic priest, a nosy anthropologist, or a curious tourist.

In earlier times, Tewa clowns engaged in extraordinarily licentious and destructive behavior. In the twentieth century, clown performances have become much less sexual and violent, because of years of pressure from neighboring Hispanics and Anglos and from missionaries who failed to understand that clown behavior reinforces acceptable social norms through negative example. Tewa clown performances in fact provide social control by demonstrating how *not* to behave.

Clowns also help integrate foreign institutions, objects, and people into the Tewa world through pantomime and humor. They may poke fun at the Catholic Church by staging a mock Holy Communion during a village ritual performance. After lining up a group of Tewa and non-Tewa observers, they tell each "recipient" to "open your mouth and stick out your tongue." The clowns then give a candy wafer to each puzzled participant. They also play with symbolically loaded objects from outside the Tewa world. A Santa Claus doll might become the object of clown antics around Christmastime, the clown holding and rocking the doll as if it were a real baby. Then suddenly the clown may lose all interest in the doll, dropping it into the mud.

Clowns especially enjoy singling out and embarrassing Anglo tourists. During a harvest dance at San Ildefonso a clown convinced a group of Girl Scouts to join the solemn dance line. To the girls' embarrassment, the war captains immediately told them to sit back down. As soon as they had, the clown again convinced them to dance, and again the officers ordered the confused Girl Scouts to leave the dance line. The clown tried a third time, but the girls would not be convinced.

During a midday break in a San Juan performance, a clown insisted that an Anglo woman dance with him in the plaza. He wanted to "disco." After the clown showed off his version of "bumps and grinds," the woman tried gracefully to leave him. The clown would not allow it, but instead convinced another clown to perform a mock marriage ceremony for them. Only after they "took their vows" did the clown let his bewildered bride go back to her friends.

San Juan clowns also enjoy borrowing a camera from an Anglo tourist and taking pictures of each other in ludicrous poses. They may also take pictures of the tourist who lent them the camera, thus reversing roles with the outsider and subtly posing the question, "see how it feels to be photographed by a stranger?"

In the Navajo dance, all the Tewa performers engage in symbolic reversals and humorous burlesque. Santa Clara and San Ildefonso present different versions of this dance, and the following passage describes it as performed at San Ildefonso in the early spring of 1974 (see Sweet 1979).

The dance was performed by forty women, half of them dressed as Navajo men and half as Navajo women. They wore traditional Navajo clothing, including velveteen shirts and long, full skirts or loose trousers, silver and turquoise jewelry, and Navajo blankets carried over an arm or shoulder. The "women" held ears of corn in their hands and wore their hair tied back with yarn. The "men" wore jeans, Western hats, and boots or moccasins. Many dancers also wore sunglasses, and some of the "men" had fake mustaches or beards.

The performers sang as they danced to the rhythm of a single drum played by a woman also dressed in traditional Navajo fashion. Each "man" shook a rattle throughout the dance. The songs delighted the listeners with English and Navajo phrases such as:

I don't care if you've been married sixteen times before,
I'll get you anyway.

I'll treat you better than the one before.
Ya'at'eeh, ya'at'eeh, I'm a Navajo.

A "campsite" complete with tent, tethered horse, and a truck decorated with flowers and the words "Indian Flower Power" had been set up next to the round kiva. Some women in Navajo garb sat around a campfire, two of them holding Navajo cradleboards containing dolls. During the dance, they handed their "babies" to a Tewa man who rocked them, making the audience laugh.

Throughout the event, dancers held out rugs, blankets, jewelry, and ears of corn to the audience, saying "Hellooo, I haven't seen you in so long, got anything to trade? We're from Ganado" (a Navajo town with a famous trading post). Villagers who were not dancing brought bundles of food and goods to the performers, who carried these gifts of appreciation to the kiva at the end of each dance appearance. During the lunch break, a few Tewa men dressed as Pueblo women took food to the dancers in the kiva, and in the late afternoon there was a throw.

The Navajo dance itself, which included some pantomime, encompassed ten dance appearances of approximately twenty minutes apiece. The dancers began each appearance by singing in Tewa as they walked four abreast from the kiva to the plaza, not in a stylized walk but in a relaxed, comfortable stride. As they walked, the "men" sounded their rattles in accent to the drumbeat. In the plaza, the dancers formed two parallel lines, "women" in one and "men" in the other. The "Navajos" traveled down these lines from west to east, turning inward and pairing up at the end of the line, each couple then traveling back from east to west. Upon reaching the other end of the line, the partners split and repeated the whole sequence. The line formation, however, as well as the steps, gestures, and quality of movement, was completely Tewa, even in parody of the Navajos. During some appearances, a few dancers broke from the line and performed part of the *yeibichai*, a Navajo ritual dance. Even then, they did not abandon the Tewa movement style.

At the fifth appearance, the dancers passed a jug down the line and each took a gulp; some then staggered backwards as if drunk. Couples occasionally left the line to "waltz" or to have their picture taken by a friend. The Tewa audience laughed uproariously at these antics because they consider such behavior typical of Navajos but improper for themselves.

An understanding of the relationship between Tewas and Navajos is essential to an accurate interpretation of the meanings and messages of the Navajo dance. The two groups have historically been both friends and enemies, and their relationship is one of ambivalence. Intermarriage is not uncommon, and some Tewa families have long-established friendships and trading relationships with Navajo families, whom they regularly visit. Yet because of cultural differences and a history of conflicts (the Navajos were once seminomadic people who raided Tewa farmers for produce, livestock, and women), some Tewas still regard Navajos as lazy folk who lie, drink, steal, and make poor spouses. Furthermore, the Tewas have always regarded as degrading the Navajo practice of sheep herding.

The Navajo dance permits the Tewas to consider their past and present feelings about Navajos. By mimicking the Navajos, they can ritualize and defuse years of interaction, including some dangerous confrontations. Through humor, the Navajos are symbolically brought into the Tewa world. The Navajo dance also plays up the antithesis of appropriate Tewa behavior, and so reinforces Tewa standards. Through symbolic reversals and humor, the performance tells Tewa Indians not to drink and act drunk, not to get divorced, and not to be wandering herdsmen.

Besides defining the differences between Tewas and Navajos, the performance plays with male and female role assignment. Tewa women do not normally dress as men (only recently have pants become acceptable attire for Tewa women), nor do men dress as women. Women do not assume important public roles such as that of drummer, and men do not serve women food in the kiva. The dance temporarily suspends these social rules, and since this suspension is seen as humorous and ridiculous, the norm is reinforced. Village ritual performances like the Navajo dance, along with clown behavior, illuminate what the Tewas find perplexing, paradoxical, or nonsensical about themselves and others; they use humor to communicate Tewa definitions of proper behavior.

References

Arnon, Nancy S., and W. W. Hill. 1979. "Santa Clara Pueblo," in *Handbook of North American Indians*, vol. 9, ed. Alfonso Ortiz (Washington, D.C.: Smithsonian Institution).

Bandelier, Adolf F., and Fanny Bandelier. 1937. *Historical Documents Relating to New Mexico, Nueva Vizcaya, and Approaches Thereto, to 1773*, vol. 3 (Washington, D.C.: Carnegie Institute).

Carroll, Terry Lee. 1971. "Gallup and Her Ceremonials," Ph.D. dissertation, University of New Mexico.

Champe, Flavia Waters. 1983. *The Matachines Dance of the Upper Rio Grande* (Lincoln: University of Nebraska Press).

Dozier, Edward P. 1961. "Rio Grande Pueblos," in *Perspectives in American Indian Culture Change*, ed. Edward H. Spicer (Chicago: University of Chicago Press).

_____. 1970. *The Pueblo Indians of North America* (New York: Holt, Rinehart and Winston).

Eickemeyer, Carl, and Lilian Eickemeyer. 1895 *Among the Pueblo Indians* (New York: The Merriam Company).

Eliade, Mircea. 1954. *Cosmos and History: the Myth of the Eternal Return* (New York: Harper Torchbooks).

Fergusson, Erna. 1936. "Crusade from Santa Fe," *North American Review*, vol. 242, pp. 376–387.

Frost, Richard H. 1980. "The Romantic Inflation of the Pueblo Indians," *American West,* vol. 17, no. 1, pp. 4–9.

Garcia, Antonio, and Carlos Garcia. 1968. "Ritual Preludes to Tewa Indian Dances," *Ethnomusicology,* vol. 12, no. 2, pp. 239–243.

Gilbert, Hope. 1940. "Reunion at Santa Clara," *New Mexico Magazine,* May pp. 14–15, 42–43.

Harrington, John P. 1916. "The Ethnogeography of the Tewa Indians," Bureau of American Ethnology, Annual Report, vol. 29, pp. 29–618 (Washington, D.C.: U. S. Government Printing Office).

Hartley, Marsden. 1920. "Red Man Ceremonials," *Art and Archeology,* vol. 9, no. 1, pp. 7–14.

Huff, J. Wesley. 1946. "A Quarter Century of Ceremonials," *New Mexico Magazine,* July, pp. 13–15, 56–59.

Jackson, H.H. 1882. "A Midsummer Fete in the Pueblo of San Juan," *Atlantic Monthly,* vol. 49, pp. 101–108.

Kurath, Gertrude P., and Antonio Garcia. 1970 *Music and Dance of the Tewa Pueblos* (Santa Fe: Museum of New Mexico).

Laski, Vera. 1959. *Seeking Life,* Memoirs of the American Folklore Society, no. 50.

Leach, Edmund. 1976 *Culture and Communication: The Logic by which Symbols are Connected* (Cambridge: Cambridge University Press).

Lyon, Luther. 1979. "Los Matachines de Nuevo Mexico," *New Mexico Magazine,* December, pp. 72–76.

Ortiz, Alfonso. 1965. "Dual Organization as an Operational Concept in the Pueblo Southwest," *Ethnology,* vol. 4, no. 4, pp. 389–396.

_____. 1969. *The Tewa World: Space, Time, Being and Becoming in a Pueblo Society* (Chicago: University of Chicago Press).

_____. 1972. "Ritual Drama and the Pueblo World View," in *New Perspectives on the Pueblos,* ed. Alfonso Ortiz (Albuquerque: University of New Mexico Press).

_____. 1977. "Some Concerns Central to the Writing of Indian History," *Indian Historian, vol.* 10, no. 1, pp, 17–22.

_____. 1979a. "Oku Shareh: Turtle Dance Songs of San Juan Pueblo," New World Records, no. 301.

_____. 1979b. "San Juan Pueblo," in *Handbook of North American Indians.* vol. 9, ed. Alfonso Ortiz (Washington, D.C.: Smithsonian Institution).

Parsons, Elsie Clews. 1929. *Social Organization of the Tewa of New Mexico,* American Anthropological Association Memoir 36.

_____. 1939. *Pueblo Indian Religion,* 2 vols. (Chicago: University of Chicago Press).

Philip, Kenneth R. 1977. *John Collier's Crusade for Indian Reform, 1920–1954* (Tucson: University of Arizona Press).

Rappaport Roy A. 1979. *Ecology, Meaning, and Religion* (Richmond, CA: North Atlantic Books).

Roediger, Virginia M. 1961. *Ceremonial Costumes of the Pueblo Indians* (Berkeley: University of California Press).

Schechner, Richard. 1977. *Essays on Performance Theory, 1970–1976* (New York: Drama Book Specialists).

Sergeant, Elizabeth. 1923. "Death to a Golden Age," *New Republic*, vol. 35, pp. 354–357.

Simmons, Marc. 1979. "History of the Pueblos since 1821," in *Handbook of North American Indians,* Vol. 9, ed. Alfonso Ortiz (Washington, D.C.: Smithsonian Institution).

Sloan, John, and Oliver La Farge. n.d. *Introduction to American Indian Art* (New York: The Exposition of Indian Tribal Arts).

Spicer, Edward H. 1954. "Spanish-Indian Acculturation in the Southwest," *American Anthropologist* vol. 56, pp. 663–678.

Spinden, Herbert J. 1933. *Songs of the Tewa* (New York: The Exposition of Indian Tribal Arts).

Sweet, Jill D. 1975. "Dance of the Rio Grande Pueblo Indians," M.F.A. thesis, University of California, Irvine.

_____. 1978. "Space, Time, and Festival: An Analysis of a San Juan Event," in *Essays in Dance Research,* ed. Dianne L. Woodruff, *Dance Research Annual,* 9 (New York: Congress on Research in Dance).

_____. 1979. "Play, Role Reversal, and Humor: Symbolic Elements of a Tewa Pueblo Navajo *Dance,"* *Dance Research Journal,* vol. 12, no. 1, pp. 3–12.

_____. 1981. "Tewa Ceremonial Performances: The Effects of Tourism on an Ancient Pueblo Indian Dance and Music Tradition," Ph.D. dissertation, University of New Mexico.

_____. 1983. "Ritual and Theatre in Tewa Ceremonial Performances," *Ethnomusicology,* vol. 27, pp. 253–269.

Thomas, D.H. 1978. *The Southwestern Indian Detours* (Phoenix, AZ: Hunter Publishing Company).

Vogt, Evon Z. 1955. "A Study of the Southwest Fiesta System as Exemplified by Laguna Fiesta," *American Anthropologist,* vol. 57, pp. 820–839.

Chapter 2

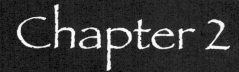

Mexican and New Mexican Dances

A Brief Historical Introduction to Mexican and New Mexican Folk Dances

Bridgit Lujan and Marcela Sandoval

In the sixteenth century, at the time that the Spanish colonized America, dance held a pivotal role in the lives of people from Spain and the Americas. When these two cultures met in Mexico, dance developed as a central activity. Still today, traditional social dance plays a primary role in Spain and Mexico, but perhaps less so in New Mexico. Most men of these cultures dance proficiently since the ability to dance well develops the male's sense of identity and brings him esteem in the community. With Americanization, the folk, social dance legacy has declined in New Mexico, especially in the younger generations. Currently interest in dance folk groups are declining in Spain and Mexico as well. Globalization of the American culture is thought to be one of the key catalysts in this decline.

In Latin cultures, men have played a dominant role in the arts. Until recently, women directed dance companies using their husbands' or fathers' names so that they received credit for the work that women in many cases created. Laws and politics have changed in Latin America and Spain and this no longer remains true. Still, today the male's presence greatly enhances and completes the *baile* (dance) regardless of who is choreographing or directing.

Mexican folkloric dance includes dances developed from the sixteenth century to the Mexican Revolution in 1910. Present day Mexican folkloric dance finds its sources in traditional events of the past since the costuming tends to reflect the period of the late 1800s in Mexico or earlier. As it evolved, Mexican folklorico assimilated music and dance styles from Europe, from the indigenous people of Central Mexico and from African slaves. The goal of most performing groups today is to preserve the creations of the past dance, music and costuming. Although the music and social dances continue to modernize, Mexican folklorico has developed into an art form performed for the purposes of celebration, preservation, pride, art and expression.

The Spanish conqueror Hernando Cortés overcame the Aztec Empire between 1519 and 1521 and shortly after, in 1540, Francisco Vásquez de Coronado came to New Mexico. The year 1610 marked the establishment of the Palace of the Governors in Santa Fe, New Mexico. At this time New Mexico would have been considered part of the *frontera* or *norteña* states of Mexico while the so-called "civilized" lands surrounded the area of Mexico City. The areas that lie farther away from Mexico City were not considered part of "real" Mexico, falling to the wayside. Even today Mexico City is not Ciudad México; it is called México. Being part of the *frontera* has great significance to the Mexican people and so New Mexico, located at the edge of the *frontera* , suffered as part of the forgotten *frontera*.

The Inquisition had a profound and lasting effect on colonial Mexico. Non-Catholic people fled Spain only to find the Inquisition strong and active in the New World, and they moved north to escape the virulent strength of the Inquisition. Many individuals who inhabited the area of New Mexico practiced Protestantism or Judaism *(conversos)*, as well as Catholicism. New Mexico provided an excellent refuge for the persecuted because the area held few ties to New Spain. The isolation of the residents in New Mexico led to the preservation of seventeenth-century Spanish and Ladino words and some customs that were brought by the original conquistadors. Seventeenth-century Spanish continues to be spoken today in parts of New Mexico as well as the concealment of Jewish traditions. People born in the New World not only hid their Jewish ties, but also denied having any Native American relatives so as to protect their property rights. Spanish law forbade people of mixed heritage in New Spain from owning property. Native American dance, despite many fusions with Spanish traditions (Matachines dance), tends to remain quite separate and not integrated into "New Mexican" dance, in contrast to Native dances in Mexico.

When Mexico won its independence from Spain in 1821, its vast areas encompassed present-day Mexico, California, Texas, New Mexico, Colorado and Arizona as well as parts of Utah and Nevada. This victory allowed the Mexican people to embrace their mixed heritage and culture. Before 1848, when speaking of Mexico, one was also speaking of New Mexico and the present Southwestern United States, as no border yet existed. New Mexico originally was part of the state of Chihuahua and received news six months to several years later from the major cities farther south.

The development of a "New Mexican" dance form, different from "Mexican" dance, began after 1848 when New Mexico became a territory of the United States. During this same period, Mexico was undergoing its own political upheavals. In 1863, the Mexican people faced occupation by the French; Maximilian was crowned emperor in 1864. The occupation by the French led to the practice of dances with a strong French aristocratic influence. After the removal of the French, dictator Porfirío Díaz ruled Mexico from 1876–1880 and 1884–1911. The outbreak of the Mexican Revolution in 1910 led to the overthrow of Díaz and the draft of a new constitution in 1917; it was modeled after the constitution of the United States. Díaz, a strong supporter of the arts, erected the Palacio de Bellas Artes building in Mexico City, which is still in use today. On a bi-weekly basis the "Nacíonal Ballet Folklorico de México" presents the revolutionary dances, among others, at the Palacio de Bellas Artes. Ironically, the revolutionary dances were developed in celebration of the strength and rebellion against Díaz and are now performed regularly and preserved in the building Díaz built.

On becoming a state in 1912, Hispanic New Mexicans were anxious to prove their loyalty to the United States. Most Hispanic males volunteered for military service during WWI and WWII in an effort to show their patriotism. New Mexicans then shunned anything that identified them as Mexican, and quickly adopted western music and cowboy dress.

When New Mexico gained its statehood and Mexico wrote its constitution, the literacy rate hovered at a mere twenty-five percent. This rate contributed to difficulties in understanding the traditions as well as accurately archiving the dances and customs of Mexico and New Mexico. Generally, they are passed down through practice and oral tradition.

Dances of Mexico

The dances from the states of Chiapas, Jalisco, Veracruz and El Norte have had a wide spectatorship and are considered fundamentally Mexican. Groups such as the Ballet Folkloríco de México have added re-creations of Aztec dances to their repertory, as well as dance dramas to the standard mestizo or folkloric dances of Mexico that are performed by most Mexican Folkloric groups. The Ballet Folklorico de Mexico, directed by Amalia Hernández, sets the standard and serves as a benchmark for all Mexican folkloric dance troupes within Mexico and abroad. Most of the professional and community dance groups of Mexico and the world model their dances and costuming after Hernández's choreography.

Indigenous music and dance forms, including sixteenth-century Spanish music introduced by the conquistadors, were incorporated into both sacred and social festivities. The Catholic Church encouraged and incorporated music into the Catholic rituals. Priests would host dances for the community and in some communities incorporated dance into church services. Both the movement and the music of folkloric dance hold special, almost spiritual, meaning to the people that transcends generations. Handmade instruments create a distinctive sound, giving Mexican music and dance its original character.

Spanish law governed the clothing and costuming of New Spain. A man's attire represented his caste and his position within the social unit. Lavishness of dress was based upon military distinction and was prohibited for the nonruling classes. Not even nobles or their sons could wear mantles adorned with colors, jewels, or plumage unless they had committed some valorous act, such as killing or capturing a man in battle. Economic and work factors influenced the evolution of masculine dress as well. Religious customs also affected masculine dress in cases where men dressed as the patron saint of their town. Women's dress, however, rarely had political significance and consequently retained an indigenous character because it was generally more modest. Only mestizo women and the Indian women who lived close to urban centers added European elements to their attire.

If we were to propose a Mexican style of dance, it would certainly presuppose a proud and long torso, with most of the movement for the man coming from the knees down. The body bounces up and down with fast and rhythmic footwork. The woman has much more freedom to use her arms and manipulate her skirts as she too creates rapid foot patterns. Folk dances from Spain served as a basis from which Mexican dance evolved. Even though Mexican folklorico dance is commonly compared and confused with Spanish dance, the technique of the limbs and stylistic bouncing is distinctively different. It is not clear to what extent the art of flamenco has influenced Mexican folkloric, but Spain's practice of bullfighting with the toro and the torero, provides many gestures and symbols in Mexican dance.

The admiration and imitation of the horse and its caballero rider (and his clothing) also exist in the dance culture in Mexico. Native Indian and African influences are also present with the imitation of other types of animals such as birds, deer and reptiles. We will now begin our dance journey through Mexico, beginning in the southern states, proceeding north, and ending in modern day New Mexico.

The Yucatán Peninsula, a southern state located the farthest east on the Peninsula of Mexico, contained the largest concentration of Mayan population during the pre-colonization period. The most festive expression of Mexican folkloric dance in the Yucatán is the *Jarana* that belongs to the original *sones* brought from Spain during colonization. The *sones, jarabes,* and *fandangos* are sung and danced all over Mexico. *Sones* derive from the Spanish *jota,* so that the male dancer snaps his fingers imitating castanets and the movements of the bullfight. He manipulates his handkerchief as a *torero* would his cape. Meanwhile, the female dancer weaves back and forth representing the bull, the couple remaining a discreet distance from one another. The performance of the *Jarana* celebrates the *vaquería* (roundup), a traditional Yucatecan postcolonial festival. The *vaquería* originated from the party held at the *haciendas* after the branding of the cattle. After dinner, old Mayan tunes, adapted to Spanish influences, rang out. The people celebrated for three days in honor of the *patron* (land owner) of the *hacienda*.

The costuming of each dance and of each region of Mexico uniquely describes historical and cultural events. The woman's costume in the Yucatan, called the *terno,* derives directly from the Yucatecan mestiza woman's cotton *huipil,* a rather long, very ample shirt that hangs below the knees. The *terno* itself consists of three parts: the *huipil,* the waist and the petticoat and is constructed of fabrics such as cotton or pure silk. Gold jewelry, a rosary, fan, *rebozo* (shawl) and white-heeled shoes are worn with the *terno* dresses, which enfold rich embroidery of bright flower patterns.

In the state of Chiapas, located in the southernmost part of Mexico, Spanish influence on the music, dance, and costumes is less pronounced, while indigenous influences abound. The majority of the dances are named after some type of animal, demonstrating the influence of the native Indian culture and animism. Some examples of these dances from Chiapas are *El javalí* (the boar), *El alcaraván* (an extinct type of love bird), *El gallito* (the little rooster), and *La tortuga del arenal* (the sand turtle). The most

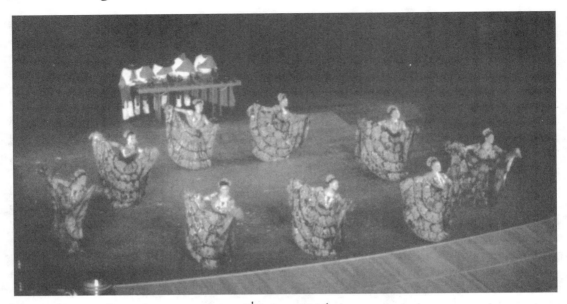

Chiapas, 1996.

Courtesy of Bridgit Lujan, taken in Mexico City of Amalia Hernandez Folkloric Ballet of Mexico.

famous dance of Chiapas, however, is *Las Chiapanecas*, which means the women from the state of Chiapas. In the dance the audience joins in by clapping during a certain part of the dance to a very well known tune. New Mexicans often identify *Las Chiapanecas* as theirs because it enjoys such popularity in New Mexico. The dance is performed in heeled shoes and contains typical patterns and footwork that is highly influenced by Spanish dance.

Another popular dance of Chiapas, *El Rascapetate*, centers on the man and the woman wrapping and unwrapping each other in and out of a *rebozo*. Like a Mexican courting ritual, the man continually flirts with the woman, while the woman gently encourages him. At the end of the dance the man finds himself completely wrapped in the *rebozo*, or tied to her for life.

Generally in regions of high temperature and humidity, lightweight white clothing dominates because white maintains a cooler temperature and helps repel mosquitoes. Despite the intense tropical weather in Chiapas, one of the featured costumes uses black netting as the base of the dress that also features large, colorful flowers. A legend says that Indian women wove the colors of the rainbow and peacocks into the embroidery of their dresses.

Oaxaca, located in the southern part of Mexico, bordering Chiapas, contains mountains known as Zempoaltépetl. They provide an exquisite and imposing backdrop for the Zapotec people who inhabit the highlands and zealously preserve the dances and costumes of pre-colonized Mexico. The dances are performed in bare feet and often have religious significance. One of the most popular dances from this region, *Lucero de la Mañana,* creates different geometric designs by hooking *rebozos* together.

The Tehuana people of Tehuantepec, renowned for their graceful and elegant carriage, always wear their native dress, even when they reside in large cities. Like the Zapotecs, the Tehuanas traditionally go barefoot, even when dressed for festive occasions. Their costume contains garland motifs crocheted in gold silk thread and skirts embroidered with large, brightly colored flowers. The skirt includes a well-starched edge and a pleated white border. The Tehuanas typically wear gold jewelry at all times due to the abundance of gold during pre-colonization.

A popular folk tale of the region speaks of a fleet of ships from Spain, en route to Mexico, shipwrecking; the ships' cargo then washed ashore, laden with trunks of baby baptismal dresses or *repones* (long, lacy white dresses). The native women discovered these dresses, not knowing what their use was, and wound them around their heads. When worn in church, the dress is tied under the chin and when worn for dance fiestas, they are tied behind the head.

Although Puebla is located near the large urban cities of Mexico City and Veracruz, their ceremonial practices still have strong native Indian influences, especially in men's costuming. One of the most colorful dances of this region is *Quetzal,* whose origins are unknown. Some sources speculate that the name of the dance comes from the quetzal bird and the headdresses used in the dance resemble the bird's plumage. It is more likely however that the name of the dance refers to the town Quetzelana where the dance is performed. The dance features a spectacular headdress with a wheel framework of reeds interlaced with multi-colored paper strips or ribbons, each spoke ending in a feather. The rest of the costume consists of short, red pants edged with yellow fringe, a jacket or two shawls crossed over the chest, and a red or yellow cape. The dancer carries a *sonaja* or rattle in one hand and a fan or bandanna in the other. The dance traces distinct designs in the form of a cross (the cardinal points), as well as the circle, which is a symbol of the rotation of time and the universe in native religions.

Another variation of the *Quetzal* is the *Guaguas* and is danced in the Totonac region near the coast. With every step the performers execute an imperceptible sign of the cross with the right foot. The dance ends with four dancers mounted on each of the legs of the great wooden cross, set on a post revolving slowly, with their plumed headdresses swaying majestically. *Guaguas* presents the ritualistic elements of the "Dance of the Flying Pole" and is accompanied by one musician playing both a reed flute and a small drum.

Veracruz, located along the Gulf of Mexico, served as one of the main ports of entry for the Spanish. *Jarocho,* the term used for the people living in Veracruz, also refers to the music and dance of the area. Other regions of Mexico have a mix of styles from both Spanish and indigenous peoples, while Veracruz has primarily Spanish folk influences in their dances. Additionally, this coastal port served as a key entryway for the slave trade. The footwork patterns of these dances contain the most complicated

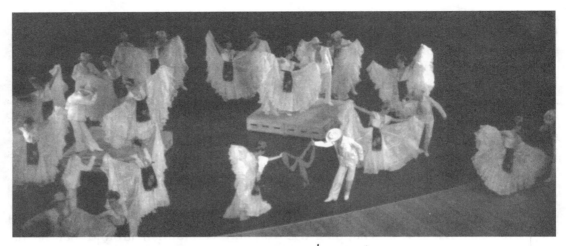

Vera Cruz, La Bamba, 1996.

Courtesy of Bridgit Lujan, taken in Mexico City of Amalia Hernandez Folkloric Ballet of Mexico.

combinations of all the dances in Mexico. Both the musicians and the dancers use improvisation, while challenges or tricks like balancing glasses of water on their heads is common. Improvisation no longer remains part of the dance, as set steps and tricks replace the creativity of the past and now must be mastered.

The most renowned dance of this region is *La Bamba*. In 1863 a famous pirate, Lorencillo, took over the port city of Villa Rica de la Veracruz. After three days of destruction and desolation without any protection from the authorities, the Jarochos became angry with their leaders. When Lorencillo arrived, help was nowhere to be found; the song *La Bamba* cynically refers to the governing troops arriving to defend the port after Lorencillo and the danger were gone. The dance itself tells little of this event, but rather speaks of a young couple in love. They carefully manipulate a ribbon with their feet so that it miraculously becomes a bow, symbolizing the joining of their lives. Failure to tie the bow foretells of gloom in the couple's future and dooms lasting love. The musicians today still improvise in *La Bamba* and construct ridiculous verses as they go along.

The most typical dress of Veracruz, known as the *Veracruzana,* resembles the dress of the region of Valencia in the province of Catalonia, Spain. The woman's skirt and ruffled train, created from organza, contains lace and ribbon intertwined within the fabric. The black velvet apron, lace shawl, fan and thick-heeled shoes are all essential elements of this traditional costume. Local influences can be seen in the lightweight, white fabric of the dresses as well as the wide neck and open shoulders of the peasant blouse. Headpieces are made of ribbons, flowers, and additional fake, braided hair. They mirror the Spanish-style *peinta* or comb, worn along with long earrings, necklaces and a large broach. The man's costume features a white shirt known as a *guayabera;* it is finely-pleated and is worn outside the pants which fit loosely and are always white. They also wear white ranch-style *botines* (half boots), a neckerchief, and a small palm hat, all of which are unique to Veracruz.

Jalisco borders seven other Mexican states and the Pacific Ocean. It has one of the most diverse climates, from hot, dry desert to lush tropical forests to arid coastal land. The name Jalisco originated from the Náhuatl word *Xalisco,* meaning sand. Jalisco is a region renowned for its production of leather, glass, palm products, soap, gum, sugar, candy and nuts. The music most closely associated with Mexico, mariachi, also originated in Jalisco.

Mariachi music, often pronounced a music of delight, gusto and joy, realistically reflects the unhappiness of people reduced in the racial caste system of post-conquest Mexico. Like the gypsies, they were unable to mingle with Spanish society, to own land, or to develop themselves as individuals. Consequently, they reflected an impersonal suffering, wearing a stoic mask, which was presented to all outsiders. The release of these sad and pentup feelings would occur with friends at social gatherings and from this, mariachi music emerged. Similar in many ways to Spanish music, it also draws upon the sound and rhythmic patterns of the central western mestizo culture. Their feelings pour out in nostalgic ranchera songs, *gritos* (yells) and in violent frustrated *zapateados* (footwork). Veracruz's footwork tends to be more intricate while Jalisco's produces a stronger, more driving sound. In Jalisco, the male dancer, the aggressor, strives to demonstrate his machismo and dominate the woman, who responds with coy flirtations. The man performs for her with assertive movements, loud *zapateados,* and the handling of knives or ropes. They also demonstrate their adept use of the *machetes* (large long knives) in a dance that requires them to hit the *machetes* together over their heads and under their legs, with an added blindfold at the end of the dance. The woman waits modestly, content knowing that the show is for her. She turns her shoulder to him, lifts an arm, creating a barrier, and turns away just as a resolution nears; however, she continues to entice her partner with her eyes.

The songs generally tell stories of ranch life through movements and gestures. The horse serves as a symbol of power, wealth and manhood to the Indian and mestizo, thus the *zapateados* (footwork) simulates the sound of the galloping horse. The gestures of the legs mimic the horse while the arm and skirt movements of the woman imitate twirling imaginary lassos.

Jarabe Tapatío, the most renowned dance from Mexico, also known as the "Mexican Hat Dance," uses a stylized form of the old folk *jarabes.* The name of the dance derives from *Tapatío,* a person from the state of Jalisco and Jarabe, meaning mixture. The *jarabe* of the colonial period contained a hopping step that resembles Andalusian folk dance. *Jarabe Tapatío* combines colonial steps as well as steps and tunes from all over Mexico, thus explaining why it is a *jarabe.* The man's steps are vigorous and showy. He constantly pursues his partner, trying to gain her attention. Nearing the end of the dance, the man throws his hat on the floor and the woman dances inside the brim. If the woman tips the hat, the man buys a round of drinks for everyone. At the end of the

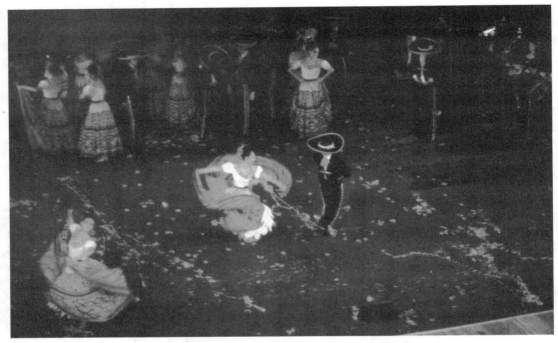

Jalisco, Jarabe Tapatio (Mexican Hat Dance), 1996.

Courtesy of Bridgit Lujan, taken in Mexico City of Amalia Hernandez Folkloric Ballet of Mexico.

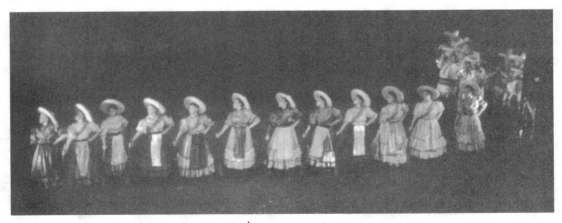

El Norte, 1996.

Courtesy of Bridgit Lujan, taken in Mexico City of Amalia Hernandez Folkloric Ballet of Mexico.

dance, the woman picks up the hat, symbolizing her reciprocation of the man's amorous feelings. They then dance together as the woman holds the hat high and modestly covers themselves with the hat and kiss.

The traditional *charro* attire of Jalisco originates from the suits worn by *haciendados* and the hacienda cowboys of Spain. The *charro*, evocative of the Spanish *traje corto*, served as the dress for the native *haciendados*, who were land owners of noble birth or descendants of the conquerors who became nobility through glorious deeds that took place during the conquest. *Haciendados* wore only the best clothing with the finest silver buttons and decorations on their jackets and hats; they are often called *plateados* (silverplated ones). The complete *charro* outfit consists of a large decorated sombrero, a cotton or linen shirt, a silk cravat (usually green or red) tied at the neck in a bow, close-fitting pants with decorations or embroidery down the sides of the legs, and a short jacket with matching decorations. Leather shields called *tapabalazos* and *chaparreras* (chaps) are sometimes worn over the pants along with boots and spurs. The women wear long, full, heavy, colorful skirts with ruffles, ribbons, lace and a blouse that matches. They also wear a *rebozo* and flowers or ribbons in their hair, long earrings and necklaces.

Another fiesta costume, the China *Poblana*, has become a national symbol of Mexico and boasts a beautiful sequined and beaded skirt. The skirt's decoration is sewn into various figures and themes. The embroidered blouse, *rebozo*, satin slippers and filigree earrings add even more splendor to the costume.

The legend of the China *Poblana* costume comes from the eighteenth century, recalling the kidnapping of a Mongolian or Asian princess by Portuguese sailors. The princess was brought to Nao de Filipinas or Nao de China in Acapulco, Mexico, and subsequently sold into slavery. She was forced to adopt the dress of a Mexican servant. The princess's memories of her former glory served as inspiration to collect and sew different shiny objects onto her skirt, hence creating the China *Poblana* costume.

El Norte includes the Mexican states of Tamaulipas, Nuevo León, Chihuahua, Durango, Sinaloa, Sonora, and Coahuila. During pre-Columbian times this land was largely uninhabited because of the severely limited water supply, and as a result, less Indian folklore existed in the area. The Tarahumara Indians, who continue to dress in ways similar to the pre-conquest, still inhabit the Cañon de Cobre (Copper Canyon) in Chihuahua.

The deer dance from Sonora is one of the most elegant and difficult dances of all folkloric dances. Dancers today who perform the deer dance must be trained in contemporary techniques, and be in excellent physical shape. The dance symbolizes the struggle between good, represented by the deer that is held sacred by both the Mayan and Yaqui Indians, and evil, represented by the coyote that is known for his awesome powers. At the beginning of the dance, two coyotes begin to dance. They wear tiny rattles made of butterfly cocoons filled with pebbles. The deer dancer stands in the center wearing a dried deer's head as his headdress. The deer then shakes the two rattles while other musical accompaniment is played on the drum and a five-tone reed flute.

When the coyotes move stealthily and threateningly, sounds of the European harp and violin are heard. The deer dancer senses danger as the coyotes draw near. His movement and rhythm become more agitated as the coyotes try to capture him. At one point, the coyotes finally corner the deer, but he escapes, attacks and kills one of the coyotes. Too quickly, the spectators all rejoice, as the coyote suddenly comes back to life in the form of a hunter who kills the deer with a bow and arrow. The death of the deer is the most difficult section of the dance and is regarded by audiences as the most beautiful part.

European dances, brought by the settlers to the United States and the French occupation, took root in northern Mexico. Some examples of these dances are the contradanza, a variation on the English country dance, the polkas and mazurkas from Poland, and the schottisches from Germany, France and Finland. Rancheras, a very popular style in New Mexico, developed while similar norteña dances developed in Mexico.

Despite hostility toward the French, *norteños* decided to keep French dances and other influences that pleased them. The Mexican Revolution reduced the isolation of "El Norte" from the rest of the country, as Pancho Villa's troops moved into the northwestern part of Mexico. Catchy tunes such a "La Cucaracha," the cockroach, were really revolutionary songs that were put in code, similar to the slave songs of the southern United States. The *soldaderas,* women who fought next to the men, cooked and nursed the wounded and received great admiration. Dances and songs such as "Jesusita en Chihuahua" and "La Adelita" are dedicated to *soldaderas* and are some of the best known songs and dances of the region and era. Despite the repetitious structure of the music, the dance has tremendous variety, enthusiasm, energy and spirit.

The men's costumes imitate the clothing of a working cowboy: dark pants, bright shirt, neckerchief, cowboy hat, boots and possibly a fringed leather or suede jacket. The women wear a modest cotton dress or skirt and peasant-style blouse in a variety of light colors. A petticoat and square dance bloomers are worn along with boots to the knee or short boots in black and white. The skirt generally hangs just below the knees, in some cases, longer.

Dances of New Mexico

The dances of New Mexico generally serve social or recreational purposes, enhancing the sense of community in small villages as well as in larger urban communities. Anglo-American visitors entering New Mexico via the Santa Fe Trail in 1821 began recording the dances in their journals while introducing new dances, such as the quadrille, waltz and two-step as well. Dances such as "La Carcoviana" and "La Varsoviana" come from Polish court dances, "Krakoviak" and "Warszowanka," and are named after the Polish cities Kracow and Warsaw, respectively. During territorial days, local musicians adopted the European music of square dances, Irish jigs, Scottish reels, and American favorites. The Mexican polka grew in popularity in the twentieth century as well, using a side-to-side step rather than the standard ballroom position. In the 1920s the foxtrot, tango and Cuban bolero temporarily took over the New Mexican dance scene. Today, traditional dances are rarely practiced, as young people do not know the steps or recognize the tunes.

The most familiar and popular dance of New Mexico is *La Marcha* and is considered essential to a traditional New Mexican wedding. *La Marcha*, or the wedding march, contains elements unique to New Mexican dance and is an integral part of the wedding reception. The tune for *La Marcha* originated from deep in central Mexico, the state of Zacatecas. New Mexican tradition requires the groom to pay entirely for the wedding and the fiesta (party), as this indulgence proves the groom is a worthy husband. A designated couple, known for their knowledge of *La Marcha*, will lead. The music of *La Marcha* pulses 2/4 time and the basic step of *La Marcha*, a shuffle step, alternates from the right to left foot, dragging the ball of the foot along the floor. The men line up on one side, usually on the left, and the women on the right. The people who form pairs do not have to be of any relation to each other; they can be a grandfather and his grandson, two sisters or two strangers. The intent is for everyone to join in. As *La Marcha* starts, the couples form a line, the lead couple first, then the bride and groom, followed by the wedding party and then the rest of the guests. This line will be central and principal to the rest of the dance. Whichever direction the line is facing becomes the front of the room for the dance. After the dance has taken place, guests from both sides of the family pin money on the bride in exchange for a dance. In some instances the groom's immediate family pins money on the groom as an additional sign of closer social relations. The money is a gift to enable the bride to start her new home. La Marcha serves as a community blessing for the couple and the bride's honored position in the home and community. Those weddings which do not perform *La Marcha* are regarded as illegitimate marriages of unhappiness, unsanctioned by the community or God according to traditional customs. The steps, designed simply, create an atmosphere of full participation. *La Marcha*, the high point of the wedding dance, creates honor, good spirits, harmony and fun.

Another well-known dance of New Mexico is *Valse de la Escoba* (Broom Waltz). Any number of dancers can participate, but there must be one extra man. The dance initiates with the participants lining up facing each other, men on one side, and women on the other. The "extra" man dances between the lines with the broom. He will spontaneously drop the broom and quickly select a woman to waltz with. The other men scramble to find a partner also. The man without a partner has to dance with the broom. The dance progresses in two ways from this point: either the group lines up again and the sequence is repeated, or the dancers continue in pairs until the broom is dropped and everyone switches to a new partner, careful not to select a repeat partner. A similar dance has been traced to rural France.

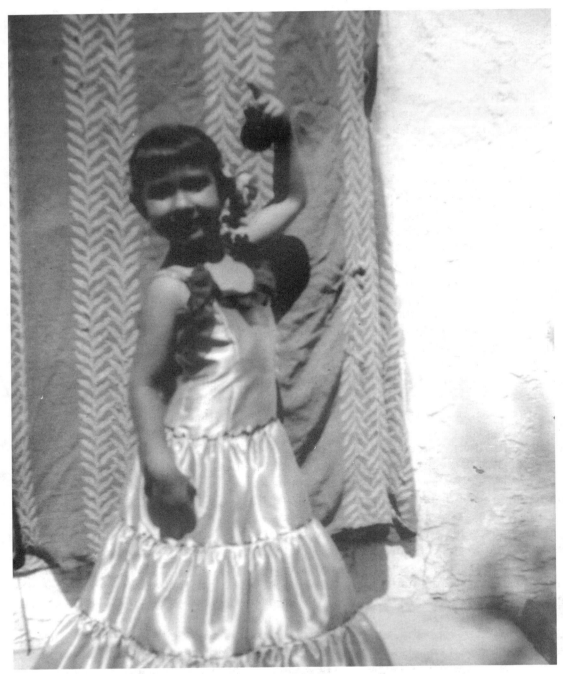

Lorraine Saavedra performing for fiestas in Albuquerque, 1954.
Courtesy of Bridgit Lujan.

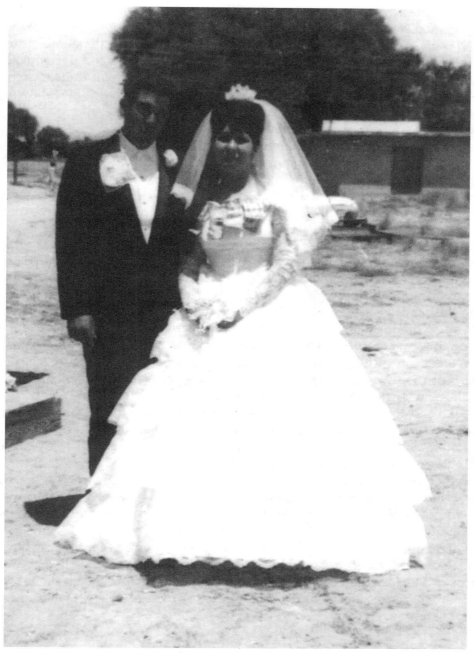

Mr. and Mrs. Felipe Lujan after La Marcha (pinned with money), 1966. Courtesy of Bridgit Lujan.

Baile de Compadres, considered a traditional dance, is more of a game. Men's ties and women's aprons are distributed to the men and women respectively. Each tie has an apron of the same fabric pattern and those who receive the items must find their coordinating partner. The two people then become *compadres* (special friends) for one year. After they find their *compadre,* the women form an inner circle while the men form an outer circle facing one another and the dance begins. Throughout the following year the *compadres* acknowledge their special association by addressing one another as *compadre* or *comadre,* rather than by their given names.

The clothing of the *bailes* is different in New Mexico from that of Mexican dress, which includes bright colors, elaborate embroidery and large gold jewelry. New Mexican dress, on the other hand, upheld conservative European styles. In the nineteenth century women wore large fitted sleeves and short-waisted dresses with no bustles. Men wore colored cotton trousers, leather belts and jackets. In the early twentieth century women wore sleeves to the wrists and a collar that fitted closely around the neck, know as *bien cerrado* (well closed) or high-necked blouses combined with dark colored dresses or skirts to the ankles. These outfits were standard for Catholic Hispanic families until the 1960s in New Mexico. Hispanic native New Mexican women generally did not wear pants until the 1960s or 1970s. With time, New Mexican women began wearing shorter dresses of lighter colors. For *bailes,* the clothing standard is now "Sunday's best," which usually encompasses a wide variety of colors and current styles. Men used to wear whatever they could afford, from suits to bib overalls with big hats and ties. Later three-piece suits became the standard.

Live music is always played for the *bailes.* Bands generally consisted of a violin and guitar player who also sang; sometimes a *tombé* (Indian drum) would also be part of the group. Later the accordion was added and is now one of the most important elements of *ranchera* music. Years ago schoolhouses served as locations for dances, however, as more and more community structures were built, dances took place in any large place suited for a party.

With increasing intermarriage, traditional dances of Mexico are being assimilated into New Mexican church fiestas and parties, and the old New Mexican dances are becoming forgotten and unknown. Salsa music and country western music, as well as DJs, are taking over where live bands once performed.

The diversity of styles in costuming, music and movement continue to hold sway over the traditions of Mexican folklore. New Mexico's dances inherited the beauty and dynamics of Mexican dance while establishing their own approach to their style and costuming. The dances themselves, however, are in a current state of decline. *La Marcha* is one of the few survivors.

Bibliography

Aguirre Cristiani, Gabriela and Felipe Segura Escalona. *Amalia Hernández' Folkloric Ballet of México.* México D.F.: Fomento Cultural Banamex, A.C., 1994.

Covarrubias, Luis. *Mexican Native Costumes*. Mexico: Fischgrund.

Covarrubias, Luis. *Regional Dances of Mexico*. Mexico: Fischgrund.

Espinosa, Aurelio M., and J. Manuel Espinosa, ed. *The Folklore of Spain in the American Southwest: Traditional Spanish Folk Literature in Northern New Mexico and Southern Colorado*. Norman: University of Oklahoma Press, 1985.

Lucero-White, Aurora, Eunice Hauskins and Helen Mareau. *Recuerdos de la Fiesta Santa Fe Folk-Dances of the Spanish-Colonials of New Mexico*. Santa Fe: Examiner Publishing Co., Inc., 1940.

Montaño, Mary. *Tradiciones Nuevomexicanos*. Albuquerque: The University of New Mexico Press, 2001.

Sandoval, Marcela. *Mexican/New Mexican Folk Dance*. Albuquerque: Hispanic Culture Foundation, 1994.

Sedillo, Mela. *Mexican and New Mexican Folkdances*. Albuquerque: University of New Mexico Press, 1945.

Interviews and Other Sources

Alarid, Elaine. Director of Ballet Foklórico de Del Norte High School, Albuquerque, NM.

Caro, Miguel. Director of Miguel Caro Mexican Fiesta Co., Albuquerque, NM.

Chavez, Regina. Director of Regina's Dance School, Albuquerque, NM.

Kessell, John L. Professor Emeritus History, University of New Mexico.

Luján, Frances. Director of Ballet en Fuego-Latin Dance Review, Albuquerque, NM.

Sanchez, Anita, *La Marcha* Procession Leader, personal interview, Albuquerque, NM, 22 April 2002.

Appendix 1

The couples separate, men going left and women to the right as they reach the front of the line. The men and women travel toward the back of the line, rejoining in the back of the line and the line starts over. The lead couple is now in the front of the line, and again the line splits in couples as each reach the front. It starts with the lead couple going right, the bride and groom left, the third couple to the right and so forth. As the couples meet each other in the back of the room they drop hands and pass between each other. They rejoin hands, go around the room and do the same in front of the room. Now the lead couple creates a bridge by holding each other's hands facing one another and lifting their arms high. The second couple goes under the arch of the first. The second couple then stands adjacent to the first couple and so forth until all the couples have formed a long bridge and the lead couple arrives at the end. The lead couple then goes under the bridge and quickly pulls all the other couples inside the bridge until the bridge is undone and the line of couples remain holding hands again. The lead couple then raises their arms, allowing the second couple to go between them, and then the third couple raises their arms, allowing the lead couple to pass under them backwards, so on and so forth. Each couple will be traveling backwards until the lead couple is in the front again. The couples then break off right and left again and join in the back as groups of fours. Then the groups go right and left and join in the back of the room to form groups of eight. The couples then line up in a line behind each other in groups of eight couples. The lead couple then makes a sharp right turn, picking up each couple as they pass. The line is then single file and forms a circle resembling a snail shell. It then flips around, turning the opposite direction, unwinding itself into a large circle with the bride and the groom in the middle. The circle then moves in and out around the couple.

The Dance of My People: Los Matachines

Jo Marie Griego Lubarsky

We saw twelve masked men in colorful costumes, their ribbons and fringed shawls flying out as they turned and stamped in unison. It was like a colorful, well-rehearsed ballet.[1]

The Matachines dance has been performed for the Fiesta de San Lorenzo (the feast of Saint Lawrence) in Bernalillo on August 10th for an estimated two hundred years. I remember watching the dance as a child and wondering why the Matachines dance was such an integral part of the fiesta. A little girl, called Malinche, danced with a man who wore a white suit, shiny shoes and a mitred headdress with rainbow colored ribbons flowing down the back. There was also a fringe over his face to conceal his identity. According to my mother, Mercy Griego, the little girl represents the Virgin Mary, and the man dressed in white represents San Lorenzo[2] or Monarca.

In Bernalillo, the dance takes place on the anniversary of the first feast of San Lorenzo after the Romans killed him in 258 BCE. The Mayordomos keep the tradition by housing San Lorenzo in a decorated altar where church and community members say the rosary every month for a year until the celebration dance. A donation box provides funds for an impressive feast at the home of the Mayordomos. If people are unable to donate money, they bring food and help serve the guests. On the evening before, Vespers begin the fiesta in the old Chapel of Saint Lawrence on Main Street. The community prays the rosary until midnight. Early the next morning, Mass is celebrated and there is a procession led by the Matachines and the Mayordomos who carry the Santo.

The Matachines has been handed down from generation to generation through oral-tradition; none of the steps or songs are written down. In the Native American pueblos of Taos and San Juan, the dance is performed on Christmas Day. In some places, a pantomime of childbirth is enacted that represents the birth of Christ and explains why it occurs on Christmas Day. Many agree that it is a day of thanks to San Lorenzo from all in the community. My mother thought that the dance was clearly a pantomime of the religious battle between the early Christian church and Ancient Rome.

The Matachines begins in dreamlike motion, very slow and deliberate. Two rows of danzantes or Matachines face one another with a slight gap in the middle. Wearing black

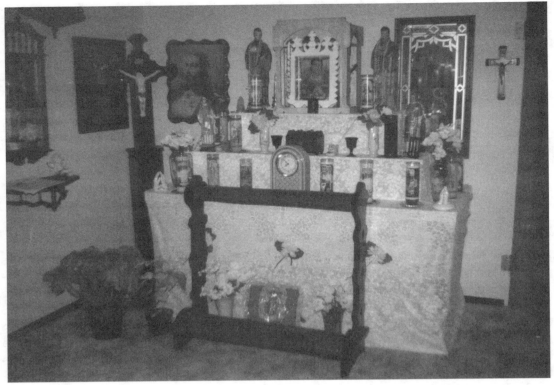

Altar with statue of San Lorenzo.

Courtesy of Aline Chavez.

from head to toe and sunglasses, the Abuelos (grandparents) carry long leather whips that they prop on their shoulders. The ribbons of San Lorenzo's headdress blow in the breeze while the sound of gourd rattles being shaken in perfect rhythm is heard. Also, there are two guardians of San Lorenzo and a Toro who wears a headdress with a fringed veil and many roses grouped together like a funeral bouquet. A pair of bullhorns protrudes from the roses in a taunting way. As the Toro or bull, he holds two black canes and walks around on all fours. The Toro taunts the Abuelos who keep him away with their whips, cracking them against the two canes that represent the Toro's front hooves. Malinche dances between the lines of the Matachines as the Abuelos keep watch that the Toro does not disturb her. At one point in the dance, a pantomime between the Abuelos and the Toro takes place and the Toro may be slaughtered. But in Bernalillo they stage a stand off between the Abuelos and the Toro who tries to attack San Lorenzo. The community eventually joins Los Danzantes to dance the promesa or promise dance. Promesa can be compared to tribal dances of the Pueblo Indians. The steps are a series of stomps and kicks in many of the sequences. The drum is not used in this dance. Instead, the dancers use gourd rattles, called guajes, to mark the rhythm of the dance. In addition to the rattles, the tunes of fiddles and acoustic guitars fill the air.

There are many other dancers who participate, including Los Danzantes. These characters are usually dressed in black pants and white shirts and wear a headdress much like that of San Lorenzo, with ribbons flowing down the back. They also wear a flag portraying a picture of a saint or the Sacred Heart of Jesus. Many choose to wear the flag of the patron saint of Mexico, Our Lady of Guadalupe. They hold a palm-like wooden trident in one hand and wave it as they keep in step with the music while they shake a gourd rattle in the other to keep time.

A common theory about the origin of the dance attributes it to the Aztec King Montezuma, whose daughter was named La Malinche. According to Sylvia Rodriguez, the Taos Indians believe that Montezuma taught the dance to the pueblos.[3] The Evans sisters compare Monarca with Montezuma as his costume rivals any great monarch's. "The headdress of Monarca . . . is called a corona or crown. The corona is fashioned of a leather ring, or headband, that fits snugly on the dancer's head.[4] Like a Bishop's mitre, it sparkles with ornaments and culminates at the apex in a radiant cross.[5] It is

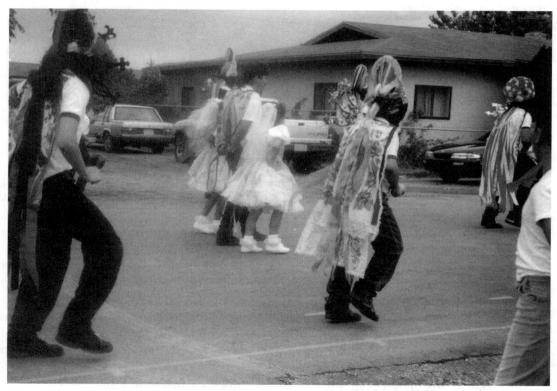

Matachines practicing in front of home (back view).
Courtesy of Aline Chavez.

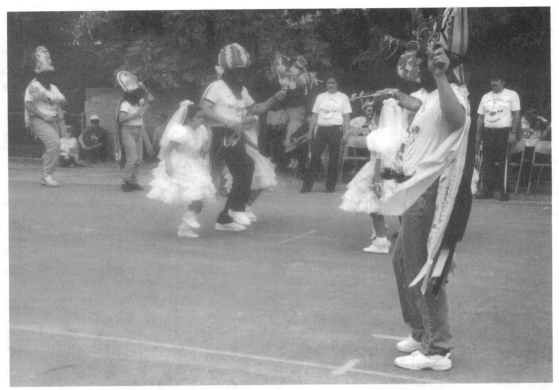

Matachines practicing in front of home (front view).
Courtesy of Aline Chavez.

entirely possible that the cross signified Montezuma's conversion to Christianity. Several other communities share this notion. Gertrude Kurath explains how the Tewa people of San Juan accepted this drama as part of their ceremonial calendar. The Tewa believe that the ceremonies involved in the Matachines dance were introduced by a mythological figure from the south (Montezuma), a fearsome Indian god who wore European clothes. Perhaps the Matachines is performed as a way of appeasing the god of Christianity, much the same way that the Native Americans appease the forces of nature. Theories abound. A tale from the pueblo of Santa Clara claims that an old man, Oyesemo, created the dance. Oyesemo is said to be the poetic representation of the Aztec word for Montezuma.[6] Also, the word *matachin* has been associated with the Arabic "mudawajjihin," an Arabic word meaning "maskers" or "assuming masks."[7] Kurath observed that double file dances and stringed instruments were common in Arabia and Spain.[8]

If the dance originated in Spain, it may have evolved from the European drama *los moros y los cristianos*. Rodriguez attended a performance at Arroyo Seco, where the program specified that the Spanish conquerors brought the play to Mexico in 1530 and performed it for the Native Americans in order to convert them. It seemed that the decorative costumes and headdresses made a fine impression on the Aztecs, causing them to include the dance as part of their religious calendar. Using dance and theatre to teach and to persuade the Native Americans was a common tool in the narrative of Spanish conquest. In her focus on the Maya myths and rituals in Chiapas, Victoria Reifler Bricker tries to show how rituals transcended a specific moment in time.[9]

In the Pueblo Indian Matachines dance, there is a touch of contempt and dismay during the dance as we can't escape the fact that it was forced upon them. The origin of the dance in Bernalillo may be associated with the anniversary of the Pueblo Revolt, which is also on August 10th. The tradition attributes the dance to the only Spanish survivors of the revolt at Sandia Pueblo. Those few people were at Bernalillo. The dance continues to have great resonance in Bernalillo because it represents a deeply religious expression of worship. Each character brings alive a certain principle of life. The Toro represents all that is evil in the world, while San Lorenzo represents all that is good. Malinche offers the innocence of a new person in the world, while the Abuelos are the angels of God. Whatever the origin of the dance, the dancer or Danzante gives God great honor by making the sacrifice of dancing Los Matachines.

Notes

1. Flavia Waters Champe, *The Matachines Dance of the Upper Rio Grande: History, Music and Choreography* (Lincoln: University of Nebraska Press, 1983), XI.
2. Interview with Mercy Griego, August 17, 2002.
3. Sylvia Rodriguez, *The Matachines Dance: Ritual, Symbolism and Interethnic Relations in the Upper Rio Grande Valley* (Albuquerque: University of New Mexico Press, 1996), 18.
4. Champe, 8.
5. Bessie Evans and May G. Evans, *American Indian Dance Steps* (New York: A. S. Barnes and Company 1931), 73.
6. Gertrude Kurath with the aid of Antonio Garcia, *Music and Dance of the Tewa Pueblos* (Santa Fe: Museum of New Mexico Press, 1970), 265.
7. Evans, 76.
8. Kurath, 266.
9. Victoria Bricker, *The Indian Christ, The Indian King: The Historical Substrate of Maya Myth and Ritual* (Austin: The University of Texas Press, 1981), 129.

Bibliography

Bricker, Victoria. *The Indian Christ, The Indian King: The Historical Substrate of Maya Myth and Ritual.* Austin: University of Texas Press, 1981.

Champe, Flavia Waters. *The Matachines Dance of the Upper Rio Grande: History, Music, and Choreography.* Lincoln: University of Nebraska Press, 1983.

Evans, Bessie and May G. Evans. *American Indian Dance Steps*. New York: A.S. Barnes and Co., Inc., 1931.

Fergusson, Erna. *Dancing Gods: Indian Ceremonials of New Mexico and Arizona*. Albuquerque: University of New Mexico Press, 1957.

Griego, Mercy. Interview by JoMarie Griego-Lubarsky, August 17, 2002.

Gutierrez, Ramon. *When Jesus Came, the Corn Mothers Went Away*. Stanford, California: Stanford University Press, 1991.

Hoever, Rev. Hugo and S.O. Cist. *Lives of the Saints: For Every Day of The Year*. Revised ed. New Jersey: Catholic Book Publishing Company, 1999.

Kirstein, Lincoln. *Dance: A Short History of Classic Theatrical Dancing*. Pennington, NJ. Princeton Book Company, 1935.

Kurath, Gertrude with the aid of Antonio García. *Music and Dance of the Tewa Pueblos*. Sante Fe: Museum of New Mexico Press, 1970.

"The Matachines Dance," *The Santa Fean Magazine* v.3 #1 (Dec.-Jan 1975): 26–27. Courtesy of the Museum of New Mexico.

Rodriguez, Sylvia. *The Matachines Dance: Ritual Symbolism and Interethnic Relations in the Upper Rio Grande Valley*. Albuquerque: University of New Mexico Press, 1996.

Romero, Brenda. *The Matachines Music and Dance in San Juan Pueblo and Alcalde, New Mexico: Context and Meanings*. Ph.D. Diss. Washington D.C.: Smithsonian Institution Press, 1979.

The Midnight Rodeo: A Virtual View of Country Western Dance

Barbejoy Ponzio

"... by wearing his clothes, listening and dancing to his music, we touch his spirit and through association share in the virtues of independence, courage, and freedom."

Country Western Swing and Western Dance and a Bit About Cowboy

To enter a country western dance club is to step back in time to a former era and begin an imaginative journey to America's mythic Western frontier. Formed over a long period of three centuries and expressed through literature, folklore, ritual, and historiography, the myth of the frontier is America's oldest and most characteristic story. The hero of this story is the cowboy, who represents the simplified social and historical experiences of the myth.

The Midnight Rodeo, located in Albuquerque, New Mexico, utilizes the cowboy myth of the Western frontier by incorporating legendary themes and motifs such as the cowboy, the frontier landscape, the horse, and the six-shooter. Dancing at The Midnight Rodeo is an expression of the original mythic story of the cowboy.

To coax the country western dancer's personal and social remembering, the dance space at The Midnight Rodeo is filled with properties and musical sounds of the "good old" western days, adding a historical flavor to the dance and evoking an immediate photoplay that belongs to the cowboy event. It brings the mystique of the Western frontier to the dancer, offering a glimpse of Western trails and fantasies. This popular dance club is a place of refuge and escape from contemporaneous problems. It brings western fantasy and reality together under one roof.

As soon as one enters, the sights and sounds hurl one back to a former dimension— a frontier town of the Old West. The false front of a Western town looms across from the east side of the dance floor. It features the Last Chance Hotel, Cactus Jack's Saloon, Black Smith & Livery Stable, Wild West Cantina, and the Bernalillo County Cooler. Perpendicular to the town stands Rodeo Plaza, a shopping arcade which houses Lilly Langtree's Social Club, Momma Feelgood's Photo Fantasy Parlor, Levi's Hattery, and the Stitchen Post, that actually sells Western apparel, including wedding dresses. One can glance at the row of buildings and quickly imagine gun battles, frantic chases on horseback, and the final showdown between the cowboy hero and the villain, which are depicted in almost every Western film. Many other symbolic distractions offer a virtual view of cowboy reality: two large video screens picturing rodeos, five saloon-type bars, a pool room, and a roping pit with a mechanical horse and calf.

The dance floor looks like the Astrodome, where as many people as possible are squeezed onto a circular, railed-in dance floor. Tradition requires that everyone dance in a counterclockwise direction around the floor. In earlier days, when women wore trains, the man had to dance backward with the lady following, in order not to step on the trailing material. After dress styles eliminated trains, it became customary for the men to dance forward so that they could see where they were going and head off collisions.[1] Although there isn't any corn meal spread atop the concrete to make it easier on the boots, as happens at the famed Gilley's in Pasadena, Texas, where *Urban Cowboy* was filmed, the crowd here is whirling up a storm on a beautifully maintained wooden surface. Scores of other men and women watch from the tables along the perimeter of the dance floor.

The dancers are garbed in the typical Western attire: broad-rimmed cowboy hats, stiff leather boots with low heels, starched jeans, a concha belt, although some accent their look with twenty-first century devices—pagers and cell phones. Ranging in age from the twenties through the sixties and adorned in all the Western ceremonial attire, the dancers become involved in a social event embodies vast lands with heroes, freedom, and the spirit of the frontier. Dancing the Cotton-Eyed Joe, the Texas Two Step, the Western Swing, and the Cowboy Waltz, listening to the sounds of top country western recording stars played by a disc jockey whose booth rests upon an old rustic frontier wagon, and attempting to rope a calf while riding a mechanical horse—all of these activities provide and bombard patrons with metaphorical images and icons of the rugged West. While engaging in the dance, the country western dancer partakes in an imaginative journey to the premodern West—a West where life seems simple and basic.

A Real Cowboy's Dance

In the imagined West, time brings no essential change. Myth chases events out of context and drains them of their historicity. The cowboy is a pervasive cultural symbol, which explains and validates traditional American ideals. For example, how a cowboy acts in myth is how an American male should act regardless of time or place. A man has to do what a man has to do.[2]

A return to life in the West restores authenticity, moral order, and above all, masculinity for the male country western dancer. By participating in the dance, he gets to look and feel like a cowboy, the epitome of manhood.

The dialogue exchanged between two country western dance instructors at The Midnight Rodeo suggests the masculine potency evoked by the legendary cowboy hero. "The two-step is a real cowboy dance," says the male instructor. "They like to have a real hold on their woman and control her." His female partner laughs. "Yeah," she says, "the only time they can control her is on the dance floor."

If cowboys like to hold on to their women and control them, it certainly comes across through the dance. Ladies move backward, men move forward. The man is in charge. It is always the lady who turns, moving fast so she is back in position when he reaches for her hand, always the lady who moves her cowboy boots double time; backing away from her gent to await the slight tug of her hand that cues her for the 360 degree whirl. The woman knows that when the man pulls her toward him, he is getting ready to fling her out. To execute the turn, the woman bows her head and casts her eyes down at the floor while the man, pressing his hand on her shoulder blade, leads her through the turn. Yet, this position is not as degrading as that of the *Urban Cowboy* dance era of the early 1980s, when the closed position consisted of the man holding the back of the woman's neck instead of placing his hand upon her shoulder blade. The men dance with hats on, the ladies without. The way the lady ducks and tucks, a hat would fly across the dance floor.

Undermining Traditional Dances

The tucking, ducking, swinging and whirling began as a result of the cowboy's adaptation of the American square dance.[3] The cowboy's love of freedom, space and experiment helped to gradually undermine Old World traditions and create the distinctive style of modern western dance.[4] This rambunctious cowboy dance style was a spontaneous adaptation of traditional moves brought West by various immigrant cultures.

During the late 1700s through the mid-1800s, diverse cultures migrated west across the plains to the promise of gold, farmland and ranch land waiting to be developed. The earliest settlers came on ships from Germany, England, Ireland, France, or Spain and on horseback from Mexico. They also came by ship or oxcart from the Eastern and Southern states, where they paused for a time after leaving the Old World. Later, after the close of the Civil War and with the passage of the Homestead Act of 1862, war-weary soldiers and people uprooted by battle headed to other states in the West with the hope of building a new life on free soil. Widely differing people, who had had little or no previous exposure to one another, gathered and danced on common ground.

Because the people were of diverse origins, few knew the same steps. They brought with them the style of dancing which predominated in their hometowns. They added or subtracted dance elements they preferred to keep. A particular dance may have been drastically different from one town to another, from one year or from one generation to the next. Thus the four men in a single set usually had four different styles and each tried to dance the other three.[5] To prevent chaos from dominating the dance floor, the caller's job was to orchestrate the heterogeneous crowd into harmonious movement. Working with the steps of formal quadrilles and folk dances, the caller told the dancers what to do next, and was able to create the dance by juggling the order of the figures. The American pattern dances, with the caller, became known as "square dances." While the European pattern dances required dancers to know the exact patterns of each dance, and to dance precisely through them from memory, Americans developed the idea of having a caller who hollered out the dance instructions to the rhythm of the music.

Catherine Cavender, stationed in Hays, Kansas, with her family in 1860, vividly recalls the fun of having a cowboy caller while attending a grand ball given by the commander of the nearby fort; it was the highlight of one year's social season:

> The square dances held the most fun for the older crowd, and a good caller was always a thing of joy. The night of this ball they had coaxed or bribed a cowboy to call a few sets and show the soldiers from Dixie just how it was done in the wild and wooly West . . . I wish I had the calls he called, most of them impromptu, I think. The first was: 'Git your partners for a Quadrille, Spit out your tobacco and everybody dance. Swing the other gal, swing her sweet! Paw dirt, doggies, stomp your feet.' This was mighty embarrassing to the uninitiated, as they did not know how to 'paw dirt' or 'stomp,' which simply meant to do a sort of jig step and lift your feet high.[6]

The cowboys' dancing was an untamed mix of reels, balances and swings, tempered with some waltzes.[7] The dancing of the cowboys was considerably more casual than that of other settlers; for the cowboys took a particular delight in swinging, since they could break away from the called patterns and swing their partners around the dance floor. Folklorists have said that it was well-known that swinging formed the major part of the dance.[8]

In 1874, Joseph McCoy, the first great cattle baron, wrote in *Historic Sketches of the Cattle Trade of the West and Southwest,* a vivid description of these dancers with questionable finesse:

> To say they danced wildly or in an abandoned manner is putting it mild . . . The cowboy enters the dance with a particular zest, not stopping to divest himself of his sombrero, spurs or pistols; but just as he dismounts off his cow pony, so he goes into the dance . . . With the front of his sombrero lifted at an angle of full forty-five degrees, his huge spurs jingling at every step or motion, his revolvers, flapping up and down like a retreating sheep's tail, his eyes lit up with excitement . . . he plunges in and 'hoses it down' at a terrible rate in the most awkward yet approved country style, often swinging his partner clear off the floor for an entire circle . . . [9]

Women's Role in the Dance

Women were handled as if the cowboy were still rounding up the cattle and getting it ready to be branded. One observer commented, in 1873, that some cowpunchers danced like a bear round a beehive that was afraid of getting stung. Others didn't seem to know how to handle a calico (a woman), and got as rough as they did handlin' cattle in brandin' pens.[10] Livingston claims that this distinctive style resulted from the cowboy bringing to the dance floor those roundup actions he used on the range:

> The habitual swing of the leg when dismounting from a horse became a mighty polka gallop . . . the 'double arms over' move [actually an overhead double turn], is reminiscent of the final 'tying off' of a calf's legs prior to branding.[11]

Being outnumbered on the dance floor and surrounded by men (mountain men, cowboys, trappers, miners, and soldiers) most of whom did not possess the social graces nor the knowledge of specific dances, the frontier woman was subjected to a variety of outlandish behaviors and movements. After long days on the range, cowboys were ready to cut loose. Their reckless deeds on the dance floor were reactions from months of loneliness on the ranch and on the trail. [12] In his eagerness to get a partner and celebrate his time off, the cowboy paid no attention to traditional dance forms. The polka and square dance were transformed into an eccentric pantomime of movements the cowboys knew best.[13] The cowboy's eccentric movements also influenced the waltz, which traveled across the continent in the 1850s. After this elegant, urban dance reached the isolation and expansiveness of the West, it was soon almost unrecognizable.

The woman involved in the westward movement during the nineteenth century did not have much influence on the development of country western dance due to her cultural predicament. For the woman who migrated to the West, her social status became critical, because she lived in a part of the country where she was outnumbered. Thus, her scarcity became a handicap. She was now a commodity—an exciting and attractive figure in the Wild West, although for sale.

The female shortage was felt most acutely at dances or other gatherings where the gaiety depended upon an even number of partners of opposite sexes. During the early periods of western migration—the 1840s and early 1850s—women were in an extreme minority. Among the members of the largest wagon company journeying to the Pacific Coast in 1841, there was but one woman; and only two were included among a similar party in 1844 traveling from the Missouri river to California. Georgia W. Read's article "Women and Children on the Oregon-California Trail in the Gold-Rush Years" estimated that the number of women who traveled westward in 1849 was 10 per cent of a total number of 50,000 emigrants—roughly 5,000 women, 2,500 children, 42,500 men.[14]

In the cattle country of western Washington, one rancher recalled attending a dance where there were sixty cowboys and three women. It was a common sight to see cowboys resort to the old trick of tying handkerchiefs to their arms to designate some of them as females. Also, a man bringing one girl to a dance got a free ticket. If he brought two girls, he would receive 25 cents.[15]

Eleanor Alice Richards, daughter of a Wyoming governor, recalled that during one winter when she was a girl of eleven living in the Bighorn Basin, there were a hundred men in the Basin and seven women, if she included herself. She attended the all-night dances with her parents:

> The men were very respectful and well behaved. I remember at one dance that a couple of the boys who became intoxicated were taken out, placed on their horses and shown the way home. There were so many men and so few women; they knew that they must behave if they wished to have a good time.[16]

The cowboy has been immortalized in song and story. The pioneer woman has been remembered with a flicker of association to the cowboy's West. For this reason, it is difficult to find a good historical account of women's influence on country western dance. Despite this, their own personal portrayals of their lives help to illuminate the role dance partook in their everyday activities. To understand the relationship between the woman and the dance and to understand the lack of historical documentation of the woman's contribution to the dance is to understand their cultural predicament in the nineteenth century.

Social historians have emphasized the fact that the nineteenth century was a lamentable time for women in general.[17] In Western Europe the peasant woman worked equally hard but with less hope. The low-class city dweller in Europe or America was subject even more to tuberculosis, skin eruptions, and social diseases and also had little hope for bettering her place in life. Only middle- and upper-class women had leisure and luxury. However, they were expected to live in almost total subservience to the male society. The nineteenth century was an extremely patriarchal society. For many of them, the search for meaning in life must have been long, frustrating, and depressing. They had no status in the law, no property, and no possession of their children should the husband leave or sue for divorce.

Country western dance is associated with the West of popular myth and imagination, usually told through the heroic adventures of trappers, cowboys, prospectors, soldiers, or outlaws—mostly male, mostly young, mostly Anglo-American, mostly 'unfettered' by family or communal ties. Women, if they had any part in this saga, appeared in minor, supporting roles, as one-dimensional sketches.

From East to West: Square Dance to Country Western

Slowly, a dance that was specifically "western" began to evolve. Stopping over in the towns on the route of the big cattle drives from New Mexico and West Texas to Dodge City, Kansas, many cowboys introduced new dance material from the West and the South to the people along the trail. As time went on, novelty moves and styles popular in Appalachia and the South came to the West and were absorbed by the new settler. The freed Black Americans in particular exerted a stylistic influence that can still be seen in today's country swing dance. This new hybrid was considerably more casual than the traditions from which it derived, which may also be due to the way the dances were passed on from one town to another, from one area to another.

As the frontier was broken up with the settling of the west in the 1900s, dance halls continued catering to local patrons. Square dancing in the West became influenced by dances from the East coast. People turned to ballroom dancing and to couple dancing. The dance halls were seldom used for square dancing. Regarded as old-fashioned and unsophisticated, the square dance was displaced to the smaller towns where there was a strong sense of community. Instead of the American square dance being the dance performed frequently in dance halls, it was seldom seen. Consequently, the same situation existed in the West as existed in the East. In the early 1900s, the townspeople celebrated with the square dance which was only performed in town halls, grange halls, and neighborhood homes. The square dance was definitely not part of the culturally refined society.[18]

The easy, early couple dances such as the waltzes, schottisches, and polkas that went underground to be kept on hold by a few honky-tonks, clubs, and country western dance halls, were to emerge later under the name of country western, cowboy, or plain country dances. Those dance steps put aside for many years achieved national prominence because they were tied in with the burgeoning popularity of country music. Thus, dancing at the dance halls evolved from the Western square dances into couple dances such as the swing, waltz, two-step and polka, in which the couple could dance without the aid of a caller. The pattern or square dances lived on as American folk dances, but not as popular, contemporary dances.

Although some new, creative styling changes updated and modernized the contemporary country western dances, the basic dances had been well established for years. In his article, "They Swing Only One Way—Country," published in the *Colorado Springs Sun*, Michael McConnell commented on the instruction at today's country western dance establishments. "What they're learning has been around a long time. Country western dance is basically an outgrowth of the country and folk dances that have always been a part of local culture."[19]

In conclusion, the American population has become attracted to country western dance as a vehicle for socializing and for the stability, respectability, and self-esteem it offers in this age of uncertainty. The mythical illusions of country western dance symbolize order and natural unity in a perilous social world even though the myth of the Western frontier embodies the full range of contradictions. The positive concepts exemplified by the myth—autonomy, unlimited opportunity for acquisition of property, social freedom, national pride—are misrepresented by the actual monotony and conformity of cowboy life, the ruthless destruction of the Native American Indian, and the passing of the infinite landscape.[20] The nostalgia associated with the Western myth suggests that a return to the premodern world offers a superior alternative to contemporary life. When our sense of security is threatened, we often turn to our myths to rejuvenate our spirits and settle our minds.

As in so many other examples, the West became something of a national mirror. When Americans looked into the imagined West for images of themselves, their own present situation determined what was reflected back. In the dance, they found not a senseless escape to fantasy frontier adventures but an imaginative escape from the economic and cultural crisis of reality.

In an article in *New York Times Magazine,* the author describes her imaginative escape during a country western dance lesson:

> I want to be lifted off the linoleum of the gym floor and set down, dancing, on a wood plank floor while a fiddler is sawing away, keeping time with his hips, and a

little cowboy is singing the truth as he knows it. Ladies' skirts are swinging, and men are stomping, and fat, pretty babies are sleeping on feather beds in the corners of the barn, sighing in their sleep.[21]

Notes

1. Betty Casey, *Dance Across Texas* (Austin: University of Texas Press, 1985), 14.
2. Richard White, *It's Your Misfortune and None of My Own* (Norman: University of Oklahoma Press, 1991), 616.
3. Peter Livingston, *Country Western Swing and Western Dance and a Bit About Cowboys* (Garden City: Doubleday, 1983), 39.
4. Livingston, 31.
5. Robert Lee Cook, "The Frontier Dance," *Sets in Order* 23 (1971): 7, 8.
6. Joanna Stratton, *Pioneer Women* (New York: Simon and Schuster, 1981), 140.
7. Charles Harris and Buck Rainey, *The Cowboy: Six Shooters, Song and Sex* (Norman: The University of Oklahoma Press, 1976), 133.
8. Frank Dobie, *Coffee in the Gourd* (Austin: Texas Folkloric Society, 1923), 33.
9. Joseph McCoy, *Historic Sketches of the Cattle Trade of the West and Southwest* (Kansas City: Ramsey, Millet and Hudson, 1874), 139.
10. McCoy, 59.
11. Livingston, 39.
12. John Avery Lomax, *Cowboy Songs and Other Frontier Ballads* (New York: Duell, Sloan and Pearce, 1950), 1922.
13. Livingston, 39.
14. Georgia W. Read, "Women and Children on the Oregon-California Trail in the Gold-Rush Years," *Missouri Historical Review* XXXIX (1944): 6.
15. Dee Brown, *The Gentle Tamers* (Lincoln: The University of Nebraska Press, 1958), 221.
16. Brown, 221.
17. See Richard Barlett, *The New Country* (New York: Oxford University Press, 1974).
18. Patricia Phillips, A Philosophical, Historical, and Cultural Analysis of the American Square Dance (Boston: Boston University Press, 1973), 204.
19. McConnell, Michael, "They Swing Only One Way—Country," *Colorado Springs Sun.* 19 Dec (1980): 17.
20. Anne Andrews Hindman, *The Myth of the Western Frontier in American Dance and Drama: 1930–1943* (Diss. University of Georgia, 1972), 327.
21. Kathleen Dean Moore, "The Cowboy Waltz," *New York Times Magazine* 10 September (1995): 34.

Bibliography

Bartlett, Richard A. *The New Country.* New York: Oxford University Press, 1974.

Brown, Dee. *The Gentle Tamers.* Lincoln: The University of Nebraska Press, 1958.

Casey, Betty. *Dance Across Texas.* Austin: University of Texas Press, 1985.

Cook, Robert Lee. "The Frontier Dance." *Sets in Order* 23:7 (1971): 8.

Dobie, Frank. *Coffee in the Gourd.* Austin: Texas Folklore Society, 1923.

Harris, Charles and Rainey, Buck. *The Cowboy: Six Shooters, Song and Sex.* Norman: University of Oklahoma Press, 1976.

Hindman, Anne Andrews. *The Myth of the Western Frontier in American Dance and Drama: 1930–1943.* Diss. University of Georgia, 1972.

Livingston, Peter. *Country Western Swing and Western Dance and a Bit About Cowboys.* Garden City: Doubleday, 1983.

Lomax, John Avery. *Cowboy Songs and Other Frontier Ballads.* New York: Duell, Sloan and Pearce, 1950.

McConnell, Michael. "They Swing Only One Way—Country." *Colorado Springs Sun.* 19 (Dec. 1980):14–15.

McCoy, Joseph. *Historic Sketches of the Cattle Trade of the West and Southwest.* Kansas City: Ramsey, Millet and Hudson, 1874.

Moore, Kathleen Dean. "The Cowboy Waltz." *New York Times Magazine,* 10 September 1995, 34.

Phillips, Patricia. *A Philosophical, Historical, and Cultural Analysis of the American Square Dance.* Diss. Boston: Boston University, 1973. (Ann Arbor: UMI, 1973).

Read, Georgia W. "Women and Children on the Oregon-California Trail in the Gold-Rush Years." *Missouri Historical Review* XXXIX (1944): 6.

Stratton, Joanna. *Pioneer Women.* New York: Simon and Schuster, 1981.

Webb, Walter Prescott. *The Great Plains.* New York: Grosset & Dunlap, 1957.

White, Richard. *"It's Your Misfortune and None of My Own."* Norman: University of Oklahoma Press, 1991.

Chapter 3

Flamenco Dance

Dancing in the Deserts of Spain and New Mexico[1]

Ninotchka Devorah Bennahum

Gypsy, gitana, bohemien, romanichel. Egipciano, Egyptian, one from the East, foreigner.[2]

*Flamenco, a Gypsy, or caló, form of song and dance of the Gypsies of Andalusia, Spain. Flamenco is danced by the body of the **bailaor/bailaora**, or dancer, sung by the **cantaor**, or singer, and accompanied by the lyrical and rhythmically-complex rasquedo, or scaling, of the guitarist, **tocaor**. Flamenco has become an international performance form, safeguarding a modern aesthetic developed as a public performance form by Gypsy andnon-Gypsy—payo— artists from the nineteenth century to the present day.*

Gypsy Flamenco developed in the white-washed pueblos of the Iberian Peninsula.[3] At its heart, Flamenco is an improvisational form of song and dance whose choreographic shape is formed by dancers moving through space. The singer's words offer the dancer's movements an arc of meaning that narrates the performance. The design of choreography is enhanced by the singer's poetic metaphors that, together, build an architectural design of the stage.

Out of the *cante's* structure of call (*siera, llamada*) and phrasing (*letra, compás*), emerges the rhythmic shape of the song. A dancer may then choose to improvise to the music or dance choreography. This organic interplay of song and dance, performed to guitar accompaniment, shapes flamenco into one of the most powerful performance forms to date. It is in flamenco's rhythmic structure that the dance historian and ethnomusicologist discover the secret to its potency and longevity as a ritual form of performance.

One further addition to the crescendoing duet between song and dance is the dancer's ornate use of gesture, called *florea* in Spanish. *Florea* is a flowering of hands and wrists in all flamenco dances that involve sensuous, delicate movements of the fingers that recall Flamenco's East Indian origins. Traditionally, women define themselves in flamenco through the outline of their hands and arms in space that accompany rhythmic footwork sequences. This use of gesture delicately added by a dancer becomes a way of speaking to the audience and a means of cueing or calling the guitarist and singer.

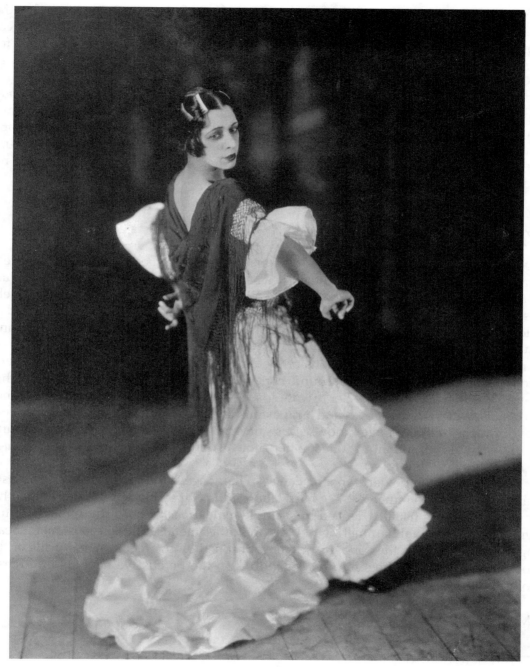

La Argentina, Antonía Merce.
Courtesy of Ninothchka Bennahum.

Three more movement qualities define flamenco technique and choreography: the use of weight; the repeated change of direction in a solo, or *soleá,* and an almost devotional focus seen in a performer's eyes. Contemplation is reflected in this internally focused expression accompanied by outstretched arms that surround and guard the face as if to hide it from spectatorship.

These technical qualities give the flamenco dancer the sensation that his/her body moves as a organic whole, a symbol of the music that travels through it to musicians on store and spectators in the audience. How the whole performance will take shape is always unknown, even for the most sophisticated of performances as Gypsies use the flamenco dance and song to speak to each other. Thus, a public performance remains a private form of communication.

The Soleá

Solo dances in flamenco are like personal prayers that begin and end in choreographic meditation, building in intensity as the dancer expands into space to the accompaniment of *cantaor,* or *muezzin,* and collapsing in exhaustion back into oneself, resonating with *desplante,* the finale of five movements of a flamenco cycle. The end of a long solo could be compared to the end of a spiritual journey taken with caller and musician. As in Persian music or calls to prayer, five movements define five places on stage and five newly begun sections of the dance phrasing. At the beginning of each movement, the *bailaora* circles around herself, at times with outstretched arms that seem to beckon audience into her private space—the space closest to her body. At other moments, with downcast eyes and a rapacious circling around herself, (as if she were devouring herself) the singer knows she signals him to sing for her. Hitting the ground with her right foot so that the nails in her shoe resound, she calls him—*una llamada*—to begin his storytelling.

One of the more powerful poetic verses in flamenco is the *Martinete.* A *cantaor* uses this serious song to remember the hard labor of the Gypsy blacksmith working at his anvil. The song is usually danced by a single male *bailaor* whose rhythmic structure symbolizes the actual hammering of nails and other metals. The sound of metal beating metal syncopates the song, its downbeat echoed by the feet in harsh drills of the floor, driving toe and heel into the stage to reap the percussive benefits of a harsh polyrhythmic flow of energy.

Martinete
　　With the weariness of death
　　I crept to one side;
　　With the fringes of my hand
　　I tore at the wall. . . .

Like the forge,
My insides glow like gold
When I remember you,
And I weep . . .

Noted twentieth century Spanish historian, Americo Castró described flamenco performance as follows: "We owe the Gypsies the building of these lyrical channels through which all the pain, all the ritual gestures of the race can escape."[4] After many minutes of dancing, a performer falls into trance, known as *cante jondo*, or deep song.

Deep Song was first defined by Spanish poet, Federico Garcia Lorca in his 1933 "Theory and Play of the *Duende*." Lorca refers to deep song as "black sounds"—"los sonidos negros"—that overtake the dancer's body and mind as he/she hammers the stage with an endless series of rhythmic sequences. Falling into an epiphenomenal state of semi-consciousness, dancers appear to lose a conscious connection with the audience.[5] Dancers in the deep song portion of a *Martinete* or a *Siguiriyas por Bulerias* describe this state as being possessed by a demon or spirit that inhabits the body, transforming corporeal form into the conduit that delivers emotion to the spectator. Later in this chapter, we will draw a connection between the flamenco dancer's ability to fall into trance and the East Indian Gypsy's belief that a similar trance-like experience called *Rasa*, pushes the body of the dancer into a quasi-religious state of mind, of being. Both the Indian *Rasa* and Gypsy *duende* ritualize the performance space, pulling spectator and performer into close proximity with one another.

Gypsies in New Mexico

It is a surprise to discover Spanish Gypsies in New Mexico, the land of Enchantment—the land of the Pueblo Indians—beating out fandango rhythms with their feet on the hot, dusty sand at the Santo Domingo Pueblo. Spanish conquistadors "discovered" the pueblo in 1540. Led by a Spanish soldier, Francisco Coronado, and eleven hundred of his foot soldiers, they entered New Mexico from Old Mexico in search of wealth. Previous expeditions, led by Cabeza de Vaca in 1535 and Fray Marcos and his Moorish slave, Estevan, in 1539, had searched fruitlessly for Cibola, the seven mythical cities of gold.[6] Some five centuries later, on a hot summer's day in 2002, the Spanish Gypsy artists known to the world as the Farrucos, arrived at the Pueblo, in peace and solidarity, bringing with them their own treasure: flamenco.

To the Gypsy mind, the Farruco name is gold currency. "Farruco" is a symbol: Sevillian timekeepers of the Gypsy treasure flamenco puro, or pure flamenco, with its thousands of song-cycles, Indo-Romani-Spanish tongue, poetry, pathos, and storytelling cantos. The Farrucos, like the Native American sand-painters, preserve time, revealing in poetic meter truths and shards of evidence, that chronicle their long, harsh road from India to Spain, from freedom to exile to conquered.

Moreno, the Farruco's *cantaor*, visited the Santo Domingo pueblo as a guest of the New Mexican-based International Flamenco Festival. As a Gypsy singer, he has inherited knowledge of the *compás*, valuable rhythmic cycles used to mark Gypsy life—songs that give musical expression to birth, baptism, marriage, and death. Walking around the earthen plaza, he begins to beat out a twelve-count rhythm with the palms of his hands. Farruco, the master of the male-dominated *farruco* dance, walks beside Moreno into Santo Domingo's modestly decorated church and then down the tiny hill to the base of the Kiva, the ceremonial hut. The pueblo appears deserted. It is silent, empty. They stop in front of a small adobe house where Moreno begins to sing a Gypsy verse, a *falseta*. Doors that were closed and windows that were shuttered are suddenly opened and Native Americans come out to greet him.

It is an encounter, perhaps one of the first peaceful ones as new Spaniards wait to see who exits the houses. One Native American, upon hearing Moreno's voice, re-enters the home, emerging with an immense drum, as if to say, "welcome." They accompany Moreno's voice as it enters the *cante jondo*, or deep song scale, the most pro-found of Gypsy verses. Farruco lifts his arms to the sky, his fingers snapping, his intense feet fighting with the earth, moving in polycentric motion to the syncretic beat of his Gypsy singer and Native American drummer. Only men stand on the dirt of the plaza, surrounded by the immense sky that wraps New Mexicans in a blanket of light.[7] Gypsies, like Indians, live as a subculture in their host country.[8]

Dancing in the Desert provides a short history of flamenco's creation by the Gypsy people on their journey from India to Spain and of the migration of the new American genre of "gypsified" Flamenco evolving in New Mexico. Inside this travel route, Gypsy Algerian filmmaker, Tony Gatlif, who in a trilogy of films, traced the history of the Gypsy migration from India to Spain, expressed the extraordinary ability of the Gypsies to carry their once native East Indian dance of Kathak from country to coun-try, adapting its rhythms and choreography to new cultures, encountered along the way.[9] The Gypsies, a willful people, have kneaded into flamenco the words, dance phrases, costumes, and song cycles that they brought with them from Rajasthan. The image of the Gypsy wandering remains in the popular imagination a subtle, seductive bohemian theme of liberation and Romanticism. It embodies a collective world history, linking eastern and western forms of music and dance inside of flamenco performance.

Theirs is a creative endurance expressed through the body of the dancer, its sinu-ous carving of space, its centrifugal power in legs and circling arms, its erect, yet fluid body stance, upper torso pulled up, head and weight thrust up and down and pushed over to the side, the twisted, disjointed, back held in an elegant, yet torqued, position. This Gypsy body, where East and West collide in the dance, recalls brilliantly their his-tory of wandering, adapting, surviving and regeneration. They are able to adapt and assimilate aspects of the host culture with East Indian Kathak traits of their own. Few art forms are as culturally influenced as flamenco. The body, the voice and the guitar, are like the pages of a book. Each time they sound or move, they inscribe on the body of the dancer or the voice of the singer a history of inter-cultural encounter.

Flamenco's History

Inside the Gypsy home, flamenco is a form of oral history, or *intra historia*, a means for parents and grandparents to pass onto their children a history of their people, struggles and persecution in host countries. Always marginalized, Gypsies have suffered in the countries through which they have passed.

In Spain, Flamenco began as a ritual form of Gypsy storytelling through song and dance, an isolated expression not shared with the outside world until the mid-nineteenth century. Protected by the mountains of the Sacromonte, the coastal region referred to by Hispanic Arabs as "al Andaluz" is today, littered with Gypsy pueblos: Almeria, Murcia, Arcos de la Frontera, Cadíz, Jerez, Granada, Sevilla. Whitewashed, flower filled, the pueblos are beautiful. One wonders whether or not the topography of southern Spain contributed to the birth of a form as intense as flamenco. The Iberian Peninsula, once inhabited by the first Iberians, then by the Carthaginians, Phoenicians, Greeks, Romans, Visigoths and Hispano-Arabs from the Middle East and North Africa, had a variety of cultures and language systems that left behind an architectural legacy.

Performed late at night in the earthen plazas of Gypsy pueblos, flamenco gave Gypsy families a cohesive, unifying means of communication through song and dance. Verse represents sung history, allowing the families to share stories, celebrate lifecycles, family deaths, harvest events, saints' days, baptisms, initiation into the clan or into the pantheon of great flamenco artists. Not every Gypsy became a great flamenco artist. But every Gypsy maintains the right to dance, sing, and play guitar, at least within the closed ritual setting of the clan-circle.

Flamenco consists of both happy and sad dances. The happy dances are explosive, allowing dancers and guitarists to show off their wares. The sad dances compose the heart, *el corazon*, of the form. Following are several coplas, or verses, from flamenco singing. It is the sheer pessimistic sadness that overwhelms. Many of these verses are about love. But, oftentimes, they are about persecution of the Gypsies, as they have always lived as second-class citizens in Spain. In fact, an interesting comparison between the thematic structures of flamenco and blues music can be drawn, as both musical forms are the expression of an oppressed people.

Siguiriyas
> I climbed to the top of the wall
> and the wind said to me:
> what is the use of sighing
> if there is no remedy?

I longed to live
To see you and hear you;
Now that you're not here
I prefer to die."

Tanguillos
"Niña, come to your balcony
I want to whisper something
To whisper something
In your ear.
The message is
That I want to lose you from sight
And that I've only come to return
The kisses you gave me.

Carceleras
Twenty-five cells has the jail of Utrera,
I have been through twenty-four
And the most painful remains with me.

They took forty men
From inside the prison of 'La Carroca'
And the work that they gave them
Was removing rocks from the water

They took me from the prison
And put me in another much worse;
And they put me in front
Of a Holy Christ of wood

I have the earth for a bed
A brick for a pillow
And to alleviate my suffering
On my feet, a pair of shackles."

Playeras
"The cart of the dead
passed by;

I recognized her
By her dangling hand.

I cry for death
But it will not come;
Even death
Finds me unworthy.[10]

Etymology

There is much to be learned from the etymological history of the words *flamenco* and *Gypsy*. Flamenco in Arabic means one who does not belong: *felag mengu*. Flamenco also means stranger, fleeing one, one without borders, without a home. Gypsy comes from *egipciano*, or Egyptian, as it is believed that the Gypsy entered Spain from Egypt, a kind of exile, like that of the Hebrews. The Gypsy represents a minority group, separated out from those who belong through language and symbolism.[11]

So, what then defines the historical relationship between the word flamenco and the word Gypsy? Do they explain a people whose art form resonates a nationless class of wanderers? When do the terms come to define the same group of people and when do they stand separately on the pages of Spanish and English dictionaries? My discussion, for the purposes of this short chapter on the history of flamenco in Spain and New Mexico, will attempt to answer these questions. Flamenco's etymological history is defined by scholars of the art form, inseparable from its proponent artists. The history of the Gypsy people is a history of struggle and migration. The Gypsy art form is represented by poetic storytelling, songs, family history, and their dancing late at night, in and outside the once Moorish and Sephardic, now Christian, towns scattered along the southeastern Iberian coastline.

An earthbound form, the flamenco dancer's lower body must look weighted so as to communicate its hard pounding, stamping, crashing of high-heeled or booted feet with nails on the bottoms of shoes, contacting the floor of a wooden stage or dirt plaza of a dusty Andalusian Gypsy pueblo. Andalusia is a beautiful place, arid, sunny, filled with hot light, mountain air, seascapes, and arid topography. Before the Phoenicians, the Iberian peoples lived along the coast.[12] They were matriarchal, farming families who worshipped a fertility goddess and lived in relative peace. Then, the Carthaginians approached from the Mediterranean Sea, as did the Romans. Finally, the Romans traveled from Italy to southern Spain in 810 c.e. where they built temples, aqueducts, canals, vineyards, and olive gardens. As in Greece, they would store their grains and harvest their wines along dry coastlines and export goods to Rome.

Cadíz, the oldest-inhabited city in Europe, was the place of the dancing girls that the Romans referred to as the Gaditanes. The Emperor would invite them to the Imperial capital to dance for him. We have descriptions of these Gaditanes by Roman

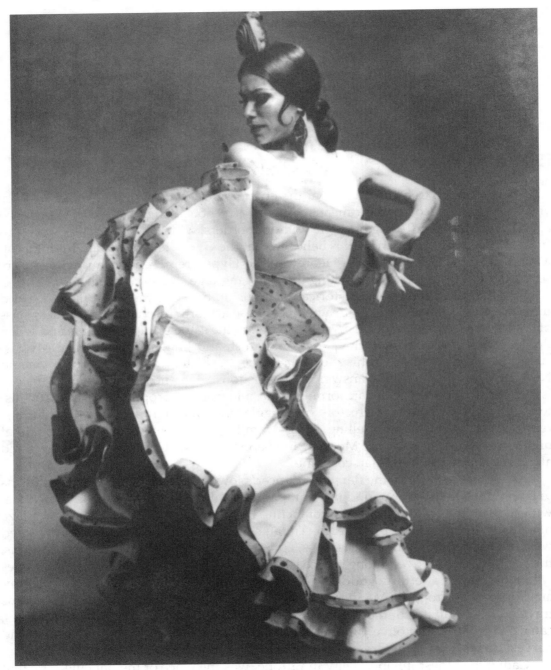

María Benítez.

Courtesy of Maria Benitez.

chroniclers that describe the dancer's tiny metal finger cymbals held between the hands, an early castanet, which they used to keep time for their own undulating hips and shoulders. Cervantes writes of the Roman Martial as having said they had "honey in their hips." This display of the female body marks the beginning of public female dancing in southern Spain.

Arab Colonialism & Orientalism

In the year 711, eight thousand Berber soldiers from North Africa invaded Gothic Spain. Led by a general named 'al Tariq, these Muslim soldiers were finally halted in the year 722. Having made it as far north as the French Pyrénées, they were met by a fierce fighter, Charles Martel, grandfather of Charlemagne. Martel pushed them back over the Pyrénées south into northern Spanish kingdoms where Spanish noblemen pushed them south of Madrid.[12]

These new Arab leaders settled in Cordoba first, building beautiful palaces and mosques with gardens, public fountains, and warm-weather date, fig and citrus trees never before grown on European soil. Mirroring the architectural magnificence of the lands from which they came—Damascus and Baghdad—they also built the largest library in Europe with books in Greek, Hebrew, and Arabic on science, theology, art, and law and translations of Aristotle, and Euclid. Baghdad, in the eighth century, was the great center of learning in the Middle Eastern world, and served as the template for the construction of a transplanted Islamic civilization in Cordoba, Granada, and Seville and throughout the tiny pueblos of southern Spain.

News of the emergence of a new Hispano-Arab culture became known throughout the Middle East, bringing scholars, court musicians, architects, physicians, alchemists, astronomers and clerics from Persian and Arabian lands. These educated Middle Easterners were deeply intellectual and curious about the world, its biology, art, and technology, and established themselves in southern Spain, further enriching the schools, libraries, and translation centers. One could argue that an orientalist mentality begins here: that of the great scholars from Baghdad who, now working in Spain, long for the East, its blues and gold, its early and prolonged first Enlightenment.

With the Expulsion of the Jews and the surrender of the last Muslim Nasrid dynasty in 1492, Spain fell into economic recession. Its labor force departed on ships bound for North Africa, Europe, the Americas, and Turkey. A tiny labor force remained to grow olives, grapes and other foods. Thus, began the importation of African slaves.

Seville became one of the largest slave ports in the world. Its Quadalquivir River became the connecting artery between the Mediterranean Sea and the city. West Africans, with the rhythms and ritual dances, were forcefully imported to pick crops and plow the fields.

With so much money being spent to fund the "discovery of the Americas" and the expulsion of the economic base—the merchant class—of the country, they could not afford to pay workers. Many poor Spaniards left for the colonies, most never to return.

The flood of gold and silver from the Americas also created great inflation. In Andalusia, crypto-Jews who had been living in hiding (behind Catholic masks), and Gypsies who had fled into the hills of the Albaicín remained. This, then, begins the story of flamenco in southern Spain.

East Indian Gypsy Migration

How did Gypsies come to live in Spain? Gypsies are not native to Spain. Flamenco historians, Ricardo Molina and García Matos, argue that Gypsies came to Spain from India, arriving as early as the tenth-century and living, at times, under the tolerant and at other times, not so tolerant Moorish Caliphate. Other Spanish historians argue that the Gypsies arrived later, around 1435, roughly thirteen years after they were first recorded as entering Rome in 1422. Whether or not they came several centuries prior to the expulsion of the Jews and the Moors is extremely important as it then influences the types of music and dance that Spaniards and non-Spaniards, forced to flee the fires of the Inquisition, might have brought with them to Mexico in the 1490s and to New Mexico on the first expedition there in 1540.

Even if the first migration of Gypsies to Spain occurred as late as the early fifteenth century, then it is possible that they had considerable contact with the Muslims, Jews, and Christians for whom they tended fields in the southern towns of medieval Spain. It is this rich inter-cultural contact that, combined with the imported East Indian dance of Kathak—the dance that the Gypsies brought with them—becomes the modern art form known as flamenco.

Hindu Influence on Flamenco

The essential difference between deep song and flamenco is that the origins of the former must be sought in the primitive musical systems of India, in the very first manifestations of song, while flamenco, a consequence of deep song, did not acquire its definitive form until the eighteenth century.[13]

Let us explore for a moment the Hindu influence on Gypsy flamenco. The potential influence of Indian dance on the stylization of upper body motion in flamenco unfolds. Professional work, religion, social status, language, dance and music are valuable ways of relating the Gypsy existence in southeast Asia to life experience in the villages and towns of once Muslim and Sephardic and, later, Spanish Catholic land.

In the third century Sanskrit text, the *Book of Manu*, a Brahmin leader called Manu, identifies a caste of Gypsies who lived in the northwestern region of India: Rajasthan. Rajasthanis, or nomads, are described as horse dealers, fortune-tellers, animal trainers, fire-eaters, and blacksmiths. Gypsy historian, Ricardo Molina, links the Spanish

Gypsy professions of singing, dancing, blacksmith work, manual field labor and, later, bullfighting as emerging out of work performed by Indian Gypsies several centuries earlier.[14]

Manu described a Hindu caste system which he referred to as the "consolidation of Brahminism". This enforced social hierarchy became a powerful weapon against continuous Muslim invasions from the North. He also identified a caste of Gypsies from Rajasthan, India. Manu placed the Gypsies one caste beneath the untouchables who, today, live somewhere between the edge of the sidewalk and the gutter; their geographical positioning symbolizes their peripheral, sub-human status.[15] One can also link flamenco to East Indian classical dance iconographically, through the actual picture or image of the dancer.

By the eleventh century, Islamic warriors conquered northwest India. The Mongols and, later, the Turks would also invade India. Because the Muslims stayed in northern and eastern India, Islam became the dominant religion of many northern Indian villages and towns, while the middle, southern, and eastern portions of the country remained largely Hindu, with the exception of East Bengal, now Bangladesh.

From their Hindu-Indian dancing origins, Gypsies believed, as did all Hindus, that the body contained the soul and, thus, was sacred, the conduit to spiritual transcendence. One way of drawing connections to Gypsies' East Indian legacies is the iconographic influence of Hindu cosmology. East Indians believe that dance is a sacred practice, a psychic and spiritual means of communing with Lord Krishna. In the Hindu imagination, a classical dancer's moving body can actually speak to Krishna, serving him, making love to him through gesture, pose, and facial expression.[16] As Hindu dancing equated spiritual ecstasy with a sexual union with Krishna, particularly for female dancers, dance movement itself was considered a holy, auspicious practice.[17]

Footwork

Kathak, from *Kathakar*, or storyteller, is the improvisational dance-song form of the Gypsies of Rajasthan, India. Accompanied by drums, *tabla* and *pakhavaj*, a double-barreled drum, the dancer creates her own rhythmic cycles, and is a metaphor for the East Indian Gypsy view of the universe. Kathak reveals, according to Indian dance historian Vatsyayan, "an organic world view," or aesthetic theory of performance textured with multiple layers of expressive meaning.[18] Kathak consists of *talas*, metrical cycles that show the dancer in various emotional states. The dance is composed of interplay between static and dynamic poses and movements.[19]

As a percussive form of dance whose fast feet are balanced by soft, lyrical arm circles and finger gestures, Kathak is also free-flowing, spontaneous, a folk dance of the people. Weaving different metrical patterns, sometimes superimposing a different rhythmic variation allows performers to show off technical virtuosity while stressing lightening-quick footwork and dazzling pirouettes.

Kathak's footwork is an intense, fiery, polyrhythmic, contrapuntal working in opposition to elegant, sinuous arm movements. This is the, perhaps, the most important element in flamenco: the tension produced by a lower torso whose motions are divorced from those of the upper body but whose movements are balanced by relationship of upper to lower halves. The Hindu-Gypsy influence on the evolution of flamenco as a technical and stylistic form of modern, proscenium performance can be most closely linked to two elements: 1. The attack of the floor by the feet; 2. The symmetry between upper and lower limbs moving in centrifugal motion to sung and string accompaniment.

Hindu-Flamenco Bodies—Kali & Madonna

Can we study a dance form by studying the shape of the body, posed in culturally significant positions that for the initiated tell a story?

Maha Kali, wife of Shiva, is Black.[20] As Hindu Goddess of Destruction and Knowledge, she is considered protector of the Gypsy people. She stands on a single leg, her gesture leg lifted high to the front in a perfectly balanced attitude. She holds her other leg (gesture leg) in a high attitude, a Vedic position. She wears a belt of severed skulls thats shifts her weight from left to right, her left leg is lifted to the front in a perfectly-balanced attitude. From India to Spain, the Gypsies worshipped Kali. Once, within Spanish borders in the fifteenth century, subjected to the religious persecution that defined the Baroque era, gypsies were forced to hide inside their dances their worship of Kali. Kali then becomes a Black Virgin, variously seen as either the Madonna or as Sara, the wife of the Hebrew patriarch, Abraham. Many flamenco verses are dedicated to a woman, perhaps Kali, a spiritual force, dancer, cosmic being.

Other influences on the heavily stylized technique of flamenco would be the tricultural environment of southern Spain: Muslim, Catholic and Jewish. While some of these influences fell, literally, on the dancing of the Gypsies, other cultural influences, such as musical accompaniment and religious chant, influenced the singer in flamenco.

When you study the body in flamenco, you see the proud torso, the sinuous, uplifted arms and fingers that make tiny circles that caress the air. Americo Castro, in *The Structure of Spanish History*, provides an excellent social history of medieval Spanish society. This 1954 book, in particular, draws substantial social and cultural connections between peoples living on the Iberian Peninsula. For the purposes of this flamenco history, I draw upon Castro's belief that Islamic-Sephardic philosophical tenets greatly influenced the Iberian continent long after the Catholic conquest of Granada.[21]

Spain, for Castro, is a unique and special country, filled with artistic potential, in some ways different from the rest of medieval Europe. Castro argues the existence of a religious and spiritual symbiosis between Muslim, Christian and Sephardic belief systems. Arab-Sephardic thought, he believes, penetrated the Hispano-Christian imagination with notions of the importance of the individual being, worship, and consciousness. I would like to draw a connection, as have flamencologists, José Molina and Angel Alvarez Caballero, between the contemplative, meditative, individualistic nature of flamenco performance art and the philosophical thinking that inspired the peoples along the Iberian Peninsula.

"The connection," writes Spanish historian Castro, "that I am trying to establish between the forms of expression of inner experience and the objective structure of society, can be corroborated in Hispano-Moslem history itself, if we remember that the Almoravids and the Almohads came to Al-Andalus."[22] For Castro, the historical connection between Muslim Hispanics and northern Hispano-Gothic society could be made through religion, literature, and music.

To survive in the many countries through which they wandered, including Islamic and, later, Catholic Spain, the Gypsies had to adapt to the customs and beliefs of their hosts in order to survive. And, thus, flamencologist Gerhard Steingrass contends that the Spanish Gypsies adopted Moorish and Sephardic musical practices and, over time, created a hybrid form of performance.[23]

Perhaps the greatest influence on the evolution of flamenco came in the form of religious chant, hence the Hispano-Hebrew word for chanter or cantor: *cantaor*. Three religious traditions are present in the deep song tradition of the flamenco: the Islamic Mullah, the Sephardic *cantaor*, and the liturgical, choral singing of the choir. Each is a call to prayer, a call to God and to one's community of worshippers to stop, pray, listen, follow, attend, participate, and know.

Religious values are embedded in the intricate, hybrid structure of the flamenco show. The Mullah's call to prayer and the cantor's Kol Nidre chant on the Jewish Day of Atonement, Yom Kippur, are heard in the Mozarabic-influenced *saeta*, one of the main musical *compás*, or rhythms, that characterize flamenco deep song.

Another multi-cultural, Andalusian influence on the evolution of flamenco is the Escuela Bolera, or Spanish Classical dance of the Castilian and Catalonian aristocratic class. There was always some form of interaction between Andalusian Christians and northern Christians living in Castile, Leon, Aragon, and Navarre. Oftentimes, dances that migrant soldiers, laborers or wealthy people learned at court in Madrid, would be imported to Andalusia, performed at a party or a function, and seen by others who danced them.

The classicism of the upper body carriage in flamenco, the erect spine, the torque in the middle back, the proud, elegant forced extension of the chest and diaphragm outwards, into space, are body positions that are western European-influenced. That is to say, they are not eastern, from India, but, rather form a piece of the history of Spanish and later, French ballet, absorbed by Gypsies living in Andalusia through folk dances like the *Sevillanas*, performed at the Easter celebration, the *Feria de Sevilla*.

Media Granaína

I have prepared for you
for whenever you want to come,
a new little cave
in the hill of the Albaicín.

I wish to live in Granada
because I like to hear
the bell of 'La Vela'
when I go off to sleep . . .

The language of flamenco songs form an oral history of Gypsy experience told through poetic, metaphoric prose, whose literal meaning must be imagined or interpreted by the listener. Flamenco singers, like Muslim balladeers, sing of love, family and identity: of being Gypsy, persecuted, and surviving. A literary connection to Islamic Spain might be made by the lyrical poetry of Arabic literature. The *Koran*, for example, is a personal book of divine revelation that is part of the existence of one person, the prophet Mohammed.

Gypsy historian Jean-Paul Clébert notes how quickly the Gypsies adapted to the customs of a foreign land. As Gypsies were illiterate, it is impossible to trace their entire history. The study of Gypsy life and performance is, thus, relegated to sparse written accounts by Spaniards who observed their dances, and to Europeanist iconography, such as the drawings of Gustave Doré.

That said, one important source remains: flamenco. Like a book or a painting, it serves as an historical document that can be studied. However, like any artistic people, Gypsy singers and dancers communicate through metaphor and it is up to the audience or *aficionado*, to derive meaning out of their poetical communication.[24]

Most Important Influences on Flamenco

Flamenco has had many religious and cultural influences that have had a profound effect on the formation of the dance and song. It is my belief that the Muslim, Jewish, and Catholic emphasis on individual consciousness as a path to spiritual enlightenment—to God—was absorbed by gypsies as an intrinsic, path to *duende* in the flamenco *cante y baile* during the *cante jondo*, or deep song. The *siguiriyas*, one of the oldest and most profound dances in the deep song vocabulary, is a quasi-religious experience for dancer and singer. The performer's emphasis is filled with frenzied, violent footwork sequences expressed in *llamadas*. They are calls to musicians to follow as her dynamic attack to the floor—that is a call to God or Mother Earth.

Coupled with the Hispano-Arab and Sephardic influence on Gypsy dance and song, an Andalusian phenomenon, was the continued influence of Hindu, Vedic valuation of the body as soulful, an embodied knowledge literally carried with the Gypsies (inside their bodies) from India to Spain. If the soul, as the Hindus believe, resides in the body, then the body is the path to God and to spiritual enlightenment.

The sacred Indian treatise on dance and music, a ninth century Sanskrit manual, the *Natyasastra*, defines three types of Indian dance: nritta, pure dancing, nritya, miming and gesture, and natya, or drama, accompanied by tala, or rhythmic sequences, charis, or movement sequences, and asthanas, or posed body positions.[25] All of these

Sanskrit words will be seen in a definition of Kathak and, thus, in the evolution of flamenco dance.

Perhaps the strongest link between Kathak as danced by Indian Gypsies, and Flamenco, as danced by Spanish Gypsies are the above-mentioned Indian Vedas, the almost literally metaphoric posing and shaping of the body into various letter-formations that stand for various words in the Sanskrit language. Kathak dancers, unlike other Indian dancers, use suggestive dance poses, an erect spine, almost no motion in the hips, lots of quick arm movements and tabla rhythms of the feet that transform the entire body of the dancer into a moving sculpture, a rhythmic visualization of Hindu mythological stories.

Although Kathak becomes a Muslim form, its essential choreographic qualities, the letter tracing of images using the hands, arms, eyes and shoulders, remains Hindu. The dancing body is used to illustrate Krishna by placing the dancer in subordinate or other narrative positions as the female dancer communicates her devotion to Lord Krishna through her body motions. Interestingly, Kathak, according to Indian dance historian Kapila Vatsyayan, is a roughly tenth century invention, developing throughout the late medieval period.[26] Thus, Kathak was already developed in Hindu script-form prior to the departure of Gypsies in the twelfth and thirteenth centuries.

What concerns us, is what dance historians, Reginald and Jamila Massey argue to be the heavy Vishnaivite influence on Kathak and the probability that anyone dancing it in the northwest of India would have had to flee to other regions to escape the censorship of Muslim conquerors and laws on public display of the body.[27] Their subcultural existence stands in relation to accepted and, therefore, dominant socio-economic groups such as the Castilian aristocracy and the Andalusian Muslim capital court.[28]

Hot Sand: **Flamenco in New Mexico**

The introduction of flamenco into New Mexico is primarily a twentieth century event. Three flamenco artists, Maria Benitez, Eva Enciñas-Sandoval and Lilly del Castillo all agreed in separate interviews that a New Mexican, Vicente Romero, brought "real flamenco" from Spain to Albuquerque and Santa Fe in the 1960s and 1970s. Because of the footwork seen at Veracruzan dances in Mexico, flamenco, as a Spanish-Gypsy dance might have made an earlier appearance in Old and New Mexico. We have the journals, correspondence, and reports of Spanish Jesuit priests describing the dance ceremonies of the pueblo Indians in the sixteenth century.[29] After the settlement of New Mexico, beginning in 1609, many of these journal entries describe a mestizo, or culturally mixed series of folk dances.

Cultural anthropologist, Sylvia Rodriguez, dance ethnologist, Deidre Sklar, and dance artists, María Benitez, Lilly del Castillo, Pablo Rodarte, and Eva Enciñas-Sandoval, all agree that some form of Gypsy dance, laced with the more European court forms—the Aragonese Jota and the northern, regional folk dances of the Basques—arrived with the conquistadors. A further musical and dance influence on the conquistadors and mercenary foot soldiers arriving from Spain would have been the influence of mozarabic music and chanting, the art of the North African and the Jews.

Conquistadors enlisted by the Spanish throne to conquer, christianize, and loot the "New World," would, through their time at court, have learned court dances and, probably, been exposed to the popular dances and musical traditions of the mozarabic world whose artistic culture dominated Andalusia for eight centuries. It is this author's contention that it is simply not possible to avoid them. The conquistadors who landed in Mexico in the early sixteenth century built the first coastal towns in the states Oaxaca, Veracruz, Zacatecas, Campeche, Merida, Monterrey, Puebla and Guadalajara, along the 425-mile coastline of the Gulf of Mexico.[30]

"I saw Mexican dancers in the Yucatan dancing zapateado, or footwork, using pitos, or finger snapping, to accompany them," said Eva Enciñas-Sandoval.[31] The dances of the Yukatan use the feet and the planta, the sideways movement of the skirt, a West African tradition imported by African slaves to Seville in the fifteenth century and, possibly, picked up by Gypsies at that time. These dances are called *Jarochos* and their musical style and dances, known as the *sones jarochos* are comprised of Spanish/Mexican music, North African and Caribbean rhythms and are accompanied by harp, not an instrument indigenous to the Americas, a *jarana*, or small guitar, akin to the North African four-stringed, later, five-stringed lute, and *requinto*, or smaller guitar. Long footwork sequences danced in conjunction with arm circles, finger snapping and head turning is danced constantly during this Mexican folk form performed on various saints' days and local feast days. The term *huagpango* refers to the *sones jarochos* and means "dance of the wooden platform," known as the *tirama*. The idea that a wooden platform would be needed to absorb and, also, resonate and amplify long footwork sequences is confirmed by Lilly del Castillo. "When I was little, my parents took me to Old Town on Saints' days. I saw people dancing New Mexico folk dances across from the Franciscan church. Sometimes they would perform in the gazebo but the wooden platforms were better because we could hear the feet stamping the wood."[32]

María Benitez concurs with Castillo, citing this Mexican-New Mexican *flamencoesque* use of the feet in northern New Mexican dance traditions. "When I was little," says Benitez, I was in public school in Taos. There we danced all kinds of local folk dances. We often did footwork passages in the flamenco style, snapping our fingers and turning the head from side-to-side. We carried fans, as in Spanish dance and we wore combs in our hair." The *Jarocho* refers to a mulatto, or mixed-race of indigenous, Spanish and African people who intermarried throughout the sixteenth and seventeenth centuries.[33]

A second Mozarabic and Afro-Caribbean influenced performance tradition to travel with the conquistadors from Spain to Mexico to New Mexico is the Gypsy-Muslim form known as the *fandango*, the Muslim dance of love. The *fandango*—"go and dance"—is one of the oldest of Spanish dances. Later, in the ninth century, it is thought that the Moorish musicians had an influence on the fandango, since the dance transformed from a court couple dance accompanied by castanets into a trio, with a man and his two female partners. From light-hearted to deep song, the fandango transformed into a chanted piece that is never danced but, rather, sung.[34]

Festival Flamenco International and the Matachines rituals represent dances of cultural hybridity in the guise of performed memory. Both are Spanish and Indian in musical and choreographic structure and help audience members to feel connected to cultures that are indigenous to New Mexico. While the Matachines dance literally reconstructs the conquest between the Rio Grande pueblo Indians and the Spanish colonists and mercenary soldiers and Jesuit priests in their entourage, contemporary Flamenco performance remains an imported art form whose appearance in the State of New Mexico represents what cultural anthropologist-Richard Schechner, refers to as a "restored behavior;" a meaningful ritual in its present geographical, repeated, and representational political place.

Flamenco as learned by New Mexicans and Mexicans, along with regional folk forms becomes a combination of foreign and indigenous. Its movements and music, like the Matachines dance, stands for journey, migration, encounter, and transformation. While there is no record of Gypsy flamenco in New Mexico prior to the nineteenth century, there is a clear pattern of northern New Mexico school children, like Veracruzan children, learning folk dances whose instrumental accompaniment is played by the castanets, the pounding feet, and the snapping figures.

Flamenco sociologist, Gerhard Steingrass argues that Gypsy music was greatly influenced by Sephardic cantors and, as Ricardo Molina and Angel Alvarez Caballero remind us, it was also heavily influenced by Hispano-Arab court sung poetry and Christian liturgical choral singing. New Mexico has benefited from colonial encounters for over four centuries long. Discovering the exact moment of encounter is impossible. However, tracing the outline of those encounters in the fierce drilling of feet into the earth, subtle head motions, shawls, combs and other Spanish dress codes in both of these performance forms gives us some notion of the historical origins of these dances.

The Interculturalism of New Mexican Flamenco

Flamenco, unlike Native American dance and drumming, an import to New Mexico, may now be considered an indigenous performance form, evolving out of the multi-culturalism of the State's triptychal cultural relationships between Hispanic, Anglo, and Indian co-existence. No dance historians and few cultural anthropologists and ethnomusicologists have worked on the possible link between Spanish dances and the appearance of flamenco in New Mexico. The reason for this is the impossibility of historical verification of sources.

We know that Spanish conquistadors and Mexicans who became conquistadors rode on horseback from Veracruz to New Mexico in 1540 in search of Cibola and the seven cities of gold. But, other than diaries and accounts kept by priests, friars and army personnel, we know little else. There is no mention of a Gypsy person anywhere in the history of La Reconquista. This raises the question—were Gypsies identified by chroniclers, during the sixteenth and seventeenth centuries throughout Mexico and New Mexico?[35] Could a Gypsy folk form of performance such as flamenco develop in parallel form in New Mexico as it had developed in Spain? Historical records aren't available.

Flamencologists who study the history of Flamenco as a culture and an art, must ask questions: If Flamenco in Spain was the result of the coexistence of Arabs, Christians, Jews and Gypsies in medieval Andalusia, what, then, is flamenco's evolution in New Mexico? How does New Mexican flamenco differ from Spanish Gypsy flamenco? Can we say the two regions produce a similar style of performance and, if true why and how? Does the New Mexican flamenco artist have either an historical or an artistic commitment to the legacy of the form as represented here in the American State of New Mexico? Lastly, in America, can women play a larger role in the singing and guitar accompaniment of the form, whereas, in Spain, women are, for the most part, discouraged, if not, excluded from *cante y toque*?

Flamenco in New Mexico is a recent development. Some New Mexican dance artists maintain that Spanish colonialism was responsible for the evolution of flamenco in the state and that Gypsies somehow boarded Spanish vessels bound for Mexico. Over time, they migrated northward with conquistadors as far north as Taos pueblo, and their children were the first *flamencos*. There is no evidence to support this assumption. However, there is a great deal of historical evidence and well-argued ethnomusicological and cultural anthropological study to connect the twentieth-century appearance of flamenco in New Mexico to the Mexican folk dances performed along the coastal regions of Veracruz, and, thus, to the New Mexican Matachines dance, performed up and down the Rio Grande river in various little Spanish towns. The Matachines dance, Sylvia Rodriguez argues, provides a significant connecting link between the importation of European court dances that influenced the indigenous population in Mexico, the Spanish conquistadors' dances imported by them to Mexico, and the meeting of these various dances in New Mexico.

Local New Mexican residents of Spanish, Mexican, and Native American origin such as Clarita Garcia de Arando Allison, Lily Baca, Vicente Romero, Lilly del Castillo, Candido Garcia, and Maria Benitez, performed and taught flamenco. In recent years, world-renowned performers such as Teo Morca, José Greco along with many other flamenco artists, have traveled to New Mexico also to teach and perform. Because of this, we now see many new flamenco artists performing in the state. Their dance is one of hybridity: influenced by the history of New Mexico and its tri-cultural dance history. This includes Native American, Hispanic (Mexican, Spanish), and Anglo American elements. Such a rich musical and dance heritage should help local teachers continue to "build" good, new choreographic talent that continues to enliven the form. No longer just an importation, flamenco is now becoming an American form, as we see in the original choreography of Professor of Dance at the University of New Mexico Eva Enciñas-Sandoval and her son, Joaquín and daughter, Marisol.

While some argue a conquest genesis for flamenco in New Mexico, others contest it. Maria Benitez, a thirty-year veteran of world tours and opera choreography disagrees. She has spent her life touring flamenco around the country and at the age of nineteen, she joined the company of Maria Rosa. In Rosa's touring company, Benitez learned a varied repertory of Spanish Classical, regional, and flamenco dances and dance-steps. Benitez was based in Madrid, Spain and benefited from the number of Spanish and Gypsy artists around her with *tablao* and main stage experience. She also took regular classes from Victoria Ohenia, the ex-artistic director of the Ballet Nacionale de España who trained Benitez in private classes at Amor de Dios dance studio. By the 1970s, under Franco, the Spanish government cracked down on foreign artists, especially American artists, dancing in Spanish companies, and many American artists, like Benitez, lost their jobs and had to relocate to America where many formed their own companies, bringing the principles of touring, regionally and ethnically-diverse dance choreography, and national profile star power to a North American public.[36]

Hence, the actual genesis of flamenco remains in dispute. Ricardo Molina argues flamenco's birth as a pre-Inquisition form. Other flamencologists, like Meira Weinzweig, trace the etymological roots of the words "flamenco" and "Gypsy" to roughly 1780, a date conceived of by Gypsy guitarist, Sabicas. If flamenco is an eighteenth-century phenomenon, it may be considered less the result of medieval tri-culturalism than the effect of the influence of the Spanish Bolero School. This is an interesting idea since today, all flamencologists, for political and artistic reasons, completely divorce flamenco from any courtly birth, an historical error on their part.[37] In Spain, Benitez learned the way to stage a story ballet, the multi-ethnic legacy of the great director-choreographer, Antonia Mercé, "La Argentina," who began the tradition of fusing Gypsy flamenco and Spanish classical dance in the 1920s and 30s, inventing a popular modern dance-theatre for the world stage.[38]

Conquistadors who arrived in Veracruz and other coastal cities performed a number of folk dances on Saints' days and other holidays carrying Spanish-influenced, European court dances as well as some form of Gypsy *zapateado*, or footwork, and snapping, or *pitos*.

As mentioned above, it is impossible to prove the existence of Gypsies in New Mexico, prior to the large summer flamenco festivals instituted by Maria Benitez's Institute for Spanish Arts in Santa Fe and Festival Flamenco International sponsored by the University of New Mexico.

"Flamenco," says Maria Benitez, "is something brought to this country via Mexico."[39] Eva Enciñas-Sandoval believes that flamenco is indigenous to New Mexico, having been imported in roughly the sixteenth century by Gypsies who traveled alongside conquistadors. Benitez disagrees with the latter view, stating that the more likely history of flamenco in New Mexico is an amalgamation of Mexican folk dances such as the Matachines with European court dance and the influence of contemporary Gypsy flamenco brought by touring Spanish and Gypsy artists to New Mexico and by her own national and international tours.

While Benitez learned Gypsy and various other forms of flamenco training and dancing in Spain in the 1960s, Enciñas-Sandoval trained locally with her mother, Clarita, a Mexican-American singer and dancer trained in regional New Mexican and

Mexican folk forms, as well as in flamenco and ballet. As Clarita was also a singer, Enciñas-Sandoval learned from the age of five the importance of the *cante* to the dance. "Clarita taught me how studying the flamenco song, the improvisational song-base of Gypsy flamenco, makes one unlimited. All variation to a certain verse, or *falsetta*, must follow the singer."[40]

Both women share a long history of training in ballet and modern dance. While Enciñas-Sandoval had the good fortune to train with three of the most outstanding modern teachers in the world, Lee Connor, Lorn MacDougal and Tim Wingerd, Benitez went to Spain, to the studios of Amor de Dios, training with Maria Alba. Both Benitez and Enciñas-Sandoval share a belief in the generative power of the *cante*, or singing, in flamenco: "Working with the *cante*," says Benitez, "is extremely important. It is the history of the form. But only certain performers become great singers."[41] Benitez has also choreographed a number of Spanish-themed operas for opera companies around the country. It is this diverse and lifelong training that illuminates her present work with her company of dancers who work in public schools and theatres around the State. "The main thing that we have to do for all of us who are involved in this art form," she argues, "is to contribute to the art form: to lend dignity to it and pass it on to children and young artists."[42]

Benitez's ballet training, unlike Enciñas-Sandoval, was local, with local dance artists in Santa Fe and Taos studios. "You have to understand," she said in a 2002 interview, "I studied ballet in Santa Fe with Louise Lichtlighter. I picked up flamenco here and there as one can. I started in Taos with a teacher, Cecilia Torres who had wanted to be a Spanish dancer and who had studied in California with the Cancino family and had returned to New Mexico to get married which signaled the end of her professional dance career."[43]

Benitez and Enciñas-Sandoval began to train in Spanish styles of movement with "a little dance teacher who had all her kids come out in capes." Lilly Baca, like every dancer in America between 1940 and 1960, was influenced by the ferocious footwork and cross-dressing of Carmen Amaya whose 1941 Carnegie Hall appearance in New York practically deified her and her accompanying sixteen Amaya cousins. Baca who taught regional styles such as the *Harapa tapatillo* and ballet, also taught flamenco and regional styles.

Eva Enciñas-Sandoval shares with Maria Benitez similar, local New Mexican training in regional folk styles, Mexican and New Mexican, and exposure to Native American pueblo dance, drumming and chant. Unlike Benitez, whose mother was a Native American and whose father was of Puerto Rican descent, Enciñas-Sandoval's mother, Clarita Garcia de Aranda was a Mexican-American, while her father, Donald Allison, was a German American chemical and electrical engineer. Eva recalls "that he bought an old army barracks in the 40s where he built a laboratory for scientific inventions and a studio for my mom. It was an extensive adobe hacienda structure on the corner of Edith and Candelaria that was later turned into a flamenco and Spanish dance studio where Clarita taught classes.[44] In 1953, my mother officially opened Clarita's School of

Dance. Our living room became the studio at night. My dad loved flamenco. He would work in his lab all day and produce my mom's shows at night at the Albuquerque Civic Auditorium. Clarita would dance with her first cousin, Candido Garcia. They were a team and Candido taught my mom a lot because he had the freedom to travel to Spain to study flamenco. He had a big professional career all over the U.S. and Europe and a duo with the well-known Luisa. He was an incredible dancer, accepted as such in Spain. But he died of AIDS. My family thought that he must have caught a 'homosexual disease' in New York.

Clarita taught Eva, her brother Tony Garcia, and many others to dance flamenco, Jota, Spanish Classical and regional styles. "The way my aunt explained it to me," Eva said, was that that "the seed of flamenco had been brought in by Juanita but that Tony went away to study flamenco and then trained his sister, Clarita in various other Spanish dances. My mother handed what Tony taught her down to me and I handed it down to my children."[45]

"I began dancing at five or six years old," said Eva, "and studied only with my mother until nine when I began ballet classes with Linda Larson. My mom also introduced me to tap, which she loved. When I was seven or eight, I also came to love tap and flamenco was just a natural for me. I learned the *Farruca*, [traditionally a man's dance,] early." Eva spoke of learning Moorish-influenced southern Spanish dances such as the *zambra mora, fandangos*, and the Sevillian folk form, *Sevillanas*.[46] "Perhaps most important in my early studies with my Clarita was fan and shawl work." The idea that gestural and stylistic accoutrements were a large part of lower body footwork and memorization of choreographic steps, were an inherently classical and studied approach to training a child the *arte* and form of flamenco. Popular in the United States in the 1950s and 1960s were big, touring flamenco companies with varied choreographies, extensively designed ballets a la Argentina. "I think that my mom had seen Carmen Amaya, if not in New York then in Los Angeles or on film."[47]

"When I was ten years old, my parents took me by ship to Spain. Perhaps my mother wanted me to be exposed to flamenco or my father wanted to take my mother to Spain. I went again when I was fourteen and when I was sixteen. And then I didn't go again until I was thirty. I remember how I loved Spain. I went to Madrid and then down to Seville. When I got back, I began to study with Teo Morca in Taos, Roberto Lorca in Santa Fe and danced as a guest artist with Maria Benitez. I also would travel to El Paso, Texas to study with Antonio Triana. I used to go down there once a month from Friday to Sunday. In Mexico, I studied with Manolo Vargas. My brother had become a very fine flamenco guitarist and he had studied with the great Juan Maya in Spain."[48]

"Clarita taught flamenco through individual choreographies, dances that you could readily put on stage. This was the style of training dancers for club work from the 1950s to the 1970s. It was, and to a large extent, remains a useful way of teaching flamenco technique. And so this is how I began to teach flamenco at the University of New Mexico, when in the 1970s."[49]

Returning again to the encounter of the Farrucos and the Morenos with the Native Americans at Santo Domingo Pueblo in August of 2001—might Gypsies have traveled with the conquistadors? No, most likely not. There is no evidence of this. But when the Farrucos and the Morenos arrived at the pueblo, they shared a perfect moment of inter-cultural dialogue, of peace and unity accompanied by the immense pueblo drum which only a man can hold and play, keeping time, beating out the rhythm of the seasons as the Gypsy male dancer claims the farruco, the solo male form of technical prowess. Clapping, eating, sharing, accompanying one another, this was the more important encounter between Spanish Gypsy artist and Native American artist, and it was peaceful, organic, intense.

What will be the future of flamenco in New Mexico? Perhaps Gypsies and Indians will merge and, together, create a new fusion form of flamenco, of Native American rhythms and storytelling legend and Gypsy rhythm, complex and layered.

To a certain extent, producer Eva Enciñas-Sandoval's Festival Flamenco International, now in its twentieth season, has answered this question in the contemporary artists who visit New Mexico during festival season, usually during the early weeks of June. Dancers like Eva La Yerbabuena, Israel Galvan and Antonio Canales hold the future in their insistent translations of flamenco songs into the steps of the dance. Other, older, more established Gypsy dancers such as Mañuela Carrasco, one generation older than Israel Galvan, balance the international contemporaneity of flamenco artists playing with postmodernist languages of choreography in their traditional performance presentation of Gypsy flamenco praxis. While highly virtuosic dancers are born into the field daily, it is the choreographic innovators like La Yerbabuena and Galvan who continue to question the powerful Gypsy drama of La Farruca and her family who also performed in New Mexico last year.

As Festival Flamenco expanded to multi-site performances—at UNM's Rodey Theatre in Albuquerque and the wonderfully-restored Lensic theatre in downtown Santa Fe in Mozarabic design (the perfect atmosphere for flamenco)—perhaps the future of New Mexico flamenco is inherent in the modernist experiments of the artists who visit. Building sophisticated audiences—*aficionados* who understand and appreciate the form—will further enrich New Mexicans love of music, dance and art. It is in the connection between audience and performer that the future of experimental flamenco in New Mexico lays.

Notes

1. The research materials used to write this chapter are the following: interviews; archival materials; dance performances; and my own multiple trips to Spain and my native New Mexico. It is dedicated to dancers who feel the rhythm travel from their feet to their necks, hands, and heads and to dance scholars whose descriptive analyses "capture the aliveness of the Spanish body and hold it in the bounds of form."

2. For etymological and social history of the Gypsy people's origins, read: Jean-Paul Clébert. *The Gypsies* (Baltimore: Penguin Books, 1961): Part I.

3. Flamenco is a complex art form that developed over centuries' time. Its music and dance rhythms and poetry require knowledge of Spanish, laced with words in Arabic and Caló, the Gypsy language. The metaphysical relationship between singer and dancer in *cante jondo*, or deep song, is mesmerizing. To understand flamenco's aesthetic power is to understand a history of the form and to learn a technical history of flamenco and also to become fluent in Islamic Spanish culture. Thus, it is to an earlier time that we travel to consider the root sources of the form, its aesthetic and spiritual philosophical base.

4. Americo Castro. *The Structure of Spanish History* (Princeton: Princeton University Press, 1954): 326.

5. Federico García Lorca. *Deep Son and Other Prose* (New York: A New Directions Book, 1975): 43.

6. Cibola, in reality, was Zuni pueblo located some hundreds of miles to the South of Santo Domingo.

7. These Indians are survivors of Spanish domination and forced labor, and is welcome into their homes, not as a foreigner but, rather, as a kindred spirit.

8. For a full argument on the performative effect of the Spanish conquest of New Mexican Indians, please read: Jill Lane, "On Colonial Forgetting: the Conquest of New Mexico and Its *Historia*," in. *the ends of performance*. Peggy Phelan and Jill Lane, eds. (New York: New York University Press, 1998): pp. 52-73. For a more comprehensive historical approach to colonial subject matter, see: Richard N. Ellis. *New Mexico Past and Present. A Historical Reader* (Albuquerque: University of New Mexico Press, 1971).

9. Tony Gatlif filmed a trilogy, *Les Princes* (1982), *Latcho Drom* (1993), *Gadjo Dilo* (1997). All three films tell intimate stories, tracing the Gypsy migration from India to Spain through the eyes of young boys. The evolution of flamenco from its East Indian origins to its present-day form is also explored, poetically, as a form of ethnic identification and modern art.

10. From a prison in San Fernando (Cadiz). These verses were given to me by Eric Patterson, guitarist and flamencologist.

11. For further etymological investigation of the roots of the flamenco term, please read Ricardo Molina: *Obra flamenca* (Madrid: Ediciones Démofilo, 1977); *Misterios del arte flamenco: ensayos de una interpretacion antropologica* (Barcelona: Sagitari, 1967).

12. *Les Ibéres*. Introduction to Exhibition Catalogue. (Paris: Galeries nationales du Grand Palais), October 15, 1997—January 5, 1998. Curators: Carmen Aranegui Gascó, Jean-Pierre Mohen, Pierre Rouillard, Christiane Eluére. For a history of the Arab conquest of visigothic Spain and France, please see: Henri Pirenne, *Mohammed and Charlemagne* (New York: Norton, 1939) and Bernard Lewis, *The Arabs in History* (New York: Oxford University Press, 1993).

13. Reginald & Jamila Massey. *The Dances of India.* (London: Tricolor Books, 1989): p. 74.
14. *Ibid*, p. 75.
15. To touch a Gypsy was to dirty oneself. To touch an untouchable was and remains unthinkable.
16. Krishna, a God represented by the "union" of Aryan and Dravidian cultures.
17. Reginald and Jamila Massey, p. 463.
18. *Ibid*.
19. In Hindu mythology, the Gods could not kill the demon Raktabija. Every drop of his blood that touched the earth transformed itself into another demon. The Gods turned to Shiva to kill Raktabija. Shiva, lost in meditation, turned to his consort Parvati, who dressed in the form of Kali to protect herself.
20. Bart McDowell. *Gypsies. Wanderers of the World* (Washington, D.C.: National Geographic Society, 1970.): p. 38.
21. Americo Castro. *The Structure of Spanish History* (Princeton: Princeton University Press, 1954): p. 326.
22. *Ibid*, p. 333.
23. Please see: Gerhard Steingrass. *Sociologia del cante flamenco* (Jerez: Centro Andaluz, 1993).
24. The issue of the Gypsy mask, a forced minstrelization of *tablao* performers with the opening of the first singing cafés in the 1840s and 1850s (historically coincidental with minstrels on the southern American saloon circuit), has profound political ramifications for Gypsy artists performing today but is too large a subject for the purposes of this short essay.
25. Kapila Vastyayan. ""History of Dance," *Indian Classical Dance* (New Delhi: Ministry of Information and Broadcasting of India, 1974): pp. 1–24.
26. *Ibid*, p. 3.
27. Reginald and Jamila Massey, p. 75.
28. It is thanks to Algerian Gypsy cinematographer, Tony Gatlif that the world's visual consciousness of being Gypsy and of the East Indian origins of flamenco as inspired by Kathak art has emerged. Please screen *Latcho Drom*.
29. The Municipal Library in Santa Fe, New Mexico holds a fine collection of early Spanish governor's and Jesuit priests' records, music and dance notations of early 17th century Spanish colonial life in New Mexico. Also see: Stan Steiner. *The New Indians* (New York: Dell, 1968); *The Waning of the West* (New York: St. Martin's Press, 1989).
30. For further reading on the *mestizo* origins of New Mexico folk dance tradition, please read: Sylvia Rodriguez, *The Matachines Dance: Ritual Symbolism and Interethnic Relations in the Upper Rio Grande Valley* (Albuquerque: The University of New Mexico Press, 1996; D.D. Sklar, *Dancing with the Virgin: Body and Faith in the Fiesta of Tortugas, New Mexico* (Berkeley: University of California Press, 2001).
31. Interview, Eva Enciñas-Sandoval, Albuquerque, New Mexico, August 20th, 2002.

32. Telephone interview with Lilly del Castillo, November 3rd, 2002.
33. Interview with Maria Benitez, Santa Fe, New Mexico, August 18th and 22nd, 2002.
34. Matteo. *The Language of Spanish Dance.* (Norman: Oklahoma University Press, 1990): p. 84.
35. The Reconquest of the southern Spanish territories—Cordoba, Seville, Cadiz, Granada—the 1492 Expulsion of all Jews from 'al Andaluz and the subsequent expulsion of the Muslims in 1508, began the Spanish domination of the world, its forced colonization of the "New World" and its Christianization of all conquered inhabitants to a Catholic God and religious system.
36. Interview with Maria Benitez, Institute for Spanish Arts, Santa Fe, New Mexico, August 21st, 2002.
37. Please read: "The Origins of the Bolero School," *The Journal of the Society of Dance History Scholars*, vol. v, no. 1 spring, 1998. Edited and translated by Lynn Garafola.
38. Please read: Ninotchka Bennahum. *Antonia Mercé, 'La Argentina': Flamenco & the Spanish Avant-Garde* (Middletown: Wesleyan University Press, 2000.)
39. Interview, Maria Benitez, Santa Fe, August 21st, 2002.
40. Enciñas-Sandoval believes that her grandmother, Juanita, who was actually confined to a wheelchair later in life, to have been a Spanish Gypsy while Clarita, her mother, was of Mexican descent. Either way, it was Clarita who danced.
41. Interview, Maria Benitez, Santa Fe, Institute for Spanish Arts, August 21st, 2002.
42. *Ibid.*
43. *Ibid.*
44. Interview, Eva Enciñas-Sandoval, Albuquerque, New Mexico, August 20th, 2002.
45. *Ibid.*
46. *Ibid.*
47. Carmen Amaya produced *Sevillanas* in 1935. The Great Antonio and Rosario starred in a series of short flamenco acts for Hollywood, one of which as the celebrated 1941 *Ziegfield Girl* in which they're shown, filmed from a bird's eye view, their flowery finger and hand work a seductive entry into their explosive footwork sequences. Such cinema brought Gypsy flamenco to the entire world.
48. Interview with Eva Enciñas-Sandoval, August 20th, 2002.
49. *Ibid.*

Bibliography

Acton, Thomas. *Gitanos.* Madrid: Espasa-Calpe: S.A., 1983.
Argentina, Antonia. *Mes Premiers Essais.* Paris: Editions Gilberte Cournand, 1956.
Balouch, Aziz. *Cante Jondo: su origen y evolucion.* Madrid: Ediciones Ensayos, 1955.
Barrios, Mañuel. *Gitanos, Moriscos y Cante Flamenco* (Seville: Editorial R.C., 1989.)
Bennahum, Ninotchka Devorah. "Flamenco," dance entry. *Oxford International Encyclopedia of Dance* Vol. 3 (New York: Oxford University Press, 1998). *Antonia Mercé*

La Argentina: Flamenco and the Spanish Avant-Garde (Middletown: Wesleyan University Press, 2000).

Blas Vega, José. *Diccionario enciclopedico ilustrado del Flamenco.* Editorial Cinterco: Madrid, 1988.

Bonald, Cabellero J.M. *La Danse Andalouse.* Barcelona: Editorial Noguer, S.A., 1957.

Castro, Americo. *The Structure of Spanish History.* Princeton: Princeton University Press, 1954.

Escudero, Vicente. *Mi baile.* Barcelona: Editiones Montaner y Simon S.A., 1947.

Grande, Felix. *Memoria del flamenco.* Two Volumes. Madrid: Espasa-Calpe, 1979.

Homenaje en su centenario. Antonia Mercé, "La Argentina." Catalogue by The Ministerio de Cultura.

Instituto Nacional de los Artes Escenicas y De la Musica. Madrid, 1990.

Jimenez, Augusto. *Vocabulario del dialecto gitano.* Sevilla, 1846.

Levinson, André. *La Argentina. A Study in Spanish Dancing.* [monograph.] Paris: Editions Chroniques du Jour, 1928.

"Argentina" and "The Spirit of the Spanish Dance," in *André Levinson on Dance. Writings from Paris in The Twenties,* 1990.

Mañuel, Peter, "Evolution and Structure in Flamenco Harmony," *Current Musicology,* no. 42, pp. 46–57. "Andalusian, Gypsy, and Class Identity in the Contemporary Flamenco Complex," *Ethnomusicology,* vol. 33, no. 1, pp. 47–55.

Matos, Manuel García. *Andalucia. sección femenina del movimiento.* Madrid, 1971. *Sobre el flamenco. estudios y notas.* Editorial Cinterco: Madrid, 1987.

Matteo. *The Language of Spanish Dance.* Norman and London: Universityy of Oklahoma Press, 1990.

Mitchell, Timothy. *Flamenco Deep Song.* New Haven: Yale University Press, 1994.

Molina, Ricardo. *Misterios del arte flamenco.* Sevilla: Editoriales Andaluzas Unidas, 1986.

Moya, Diego Lopez. *Pastora Imperio.* Madrid, 1915.

Otero, José Aranda. *Tratado de bailes de sociedad.* Sevilla: Tip. de la Guia Oficial, 1912.

Pahissa, Jaime. *Vida y obra de Manuel de Falla.* Buenos Aires: Ricordi Americana, 1947.

Pohren, Donald. *Lives and Legends of Flamenco.* Society of Spanish Studies: Madrid, 1988. *The Art of Flamenco.* Society of Spanish Studies: Madrid, 1972. *A Way of Life.* Society of Spanish Studies: Madrid, 1980.

Puig, Alfonso Claramunt. *Ballet y baile español.* Barcelona: Montaner y Simon S.A., 1951.

Rice, Cyril. *Dancing in Spain.* London: British-Continental Press, 1931.

Serrano, Juan, and Elgorriaga, José *Flamenco, Body and Soul.* Fresno: The Press at California State University, 1990.

Steingrass, Gerhard. *Sociologia del Cante Flamenco* (Jerez: Centro Andaluz, 1993).

Thiel-Cramer, Barbara. *Flamenco. The Art of Flamenco, Its History and Development Until Our Days.* Remark AB: Lidingo, Sweden, 1991.

Triana, Fernando el de la. *Arte y artistas flamencas.* Madrid: Imprenta Helenica, 1957.

Washabaugh, William. *Passion, Politics & Popular Culture.* (Oxford: Berg, 1996).

Weinzweig, Meira. Unpublished dissertation. *Border Trespasses: The Gypsy Mask and Carmen Amaya's Flamenco Dance.* UMI Dissertation Services, Temple University, 1995.

Interviews

Maria Benitez. Santa Fe, New Mexico, August 18 & 21, 2002.

Eva Enciñas-Sandoval, Albuquerque, New Mexico, August 20, 2002.

Telephone interview. Lilly del Castillo, Albuquerque, New Mexico, November 3, 2002.

Teo Morca, Washington, D.C., October 18, 2002.

Chapter 4

Modern Dance

Modern Dance—Tradition in Process*

Marcia B. Siegel

By definition, American modern dance is the art of the individual. Isadora Duncan, its acknowledged founder, did more than reject the confining costume and body-languages of 19th century ballet. With her bare feet, loosely draped clothing, and naturalistic scamperings, she brought to life the free-spirited, exploratory aspect of the American character. Through her espousal of Nietzschean philosophy—a return to Greek ideals of theater and a glorification of the creative artist—she also allied herself with an older intellectual tradition that endows a single protean genius with the responsibility and the privilege of constantly re-imagining art.

This concept dominated Western arts practice for more than a century, but nowhere was it more pertinent than in the modern dance, a medium that allows the artist not only to construct a personal view of the world, but to embody it through his or her own physical form and presence. For much of the 20th century our changing notions of body-image, technical accomplishment, choreographic structure, and theatrical themes in dance depended on these independent, often idiosyncratic and intractable spirits. American modern dance has avoided building a monolithic system of training or aesthetics. Its first generation was a mostly compatible group of individuals whose resistance to ballet bonded them together even when their concepts of their own field differed. What they wanted most of all was to move in a personal way and, through the medium of the stage, to express something about their times and temperament.

By the end of the 1920s, American culture had emerged from its early dependence on European models, had passed through a sort of adolescence after the turn of the century, during which artists self-consciously examined their work, embraced and often rejected modernist trends, and tried to determine what it meant to have an individual style. Classical examples, the academic disciplines, never disappeared, but

*Portions of this essay have been published elsewhere in slightly different form. "Art Aspiration, and the Body: The Emergence of Modern Dance" by Marcia B. Siegel from *Bird's Eye View: Dancing with Martha Graham and on Broadway* by Dorothy Bird and Joyce Greenberg, © 1997. Reprinted by permission of the University of Pittsburgh Press. The author acknowledges the United States Information Agency for use of "Creating a Tradition," written for its publication *American Dance*.

painters and visual artists rallied around pioneers like Alfred Stieglitz, whose New York gallery at 291 Fifth Avenue promoted avant-gardists from Europe and North America; and Robert Henri, the influential teacher and center of the so-called Eight or Ashcan painters, who depicted the rough and immediate realities of contemporary life. Louis Sullivan's *Autobiography of an Idea* (1924) traced the evolution of a philosophy that was to revolutionize American architecture. Poet and critic Vachel Lindsay made the first attempt at a theory of film, in *The Art of the Moving Picture* (1915), a farseeing look at the infant medium. And in 1920 the photographer Arnold Genthe published his *Book of the Dance*, a collection of images that challenged the overdecorated, codified personages of the typical ballet stage.

These pictures, made before 1916, documented what Genthe saw as a large-scale shift in the public's sensibility. In a foreword, he announced his goal of "permanently recording something of the fugitive charm of rhythmic motion, significant gesture and brilliant color which the dance has once more brought into our lives."[1] Genthe's subjects included not only the dissident stars Anna Pavlova, Ruth St. Denis, and Isadora Duncan, but a score of other exemplars, now unknown, of exotic, aesthetic, and naturalistic dance expression. These bodies Genthe captured are distinctly uncorseted, supple, curving, determined to break the sanctioned linear presentation of classroom ballet. The Duncanesque dancers look soft, filled with breath. They seem always rising upward with an open chest, taking pleasure in the expansiveness of their movement, even when they seem to be appealing to an invisible partner. Arms, heads, arching necks and rounded upper torsos follow the thrust of the legs in unbroken lines from the propelling skip or prance. The exotics, costumed as primitives, peasants, or Asiatic deities, are more flamboyant. Their eyes flash, their bodies twist and angle more decoratively, their arms frame intense faces, their hands touch their skin sensuously, suggestively.

But whether spirited or demure, these dancers revel in a prodigious release of energy. The new forms of dancing allowed them to display their femininity more openly and completely than ever before. Men too were liberated from the strict courtliness and formal virtuosity of ballet protocol; following the example of Fokine, Nijinsky, Mordkin, and Bolm, they could be sensuous, playful, earthbound. Men and women acquired dignity as they took on the character of Greek choruses or Hindu deities, but whether they portrayed imps or angels, they exuded a fierce dynamism, which still radiates from their photographs.

The release of the body in dance was linked to dress reform and physical culture, both of which were practiced widely in schools and fashion by the end of the first world war. Bodies, especially women's bodies, took on a new strength and articulateness. But the new dancers justified their work as superior to novel displays of physical prowess. It was to be aesthetic if not Art, uplifting, inspiring, at the very least a notch above recreation or exercise, and certainly more beneficial to the viewer's mind and spirit than a trip to the music hall. "Physical culture," in the words of Duncan scholar Ann Daly, ". . . accepted the body only as a transparent representation, or 'expression,' of the soul. Body-building thus was another form of character-building."[2]

Duncan and St. Denis, the most important progenitors of the modern dance, insisted above all on dancing as a serious and respectable art. However much their private lives may have contradicted it, their dancing was to be morally impeccable, a purifying flame to scourge the sins of the past. They may not have been any more secure economically than the 19th century ballet girls whose survival depended on the acquisition of wealthy lovers. Indeed, St. Denis plied the hated commercial stage to pay her bills, and Duncan had a generous paramour in Paris Singer. But their dancing, their attitude toward their dancing, was altruistic. Philosophy and form were both put to work in the service of delivering dance practice from its taint of decadence. The stigma attached to doing something for pure pleasure could be lessened by rationalizing physical practice into systematic processes leading to the dancer's higher evolution.

François Delsarte, the French teacher of rhetorical gesture, had devised an elaborate system linking life (vitality, emotions), mind, and soul in a triune scheme that was applied to the parts of the body, the way the body parts combine in movement, and the directions movement proceeds in space. To the head Delsarte ascribed functions of the mind; the torso was the emotional, spiritual and moral zone; and the limbs were the vital or physical area. All these body segments, subdivided into units like the forearm and the eyes, were assigned significance as they were combined and brought into action. In this way, according to Ted Shawn's book on Delsarte, every little movement was thought to produce detailed expressive effects.[3] Delsarte training spread widely, undergoing shifts and extensions from its beginnings in the mid-19th century, but keeping its tightly logical, Christian ethic. It promised that orators could be stirring, actors could be convincing, and stage tableaux could project emotional states as well as three-dimensional pictures. A basic configuration of Delsartism, the Ninefold Accord, was even considered "the key of the universe," as reported by Genevieve Stebbins, a principal exponent in America.[4]

Delsartism—in America this meant a system of exercises based on breathing and conscious activating of specific parts and zones of the body to convey specific expressive information—found its way into ladies' literary recitals, patriotic community pageants, and emulation of Greek statuary. It was a major item in the curriculum of the Denishawn School, founded in Los Angeles in 1915 by St. Denis and her partner Ted Shawn. Delsartian gesture undoubtedly underlay the movement in much Denishawn dancing, since both St. Denis and Shawn were devoted to the Delsartian ideal that equated movement with spiritual and mental harmony. Perhaps it was the widespread practice of Delsartian "statue posing" that inspired St. Denis to imitate other iconography, to put painted or carved East Asian goddesses and dancing girls into motion. She wasn't simply trying to re-create particular dance forms; she wanted to merge with the sacred or profane personas they suggested. She would *become* Kuan Yin or Radha— or the simple devotee of *The Incense*, the Yogi, the nautch dancer—by assuming and then animating their bodily positions. Denishawn dance grew out of the effort not merely to *look* like Greek or Indian or Siamese, Japanese, Burmese, Arabian dancers, but to *be* those figures, to take on their physicality and so to dance them.

Isadora Duncan's Hellenism floated on an even more idealistic plane. Surely she saw the Greek marbles in the British Museum, danced in the moonlight at the Theater of Dionysos. Surely she draped her body with the tunic and the Phidian curve. But whether she was wafting ecstatically to Beethoven or Chopin to celebrate the innocence of antiquity, or majestically interpreting the tragic passions in Glück's *Iphigenia* and *Orpheus* operas, she did not try to dance like a sculpture come to life—regardless of how many adoring witnesses called her statuesque, heroic, monumental. Many disciples have recorded and interpreted Duncan's teachings, but the way she transformed her notions of body use and development into stage apparitions that stunned a generation has never been explained. Her effects remain shrouded in mystique.

Perhaps she was merely an intuitive dancer responding to the rise and fall of music. But even her writings reflect the need to synthesize individual experience with a larger continuum. In 1903 she compared her ideal dance to the rhythms of nature: ". . . we must try to create beautiful movements significant of cultured man—a movement which, without spurning the laws of gravitation, sets itself in harmony with the motion of the universe."[5] Her followers codified a technique from this credo, and it is echoed in one of the most influential books on art theory to come from the early 20th century, Robert Henri's *The Art Spirit*. In 1915 Henri wrote: "It is not too much to say that art is the noting of the existence of order throughout the world . . . Everywhere I find that the moment order in nature is understood and freely shown, the result is nobility . . ."[6]

Duncan claimed to have rejected the pre-eminent approach to musical analysis of her time, the Eurhythmics of Emile Jaques-Dalcroze. Although not primarily a system of physical training, Dalcroze exercises, like Duncan's, were based on a full activation of the torso through coordinated breathing, and asked little of the lower body in the way of intricate footwork. So pervasive were the ideas of holistic, "natural" movement, and the vision of ancient Greece as a source of a purer, more elevated life, that the photographs in the Dalcroze manuals could almost be interchangeable with those of the Duncanites in Arnold Genthe's book. Dalcroze used the whole body to develop the most sophisticated rhythmic sensitivity, but neither personal interpretation nor formal composition was a major goal of his training. He felt the true realization of the artist would come through a unity of mind and body, asserting in the preface to the first volume of his *Méthode Jaques-Dalcroze* that these exercises "clearly indicate our intention of establishing through our rhythmic studies an intimate alliance between the physical and artistic faculties, and of making music, in its infinite dynamic and temporal nuances, serve the education of this musical instrument par excellence which is the human body."[7]

What Duncan, St. Denis, and Dalcroze had in common was a stripping down of movement to "motions familiar to all races, such as walking, running, skipping, jumping, kneeling, reclining and rising," as Irma Duncan characterized the vocabulary of Isadora's technique.[8] In effect, this basic locomotor lexicon also pervaded the many systems of gymnastic and body training long-established in schools, colleges, and recreational clubs. Resembling calisthenics in the abstract repetitiveness of their movement routines, these programs often used music to help students integrate moving with healthful breathing. Music also lent a degree of aesthetic sheen to what quickly became an activity attractive to women. Rhythmic gymnastics, much of it imported from Scandinavia and Germany, built strength in the arms and back, often through the use of rings, balls, and other quasi-sporting devices. It might incorporate ballet positions and even steps, it might be adapted from folk dance forms, and it might promise an improvement of social graces, but rhythmic gymnastics was not intended to train girls for the stage. Health and beauty was its mission. Elizabeth Selden, the first to articulate the principles of the New Dance as a genre in itself, saw the link between recreation, physical training, and dancing: "With the advent of barefoot dancing, the Dance has once more advanced to the rank of an educational subject . . . and it will lie with the dancers themselves to establish it as an art."[9]

The passage from physical education to modern dancing was a small step. Proponents of rhythmic gymnastics, aesthetic dancing, and other physical training for young ladies were eager for inspiration. In their perpetual quest for respectability, teachers sought out new pedagogical structures and programs of development. Many traveled to Europe to attend summer courses in folk dance and new educational practices. The German modern dance, or Ausdruckstanz, with origins in the expressionist arts before World War I, owed much to the systematic teachings and charismatic leadership of Rudolf Laban. By the 1920s his theories of Choreutics (space harmony), Eukinetics (dynamics or "effort"), and dance notation had kindled schools, creative work, and community dance activities throughout central Europe. Laban's early student, Mary Wigman, became the leading dancer and choreographer of her generation. By the late 1920s she had mesmerized audiences with her solo dances and choreographed important group works, ranging from the ritualistic (*Celebration*) to the lyrical (*Shifting Landscape*). Mary Wigman undertook her first solo US tour in 1930, Harald Kreutzberg in 1927, both to huge acclaim. Both the rigorous training techniques and the performing expertise of the Germans made a deep impression in the emerging world of American concert dance.

The Denishawn dancers toured the United States and Asia during the 1920s, mostly as a component of variety or vaudeville shows, the only venue for theatrical dancing outside the opera houses of the time. Young film actresses studied at the Denishawn school, and the whole company created the scenes of Babylonian debauchery in D.W. Griffith's *Intolerance* (1916). With its ties to the emerging movie industry and the commercial stage, Denishawn's prototypal modern dance maintained an uneasy relationship to popular culture. Its founders had higher aspirations, and most of its graduates did too.

From the first, Shawn was intent on reforming the effeminate image of the male dancer. His own dancing and choreography modeled assertive male figures, and after the breakup of Denishawn he assembled his company of Men Dancers. Based at Jacob's Pillow in the Berkshire hills of Massachusetts, the troupe danced his classical and ethnic portraits, work dances, athletes, and spiritual figures, from 1933-1940.

Periodically, after performing alongside comedians, popular singers, magicians, and dog acts, Ruth St. Denis would take a sabbatical from touring to do what she considered serious choreography. While Shawn took the main company on the road, she assembled a company of women she called the Ruth St. Denis Concert Dancers. Her interpretations of meditative poetry and musical miniatures reflected the barefoot innocence of Duncan dancing. These pieces, however, were more formally organized, according to an analytical practice St. Denis called music visualization. A close cousin of Dalcroze Eurhythmics, this scheme based movement progressions literally on the phrasing, timing, and melodic shape of their musical accompaniments, which ranged from Bach to Romantic classics to contemporary impressionistic sketches.

St. Denis's assistant and frequent co-choreographer was a young dancer-teacher from Chicago, Doris Humphrey. As she collaborated with St. Denis during this period (1919-23), and toured briefly with a group of her own, Humphrey began to cultivate her own ideas about choreographic structure and design. In 1928 she left Denishawn with two other breakaways, dancer Charles Weidman and musician-manager Pauline Lawrence, to start the Humphrey-Weidman group. Drawing on their own skills as dancers and choreographers, Humphrey and Weidman enlisted their students for concerts and soon became acknowledged leaders of the New Dance. Together they formulated a classroom technique based on Humphrey's concepts of body movement. She saw the dancer in a constant state of resistance to stasis, or "fall and recovery." Supported by the ongoing rhythm of breathing, the body moves through an "arc between two deaths," which was Humphrey's metaphoric way of depicting a dramatic, continuous adjustment to gravity. Either the mover works to achieve vertical stability, or she collapses to the ground, where inertia takes over. Dance movement is a variable passage through these two poles. Humphrey-Weidman technique comprised a vocabulary of swings, tilts, spirals, and falls of different durations, directions and intensities. In locomotion it produced a sculptural and rhythmic subtlety.

Humphrey's great dances of the 1930s, especially the *New Dance Trilogy* (1935-36), asserted her responsiveness to the behavior of groups and her confidence in a creative interaction between the individual and society. Weidman's gift for satire and physical comedy complemented Humphrey's more serious humanistic works. Humphrey-Weidman broke up in 1944, when Humphrey's arthritic hip forced her to stop dancing and she was no longer able to keep the company together. Soon after the War, her most important protégé, José Limón, formed his own company, and she served at his request as artistic director until her death in 1958. During her last years she contributed lyrical and dramatic works to his repertory, including the luminous *Day on Earth* (1947). Throughout her life she worked to articulate her theories of dance composition in written form. *The Art of Making Dances* finally appeared posthumously and became an important text until the next dance revolution deemed it too prescriptive.

Hanya Holm brought German modern dance training to New York in 1931 as an emissary of Mary Wigman. She later dropped Wigman's name when anti-German sentiment made the connection politically difficult for her to acknowledge. Holm, a revered teacher, choreographed for her own group during the '30s, reaching a peak with the ambitious choral piece *Trend* (1937). Holm was not too high-minded to accept commercial work, and she made a very successful career on Broadway, choreographing the

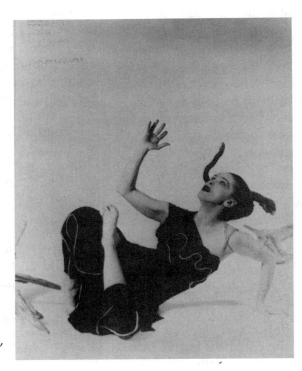

Martha Graham in *Cave of the Heart.* (1946)
Jerome Robbins Dance Division, The New
York Public Library for the Performing Arts,
Astor, Lenox and Tilden Foundations.

legendary musicals *Kiss Me Kate* (1948) and *My Fair Lady* (1956) among others. Her extension of Wigman's and Laban's theories of space and dynamics became a basis for the Nikolais-Louis school, where she remained a teacher and mentor throughout her long life.

Pedagogy was a natural and necessary component of modern dance. It is inherent in the choreographic process: dancers must be trained and proficient in a choreographer's idiom before they can execute whatever new movement patterns the choreographer has in mind. The process of dancemaking usually starts in imitation. The choreographer demonstrates what he or she wants the dancers to do, and often performs central roles in new dances. One barometer of success in the early years was an artist's ability to offer a model that others could identify with.

Martha Graham emerged from Denishawn a few years before Humphrey and Weidman, and began concertizing in 1926 with solos and a trio of women. Like Humphrey, she declared her opposition to the decorative and derivative sources of Denishawn dance. They were both determined to represent the rhythms and desires of contemporary American life, but to avoid literal gesture and over-reliance on musical guideposts. Abstraction became a device for them both. Humphrey made the sweep of choral groups in space stand for community action, and solo dancers symbolized individual aspiration, in harmonious counterpoint with the group. Graham concentrated on enlarging inner feelings into body movement filled with conflict, using controlled affect to generate activity.

The exoticisms left over from Denishawn quickly dropped away as Graham dug into her own physicality to externalize emotional states. She wrote in 1927: "Out of emotion comes form. We have form in music as the reflection of the composer's emotion. There is a corresponding form of movement, a dynamic relation between sound and motion. One can build up a crescendo either with a succession of sounds or with a succession of movements."[10] Graham's explorations of movement grew into a formal technique based on the contraction and release of breath, to create propulsive jumps, locomotion, and intricate, conflicted body shapes. The dances of this period transcended personal expression, although her presence as a performer was electrifying. Her dynamism, translated onto a group of women in the '30s, created mass energies that embodied the tangles and oppositions of modern life. *Lamentation* (1930) was not Martha Graham being a grieving person, but the embodiment of grief. The group work *Heretic* (1929) was not the story of one outsider's struggles but a depiction of the process of rejection.

Bolstered by an increasingly detailed technique and a passionate following of students and audiences, Graham developed her work from the early, impressionistic studies to the contemporary portraits and ritual dances of the '30s. Her travels in the Southwest with music director Louis Horst led to studies of American Indian culture and an appreciation of her own pioneering ancestors. As the nation was drawn into the catacylsmic events in Europe, she turned to patriotic themes, and when Erick Hawkins joined the company in 1938, followed in 1939 by Merce Cunningham, the presence of male dancers opened up new theatrical possibilities.

Graham's dance theater emerged in the 1940s after the formative group works *El Penitente*, based on the flagellant Christian sects of the Southwest; *Letter to the World*, from Emily Dickinson's poetry; and *Deaths and Entrances*, a character study of the Brontë sisters. She turned to Greek tragedy for a series of epic, psychological works centering around tragic heroines beset by sexual ambivalence and forbidden desire, jealousy, honor, and fateful choices. The archetypal characters in these works moved back and forth over time, with Graham as a central, remembering voice, and individuals and groups around her inexorably working out mythology's catastrophic plots. Her company grew into an ensemble of featured men and women, with roles handed down in repertory. Graham continued to choreograph and head the company until her death in 1991. As a choreographer, teacher, and influential theorist, Graham has been honored and written about more than any other American modern dancer. Her school and company have endured into the 21st century.

Modern dance in the 1930s was a freewheeling scene where individual expression found its outlet in solo concerts, clusters of friends made temporary alliances or presented group work in occasional one-night stands, and an important teacher could form a temporary nexus of students to try out her or his ideas. No professional structures of production, hiring, or administration existed as they are known today. The choreographer-centered companies we now think of as the bulwark of historical modern dance stayed together by their mutual dedication to creative work, with nominal paid employment, usually from touring. The dancers had to piece together ingenious solutions to making a living.

Helen Tamiris was less prominent as an innovator than as a vivacious dancer and tireless organizer. Always attuned to the concerns of workers and civil rights, Tamiris performed a series of sympathetic portraits based on Negro spirituals and protest songs beginning as early as 1928. It was Tamiris who first perceived the cost of partisanship and fragmentation to expanding the audience for modern dance. She succeeded in bringing together the Graham and Humphrey-Weidman forces to perform with her own group as the Dance Repertory Theater, for two seasons on Broadway—in 1930 and, with Agnes De Mille, in 1931. When the Federal Dance and Theater Projects were created in the depths of the Depression to give employment to artists, Tamiris played a central role, as choreographer, teacher of movement for actors, and persuasive lobbyist with funding agencies. After the highly successful show *Up in Central Park* (1945), she choreographed for Broadway musicals while continuing to present her own work in periodic concert appearances.

Larger forces were at work during the 1930s to bring about an appreciation of modern dance and its possibilities. The summer school of dance at Bennington College, inaugurated in 1934 and lasting until the early 1940s, brought together the major choreographers—Graham, Humphrey, Weidman, and Holm initially—to teach and make dances in a subsidized institutional setting. The opportunity to have their own groups in residence, augmented by student apprentices, resulted in major choreographic work: Graham's *Panorama* (1935), Humphrey's *With My Red Fires* (1936), Weidman's *Quest* (1936) and Holm's *Trend* (1937) among others. Although only one company held featured status at a time, their professional rivalries persisted. Holm was offered the chance to head a summer program at Colorado College in 1941, returning there to teach and choreograph for the next five decades.

At Bennington, in addition to the Graham, Humphrey-Weidman, and Holm techniques, the curriculum included general courses in teaching methods, dance composition, music resources, dance history, and production. Bessie Schönberg and Martha Hill devised the first Fundamental Techniques course to identify the basic principles underlying all personal styles. As described in the 1934 Bennington College Bulletin, the course would offer ". . . fundamental techniques of movement for the dance analyzed into its force, space, and time aspects; the elements of form and meaning in movement for the dance."[11] The Bennington students, from all over the country, were typically teaching in schools and colleges, and they carried their new knowledge and their enthusiasm back to their home institutions after the summer. It was they who became the loyal promoters and sponsors of modern dance touring. After its demise the Bennington School of Dance was succeeded as a summer teaching and performance center by the American Dance Festival, founded in 1948 at Connecticut College and later based at Duke University.

The first full-time dance critic in the country, John Martin, began a 35-year tenure at *The New York Times* in 1927. An outspoken advocate for the New Dance, Martin drew attention to what he considered the legitimate American dance form through his columns in the prestigious Times and in two important books of theory and description, *The Modern Dance* (1933) and *America Dancing* (1936). Martin insisted on the integrity and uniqueness of modern dance as a substantial art form, the equal of classical music and poetry. Beginning in 1931 at the New School for Social Research in New York, he invited individual choreographers to appear on a lecture series with their companies, to show and explain their work. The lecture-demonstration soon became a finely crafted device for introducing dance to the public in touring situations.

Pianist and composer Louis Horst acted as a musical mentor to many of the new dancers, eventually concentrating on Graham, for whom he served as Musical Director and advisor until 1948. Horst also taught dance composition, using specific music and art precedents as a guide to formal structuring. His courses in Modern Dance Forms, Pre-Classic Forms, and Group Forms helped give shape and clarity to the expressionistic urges of young dancers. He began to publish his classes in his own periodical, the *Dance Observer* (1933-64), and later, in book form, they were used as texts in college dance departments.

During this period of consolidation, a second generation of voices was already emerging. Splinter ensembles orbited the main companies, like the quartet of Humphrey-Weidman dancers who began touring in 1931 as the Little Group (Ernestine Stodelle, José Limón, Eleanor King and Letitia Ide). Independents and members of existing companies were trying out their choreographic ideas in studio showings. But the shadows of fascism, anti-Semitism, racism, and poverty on the world stage persuaded many dancers that bolder statements were needed. All the major innovators responded to political and social realities, but aside from the outspoken Tamiris, political activism was regarded as inimical to art dance. Those with leftist sympathies began making protest dances, often deliberately populist and ephemeral. Working in overlapping, often short-lived collectives such as the New Dance League, they appeared at benefits for labor union causes, the Spanish Civil War, and racial integration; and joined in revolutionist and anti-fascist rallies. Several of Martha Graham's dancers participated in these efforts, including Jane Dudley and Sophie Maslow, who became founders of the only coalition of radicals that held together, the New Dance Group.

Perhaps because of their principled liberalism, perhaps because world politics for them transcended any exclusive dance ideology, the leftist dancers contributed to the democratization and stylistic diversity of modern dance in the 1940s. The New Dance Group began in 1932 with classes, improvisational sessions, and naïve Marxist proselytizing in addition to sponsoring concerts by its members. Classes for nondancers were offered from the start, and both the teaching and performances embraced folk, jazz, ethnic, and even Duncan dancing as well as the three major modern styles. The New Dance Group nurtured African-American dancers when few opportunities were available to them elsewhere, awarding one of its first scholarships to the young Pearl Primus in 1941. Long after the political issues that brought it into being had lost their immediacy, the New Dance Group stayed in business as a school with a staunch commitment to inclusiveness.

Primus studied modern and Caribbean dance styles at the New Dance Group and made an impressive debut as a solo dancer in 1943. Her mature concert work combined modern dance movement and social-justice themes with folk material she collected in several study trips to Africa and the West Indies. Katherine Dunham, the other great African-American choreographer of the 1940s, had an eclectic background in Chicago as an actress, concert dancer, and interpreter of high-class exotica. She formed a company, the Negro Dance Group, but soon entered the University of Chicago to study anthropology. Dunham did extensive field work in the Caribbean, becoming interested in ritual dance forms which she later translated for theatrical presentation both on Broadway and the concert stage. Despite her glamorous reputation, Dunham preserved a strong commitment to exposing racial injustice and serving poverty-ridden communities. She established a home in Haiti but in the 1960s she returned to Illinois to found the Performing Arts Training Center, in the depressed urban area of East St. Louis. Dunham published several books of memoirs and reflections on her travels to the Islands.

Anna Sokolow, from a Jewish immigrant family, knew ghetto life first-hand and carried a fierce social conscience throughout her life. She danced in Graham's all-female company, assisted Louis Horst in his composition classes, and choreographed militant solos and group works during the 1930s. Sokolow began longterm mentoring relationships with dancers in Mexico in 1939, and Israel in 1953. Her own stark, alienated choreographic style emerged with *Lyric Suite* (1953) and *Rooms* (1955). Sokolow worked extensively in the theater and adapted the techniques of the Stanislavsky method for training actors. Echoing Graham's conviction that expressive movement came from inside, Sokolow demanded total body investment and risk from all movers.

Almost as soon as the first generation consolidated its work, a modern dance establishment became apparent, presided over by Humphrey, Graham, Limón and their disciples. As teachers in their own schools and at the new Dance Division of the Juilliard School, inaugurated in 1951, they exercised considerable influence over the field. Not only were their styles singled out for prominence, as components of Juilliard, the prestigious conservatory of music, they could recommend candidates for coveted teaching and performing jobs. As advisors and adjudicators they shaped the careers of young dancers. Louis Horst chaired the selection committee for the performance series at the 92nd Street YM-YWHA from about 1940 on. Humphrey was a mainstay of this group in its most active years along with Martha Hill, who had co-founded the Bennington School of Dance and chaired the dance program at Juilliard.

After World War II, the perceived entrenchment of the first generation was countered by new, stimulating ideas. Modern dance began lowering its ideological resistance to ballet and to the entertainment fields. Broadway had already called on venturesome talents like Charles Weidman, Helen Tamiris, and Hanya Holm from the '30s onward. Jerome Robbins and Agnes De Mille, with their eclectic backgrounds, planted American themes and energies firmly in the repertory of American Ballet Theater. As early as 1937 Lincoln Kirstein's Ballet Caravan produced a piece by Erick Hawkins, and ten years later Valerie Bettis created *Virginia Sampler* for the Ballet Russe de Monte Carlo. The barriers between genres quickly softened as modern dancers recognized the value of ballet classes for acquiring the technical versatility to get jobs in television and commercial theater. International touring and exchanges speeded up the blurring of disciplines. By the '60s a crossover assignment no longer seemed a betrayal, and as the giants of ballet choreography left the scene (Tudor, Ashton, Balanchine), the ballet repertory welcomed reinforcement from the other side. A number of modern dancers developed productive careers as fusion choreographers, including John Butler, Glen Tetley, Lar Lubovitch, and Twyla Tharp.

Among the second generation dancers there were important dissenters from Graham's psycho-sexual expressivity. Erick Hawkins had acquired a BA from Harvard and studied ballet before joining Graham. He spent an often stormy decade as her partner and finally left to find his own path. Hawkins rebelled against the specific dramatic basis of Graham's "Greek" epics and the bodily tension it required of performers. Going back to the more "organic" movement theories of Isadora Duncan and kinesiologist Mabel Ellsworth Todd, Hawkins devised his own technique to develop "flow" and spare the dancers the stressful oppositions and dynamic exaggeration he had experienced with Graham. Often influenced by American Indian ceremonials and Zen philosophy, with images drawn from nature, his meditative, poetic dances appealed to intellectuals and aesthetes as well as dancers. From his first independent concert in 1953, Hawkins found his ideal collaborator in composer-percussionist Lucia Dlugoszewski, who frequently appeared onstage playing a visually and aurally intriguing array of homemade instruments.

Before finding his way to Hanya Holm, at Bennington in 1937, Alwin Nikolais had been a musician and puppeteer in Hartford, Connecticut. Holm's analysis of the spatial and dynamic possibilities of movement gave Nikolais the grounding for a theater in which dancers of extraordinary articulateness inhabited worlds of illusion and surprise. In 1948 Nikolais acquired his own theater, at the tiny Henry Street Playhouse in downtown New York, and during the next two decades of experimentation he designed the choreography, costumes, masks, tape recorded and electronic music, sets, projections, and stage effects for a series of delightful non-narrative works. Because he often put the dancers inside costume constructions or required them to manipulate oversized props, he was accused of dehumanization, but Nikolais maintained that motion was more important than emotion. He felt he was restoring the dancer's humanity by portraying him as "kinsman to the universe."[12] His partner and principal dancer Murray Louis kept their school and companion companies in operation after Nikolais' death in 1993.

With the decline of the first generation, and the diffusion of their ideas into a more eclectic, manageable and necessarily depersonalized stage idiom, the modern dancers started to develop mechanisms for the survival of repertory and the recapture of styles. Always preferring to invest in the exhilarating process of creating new work, they have placed a low priority on maintaining repertory. But as the history of modern dance lengthens out, its practitioners recognize the need to create a more substantial context for contemporary work by bringing historical precedents into living practice. Repertory Dance Theater of Utah, the first company created specifically to undertake this task, was founded in 1965 with a grant from the Rockefeller Foundation.

The José Limón company, which survives its founder by more than three decades, has undertaken the preservation not only of Limón's work but a wider spectrum of styles in the early and contemporary modern traditions. Limón's classic version of *Othello, The Moor's Pavane* (1949), entered the repertory of American Ballet Theater in 1970, with Bruce Marks, a former modern dancer, in the choreographer's original role. Limón's mentor Doris Humphrey recognized that extraordinary efforts were required to preserve a choreographic legacy. She was the first modern dancer to allow her dances to be recorded in Labanotation, beginning in 1948 with *The Shakers*, and she had her work documented on film when finances permitted. With the development of affordable and convenient recording equipment, videotape became a staple of the choreographing and rehearsal process. Examples of the modern dance repertory since the 1970s have been professionally filmed for television, but the effort to recover or retain older works in live repertory remains an ongoing challenge.

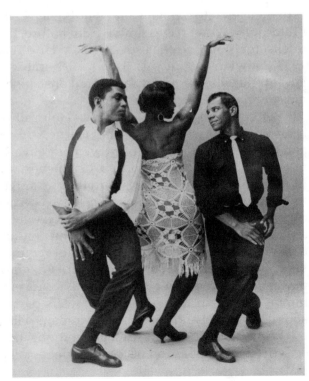

Alvin Ailey, Minnie Marshall, and Nathaniel Horne in *Blues Suite*. (1958) Jerome Robbins Dance Division, The New York Public Library for the Performing Arts, Astor, Lenox and Tilden Foundations.

A product of the multicultural Lester Horton school in Los Angeles, Alvin Ailey arrived in New York in 1954 to dance in the musical *House of Flowers*. He studied with all the major modern dance teachers and presented his first concerts in 1958. Ailey's early works, *Blues Suite* (1958) and the masterful *Revelations* (1960), established a definitive black dance image for the concert stage, perfectly combining African-American sources—jazz, spirituals, and gospel—with modern dance movement and an assortment of vernacular character types. From the inception of his company, Ailey shared choreographic responsibilities with a wide variety of artists, black and white. The company was a sensation and as it toured, Ailey set out to recover the work of black American dancers like Katherine Dunham and commission new work from contemporaries like Ulysses Dove and Donald Byrd. After his death in 1989 principal dancer Judith Jamison assumed the leadership of the company and continued Ailey's mission, providing opportunities to important African-American choreographers Dianne McIntyre, Ronald K. Brown, Garth Fagan, and Robert Battle.

The Alvin Ailey American Dance Theater had become internationally famous, with a junior company and a major school in New York. In 2005 the company dedicated the Joan Weill Center for Dance in Midtown Manhattan. The $54 million building houses the Ailey companies, offices, studios, and a black-box theater, becoming a permanent home for the country's most established modern dance institution.

Paul Taylor danced with Graham in the late 1950s and his projection of the body retains a Graham-like distortion, arms and legs rotated inward, the torso curled in on itself or spiraled outward. But Taylor's dynamics, unlike the dissonant sharpness and pressured sensuality of Graham, are softly weighted and successive, like a gymnast's. Indeed, both his male and female dancers now can do quasi-acrobatic flips, somersaults, and sculptural designs as well as speedy leaps and floorwork. Taylor's dances usually seem to be about deviant communities, cavorting in Utopian light (*Aureole*, 1962, was the prototype) or struggling in darkness (*Scudorama*, 1963). The inhabitants of these imagined societies share a language and a set of ritual practices through which they communicate their boundless physicality, their alienated kinship, their violence, lust, nostalgia, and ironic hope.

Since his retirement from dancing in 1974, Taylor has re-invented his movement vocabulary from a more detached, objective position. His choreographic tendency is inherently classical. He loves form and structure, he has a great facility for arranging groups in space, and his dance is musically sensitive. His newer works have built virtuosic changes onto basic walking, running, and gestural patterns, so that he essentially makes ballets without a technical ballet vocabulary.

Merce Cunningham's influence now extends into the second generation of so-called postmodern dancers. After his formative years with Martha Graham (1939-45), Cunningham turned against the erotic and narrative content of Graham's work. In partnership with composer John Cage, he wanted to make dance that would not be a projection of his conscious or subconscious desires. Resisting the role of the controlling artist-genius, he concentrated on pure movement, and by 1951 was trying out his theory of chance choreography. Chance procedures allowed him to substitute external structuring devices, like the throwing of dice, for making choices himself about the sequence, duration and directionality of movement phrases. For Cunningham this revolutionary system is as rigorous a working process as the personal, intuitive methods of more conventional choreographers. Not only did it allow him to abolish narrative and characterization from his dances, it bypassed theatrical notions of development-climax-subsidence, hierarchical structuring of action in the space, dependence on musical scores, and even the audience-orientation of all previous stage dancing. Cunningham, as a matter of fact, had few attachments to the stage, and considered his work as validly produced in open spaces of all kinds. Rejecting metaphor, illusion, "crisis," he wrote in 1952: "For me, it seems enough that dancing is a spiritual exercise in physical form, and that what is seen, is what it is."[13]

A Cunningham dance is a series of movement events, often layered with several different things going on at the same time. The audience is given few aids to sorting out the most important thing to watch. The sound one hears may be strange or unmusical, and is almost always unrelated to the dancing. Cunningham's movement style, based originally on his own slender, quick body, is centered in the spine, feet and legs, with little decorative detail in the arms, and a torso that tilts and arches directionally but has little sculptural mass. Over the years, as he himself has grown less agile, he has challenged his dancers with intricate spatial and rhythmic patterns, and he has eagerly incorporated new technologies of film, video, computer-animation, and motion-capture into his creative process.

Cunningham's dance is sometimes called balletic, because of the erect carriage and the virtuosic demands it places on the lower body, but, where ballet's action always implies an ideal of harmony, proportion, and aristocratic grace, in Cunningham's pragmatic universe, dancing is a matter of coping with, but never conquering, the urgent demands of the unexpected and the irrational.

While Taylor and Cunningham have worked with essentially the same concerns throughout their careers, Twyla Tharp, since establishing her own company in 1966, has choreographed for ballet companies, films, television, Broadway shows, ice dancing, and large public events. Although she doesn't now call herself a modern dancer, Tharp's constantly evolving movement style originated in her own articulate, witty and elegant performing and the distinctive personalities of her longtime partners, modern dancer Sara Rudner and ballet-trained Rose Marie Wright. Tharp dance requires maximum fluidity, speed and daring, acute musicality, and an escalating virtuosity in partner work. Her dancers, whatever their previous training, must have agile minds and quick reflexes to absorb the intricate configurings through which her choreographic process takes the movement.

In the 1960s Tharp danced with Taylor briefly, then began in the same, highly experimental fashion as nearly all the major moderns. Where Graham did shocking, jagged solos and Humphrey choreographed without music, Cunningham used a mathematical time structure in 1944 (*Root of an Unfocus*), Taylor did a dance standing still in 1957 (*Duet*), and Tharp hid her dancers behind a box in 1966 (*Re-Moves*).

After several cerebral and didactic pieces, Tharp turned to American popular culture as a source for music and movement style. The long line of extremely successful jazz dances that commenced with *Eight Jelly Rolls* (1971) was considered blasphemous by the modern dance establishment. So was the interface between her company and the Joffrey Ballet in the Beach Boys/graffiti ballet *Deuce Coupe* (1973). A phenomenal hit that made Tharp a media star, this collaboration netted her some defecting Joffrey dancers and infused elements of ballet technique into the Tharp style. During the 1970s and '80s Tharp's company represented an unprecedented fusion of modern and ballet dancers. She created some of her most innovative works for them, venturing into narrative (*The Catherine Wheel*, 1981), performance with live video (*Bad Smells*, 1982), heavy-metal, aerobicized spectacle (*Fait Accompli*, 1983), and pointe-work (*In the Upper Room*, 1987).

Even though the company was highly successful, Tharp tried a number of schemes to circumvent the intense touring and fundraising required in the not-for-profit arts climate. In 1988 she abandoned the company altogether, taking seven of the dancers into American Ballet Theater, where she had been choreographing as a freelance since her 1976 tour de force *Push Comes to Shove*, starring Mikhail Baryshnikov. Two years later she left ABT and from then on she assembled groups of dancers for limited periods of time to work on particular projects. She formally resurrected a company, entirely populated by ballet dancers, in 2000, quickly folding it en masse into her first Broadway hit, *Movin' Out*, to the music of pop star Billy Joel.

Baryshnikov's White Oak Dance Project might be seen as the inverse of Tharp's journey from experimentalist to mistress of virtuosic technique and popular forms. The great ballet dancer created a chamber company in 1990, when he no longer could dance the most exacting roles in the classical repertory. With Mark Morris as a founding choreographer, White Oak at first featured mature modern dancers, to make the point that though past the physical peak of youth a dancer still has much to give the audience. White Oak commissioned new work and revivals from some of the major modern and postmodern choreographers for a decade. In 2000 the company produced *PASTForward*, two evenings of reconstructions and new works by former 1960s Judson dancers, making a claim for the enduring influence of their experiments.

Mark Morris too has taken modern dance in a different direction from Tharp. He has created an extensive repertory of accessible, nonballetic dances whose form and musicality counterbalance their often unconventional content. Morris moved to New York from Seattle in 1976, fortified by his training in Spanish dance, ballet, and Balkan folk dance. Ignoring the closeted customs of the time, Morris made headlines by being flamboyantly gay, long-haired, overweight, and outspoken. His early company included modern dancers of distinctly nonstandard sizes and shapes, and his choreography has either avoided emphasizing gender distinctions or overturned traditional gender roles entirely. His movement, initially earthbound but later more speedy and light, seemed determinedly ordinary, with signifying gestures and action that often mirrored the texts of accompanying songs.

Less than ten years after his first concerts in New York, Morris was invited to install his company in residence at the Théâtre de la Monnaie in Brussels. The unusual arrangement, controversial on both sides of the Atlantic, lasted only three years, but the opportunity to work in a luxurious European opera house seasoned the company and greatly expanded the reach of its leader. Three of his most important works were premiered in Brussels: *L'Allegro, Il Penseroso ed Il Moderato* (1988), a full-length philosophical oratorio by Handel set to John Milton's poems; Purcell's *Dido and Aeneas* (1989), with Morris himself playing both the heroine and the Sorceress; and a modern dance *Nutcracker, The Hard Nut,* (1991) set in pop-art style with a campy 1960s family and a corps of unisex Snowflakes.

After his return to the United States in 1991, Morris's mainstream status was assured. His company toured consistently and he made commissioned works for both ballet and modern dance companies. Unlike the chameleonlike Tharp organization, Morris's company structure moved toward longterm stability. A major fundraising campaign was undertaken to acquire and rehabilitate a building in downtown Brooklyn. The company headquarters opened there in 2001, with rehearsal studios, performance space, administrative offices, and a school, a palpable message that modern dance could muster its own institutions.

The late 1950s had seen a gathering unrest among the younger modern dancers, a dissatisfaction with what they saw as a congealed and outmoded romanticism in their teachers. Cunningham, Hawkins and Nikolais led the move for renovation, but the complete overhaul was achieved by others. Musician Robert Dunn and Cunningham dancer Judith Dunn, spurred by the theories of John Cage, started a series of composition classes in 1961 with the intention of exploring and rethinking the dancemaking apparatus. They were open to influences from visual artists and musicians, Happenings, experimental theater and films, and the political protest movements. Products of these workshops were shown at the Judson Memorial Church in New York's Greenwich Village, and the revolutionary concerts that took place there over the next few years became the cornerstone of the so-called postmodern dance.

Retrospectively, the last half of the 20th century may be seen as a period during which the modern dance, drained of its original impulse, gradually settled into historical respectability. We still use the term modern dance, loosely, to refer to work produced outside of the classical ballet establishment, but two major tendencies followed Merce Cunningham. They might be distinguished as contemporary dance, which fuses modern dance and ballet characteristics in a variety of ways, and postmodern dance. As a reference to at least three interrelated phases of non-mainstream activity, "postmodern dance" is a convenient but ambiguous label.

Initially the Judson work was called postmodern as a way of distinguishing it from the Graham-Humphrey-Limón-Ailey line of development. Judson dance in the 1960s was deliberately anarchic in form, anti-theatrical but made of decontextualized theatrical elements, non-expressive on the part of the performers but intentionally provocative to the viewers. Judson dance was neither aesthetically nor compositionally consistent enough to be called a style. By the 1970s many of the Judson dancers had begun exploring certain aspects of performance and movement in a more persistent manner. The minimalist, task-oriented, plainspoken work of this phase did have a certain consistency and was more thoroughly analyzed as postmodern dance, although its practitioners tended to deny they belonged to any trend or category. In the '80s and '90s, with the idea of art itself under suspicion, the term postmodernism was being widely applied to art, architecture, and literature that borrowed ironically and almost indiscriminately from unrelated subject matter, historical forms and stylistic gestures. Gradually, many dance artists began to use their accomplishments to address and re-envision issues of community, gender, race, ethnicity, and physicality; their work has been aligned with theoretical postmodernism and post-structuralism by writers in scholarly journals.[14]

Judson dance and the whole experimental movement that followed in the '60s and early '70s deliberately rejected the technical, aesthetic and theatrical values of the established modern dancers. These avant-gardists not only disparaged the work of their predecessors but they reconceived dance as an object in its own right rather than a projection of one stellar choreographer's creative decisions. All the considerations related to that kind of leadership were re-routed. A dance didn't have to be identified by a central expressive concept with stylistically unified movements, props, sounds and stage effects. Dancers didn't have to look or move like the choreographer. Events didn't have to follow each other in any deliberate sequence. In fact, the course and the outcome of the dance could be collectively determined and could even be unknown before the dance was performed.

Many of the first postmodern works seemed like miscellaneous, uncontrolled outbursts, dadaist displays of words and outrageous props, indulgence in more or less forbidden activity. By 1965 Yvonne Rainer, one of the original Judson dancers, who had studied with West Coast experimenter Ann[a] Halprin as well as more conventional modern teachers, had assembled her thoughts into an essay that became the credo of dance postmodernism for the next twenty years.[15] Distrusting the power of theatricality, and especially the exploitation of the dancer's physical seductiveness, Rainer wrote a large NO to most of the building blocks of theater dance.

Perhaps the most drastic consequence of Rainer's tirade against spectacle was the discarding of dance technique, as an elitist and dangerous appurtenance, and along with it went the manipulative performance strategies of smiling, souped-up dynamics, streamlined bodies and the enhancing of those bodies with form-fitting dancewear. By this time, the counterculture had delivered its message of egalitarianism, and people of all kinds began dancing. Audiences were encouraged to look at and appreciate ordinary bodies moving in an ordinary way. The experimentalists made dances where people walked back and forth, sat down, moved their arms in semaphore fashion. People rolled in mud, tore up newspapers, threw paint on each other in a glorious release of inhibitions.

If performing was to be redefined, then the performance itself, including the audience, could also be put in question. Dances spilled out of stages into lofts, plazas, parks and rooftops. Deborah Hay created simple walking-dance rituals in public spaces, and invited passersby to join. Trisha Brown asked the spectator to look more closely at the performing environment, and at the act of moving itself, by devising ways performers could act normally in decidedly abnormal situations—walking down the side of a building, for instance, or doing a rehearsed movement sequence while lying on their backs. The different ways people could lean on each other or fall could be a dance. There were choreographed squads of motorcycles, and movement instructions that participants found by following a trail of clues. The Grand Union, founded by Rainer, did improvisatory performances employing movement, talking, props and music. Eventually, the group members acquired ongoing personas and did dramatic vignettes along with movement. Their performances could be inspired, or they could be boring. In the 1970s and 80s, improvisation, lightly seeded by particular "problems" or preset movement phrases, became a working process and a performative mode for several accomplished solo dancers—Dana Reitz, Sara Rudner, Douglas Dunn—and collaborative ensembles. Daniel Nagrin's Workgroup, Dianne McIntyre's Sounds in Motion, Richard Bull's groups, and the loosely affiliated artists of the early Dance Theater Workshop all brought collective improvisation to a high degree of imaginative performance.

No longer oriented toward polished, edited products, dancers offered the choreographic process as a matter of interest for the audience, and a whole array of open structures entered the compositional repertoire. Using unconventional information as "scores," new ways of making up movement appeared—dancing the shapes, colors, and objects observed on a wall, for example, or devising transitions between a pageful of photographic poses. But material derived from scores could also be rehearsed and eventually performed. Beginning in the mid-1970s Remy Charlip, an artist and former Merce Cunningham dancer, began sending pages of sketched figures to distant friends, encouraging them to make dances based on the figures. Eventually Charlip initiated a whole series of "air mail dances" in this way.

Gradually, all this experimentation became the basis for a new cycle of refinement. Though the revolution de-glamorized the performer, it soon drew attention back to the individual. Improvisation and stripped-down production revealed the differences between performers, and the contribution of each member of a group became essential to the total performance product. By the early '70s both Robert Wilson and Meredith Monk were presiding over huge, complex theater pieces made from the physical and autobiographical contributions of the performers, who also lived and worked communally. Simple movement led to intensely structured minimalism, with Laura Dean and Lucinda Childs as its main exponents. Trisha Brown developed a detailed dance style based on extremely fluid but spatially precise body movement. David Gordon, building on everyday movement and words, invented gamelike movement structures with intricate verbal and physical puns. Steve Paxton fathered the Contact Improvisation form, which spread throughout the country as a quasi-social, quasi-ritualistic activity based on the play of weight transfer between partners.

As physical dexterity re-emerged, dancers were gaining a greater awareness of the body and its functioning. What came to be called Release technique is not a single technique but an approach to movement, with its roots in the early 20th century. Combining kinesiological intelligence, relaxation principles, and an ability to visualize one's own movement process (ideokinesis), the dancer retrains his or her body to avoid stress and trauma. Release training is a companion to two other great influences that affected modern dance in the 1970s and '80s: body therapies, correctives, and alignment; and Eastern spiritual practice, martial arts, meditation and centering. Release advocates believe dance training is not solely a matter of muscular development. According to Sara Rudner, "'Releasing' has become a metaphor for an ability to access potential. 'Ideokinesis' has become for me another word for meditation and awareness in rest and in motion."[16]

Contemporary dance is built on all these approaches, but it has grown more conventional again. Like the early modern dancers and their descendants Ailey, Cunningham, Taylor and Tharp, many postmoderns eventually wanted their work to expand and to be seen by wider audiences. As in the society at large, spontaneity and risk gave way to the pursuit of a more predictable, high-tech success. Gradually the audience enticements re-emerged—glamorous bodies dancing splendidly in theatrical costumes, with elaborate staging and important music. The drastic practices employed by Cunningham and the postmoderns became integrated and eventually submerged into the look and intentions of a new generation. Nonlinearity, inclusiveness, and the objective performing style permeate contemporary dance, alongside a standard of technique boosted even higher by ballet classes.

With so many possibilities open to them, some of the most original talents in [post] modern dance drifted into closer relationships with other media. Yvonne Rainer has worked primarily in filmmaking since the late 1970s. Martha Clarke has directed a series of theatrical tableaux with narrative based on literary and visual art works. Bill Irwin built entire shows around his brilliant movement-based clown character, and has frequently appeared as an actor in television and the legitimate theater.

For the first time since before World War II, innovations in dance and movement theater have appeared in Europe and Japan with reverberations on the American

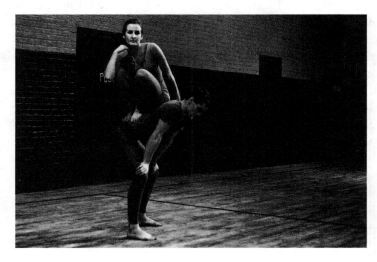

Trisha Brown and Steve Paxton in *Lightfall*. (Brown, 1963) Photo by Peter Moore © Estate of Peter Moore/licensed by VAGA, New York City.

scene. The German Tanztheater, originated by Pina Bausch in the 1970s after a period of study in the US, stages the behavior of neuroticism and sexual oppression in contemporary life as a violent and disturbing spectacle. Japanese Butoh, which creates bizarre and beautiful imagery through surreal juxtapositions and bodily distortion, suggests that life after the atomic bomb has undergone irreversible disfigurement. Tanztheater conveys its shock through expressionistic exaggeration of pedestrian activity; Butoh artists use extreme inner control and meditative imagery that does not "read" as expressive in the ways established by the modern dancers. Another European influence, physical theater, features the elaboration of everyday behavior into dancelike narrative. Because their productions often take place in highly theatrical settings and don't primarily depend on specialized dance vocabularies, these genres can engage controversial issues in a direct way. Their methods have been incorporated into the stockpile of possibilities available to modern dance choreographers.

By the late 20th century modern dance seemed more responsive to contemporary culture than at any time in its history. Virtuosity and high-tech production could be used to convey serious content. Gender roles, persistent racism, addiction, domestic abuse and the effects of globalization became themes of dances. For many, the emphasis shifted from the individual to the group, from a personally derived movement idiom to a more generic technical ability, and from metaphor and abstraction to a preoccupation with display, effect, and irony. In the late 1980s, [post]modern dance looked at its own history and at current society and popular culture with a detached, often parodistic eye. Karole Armitage simultaneously used and made fun of the balletic conventions and devices of George Balanchine. After working in Europe for more than a decade, Armitage returned to New York in 2005 with a new company and a mature, Cunningham-descended repertory.

Ambitious deconstructions and glosses on well-known works or styles relied on singing, acting, dancing, and skillful combinations of live performing with visual, scenic and recorded devices. In John Kelly's *Find My Way Home* (1988), the Orpheus legend was retold as a detective story set in the 1920s, with excerpts from the Gluck opera sung in an untrained, body-miked countertenor by Kelly. Jane Comfort's *Cliff Notes Macbeth* relocated Shakespeare's revenge murder in contemporary suburbia, and the group Kinematic did a zany trilogy of well-known fairy tales. Others whose work reflects and comments on itself include Douglas Dunn, whose seemingly reckless eclecticism covers a preoccupation with the virtuosic and comedic possibilities of awkwardness; and Yoshiko Chuma, who features the unrelated special talents of her School of Hard Knocks—torch singing, piano-playing, acrobatics—to make pieces about the problems of modern living.

Despite the theatricality, the sophisticated application of multi-media, the accommodation of so many other styles and genres, and the extension of dramatic possibilities by the use of words and symbolic gesture, modern dance remains a haven for movement exploration, and for probing the expressive power of the nonverbal. Eiko and Koma make very slow, often grotesque pieces in which they seem to evolve from primal organisms into inarticulate, sensual human beings in varying states of desire, loss or ecstasy. Movement can metaphorically depict the harmony and discord of human relationships in the dance of Susan Marshall, Bebe Miller, Stephen Petronio, Victoria Marks and others. Physical strength can be glorified in the artful mastery of trapezes and aerial equipment, and in the performance of difficult tasks on ramps, walls, or specially constructed props. Elizabeth Streb has persistently challenged the limitations of gravity, space, and equilibrium with her "pop action" training. The collective Pilobolus, founded in 1971, has created a popular repertory that draws on gymnastics, the designs of interlocking bodies, and an often scatological appreciation of the incongruous.

Recurrently, throughout its history, modern dance has served as a vehicle for social justice. The political and social activism of the '30s was silenced by World War II and the subsequent wave of anti-communism, but a new humanitarianism surfaced in the postmodern dance era. It survives into the 21st century as dancing with a social conscience and a desire to bring dance out of the professional stage and into the community once again. AXIS Dance Company of San Francisco is the best-known of several groups that made work for dancers in wheelchairs. Liz Lerman's dance classes for senior citizens led to the establishment of Dancers of the Third Age, a performing company for men and women over sixty. Ann Carlson choreographed for basketball players and lawyers, and made a series of dances with live animals. Glorifying undancerly bodies and movements, Johanna Boyce once did a dance in a swimming pool, and later she gave her baby a prominent role in one of her pieces.

The generous public funding for touring, performing, and new work that fueled the Dance Boom of the 1970s and '80s was diminishing. Government agencies such as the National Endowment for the Arts began to focus less on creative artists and more on the groups being served. Partly in response to this shift, the dancers crafted a series of strategies to investigate forgotten local histories. Outreach became an important part of their mission. Not only dancers took part in these projects. Both Liz Lerman and Ann Carlson have mobilized whole cities or members of related professions for expansive quasi-documentaries and celebratory events. Others have organized site-specific works that called attention to local landmarks or staged historical re-creations harking back to the pageantry of the 19th century. James Cunningham and Tina Croll began a series called *From the Horse's Mouth* in 1998 as a way of reuniting their colleagues of postmodern days. They devised a portable working structure to accommodate storytelling and dancing contributions by performers of all ages and backgrounds into a democratic entertainment. Each installment of the show had a new cast and became a reflection of a particular community.

Autobiographical tendencies resurfaced in a spate of quasi-narrative dances, usually with accompanying words and visual documentation. African-Americans such as Jawole Willa Jo Zollar and the Urban Bushwomen, Ishmael Houston-Jones, Blondell Cummings, Ralph Lemon, and David Rousseve have explored their own ethnicity, spirituality and social experience in different ways. Philadelphian Rennie Harris began choreographing about street and prison life, using a movement vocabulary based on the virtuosic bravado of hip hop. On the West Coast, Anna Halprin, who had never been particularly oriented toward a repertory of dances, extended her experiments with body work and nontheatrical spaces into quasi-therapeutic projects involving whole communities anxious to work on body awareness, group interaction, and healing through ritual.

Bill T. Jones took part in college athletics before he was drawn into contact improvisation training by his partner, Arnie Zane. Together they made dances of complementary opposites (black/white, big man/small man, extroverted performer/ withdrawn conceptualizer) that insisted the audience consider questions of gender and race, the nature of performing and the performer. When Zane died of AIDS in 1988, Jones carried on the company they had established together. Although he continued to choreograph group dances and perform his own seductive, talking-dancing solos, he began working with the larger community in 1990. For *Last Supper at Uncle Tom's Cabin/The Promised Land*, a full-length touring work about the permutations of slavery and freedom, he recruited large groups of men and women to join the company in a culminating celebration of nudity and difference. Jones began leading "survival workshops" for people with AIDS and other terminal illnesses, hoping to explore and validate their experience. Edited tapes of these sessions were incorporated in a large company work, *Still/Here* (1994), which touched off a nationwide debate on the relationship between art and social activism.

At the start of the 21st century, modern dance, particularly the formal stage work that lends itself to repertory performance, has gained a large audience and is presented in major theaters. Besides its nearly universal acceptance as a movement resource for ballet and contemporary dance, the concepts of modern dance have spread internationally since the pioneering travels of Graham, Limón, and Anna Sokolow. All the major modern dance companies have toured the world extensively. Merce Cunningham and the postmodern dancers have exerted major influence in Europe, particularly in France, where Trisha Brown, Viola Farber, and Lucinda Childs established productive connections. Long an advocate of cultural exchanges, the American Dance Festival under directors Charles and Stephanie Reinhart began sending teachers to the Beijing Dance Academy in the 1980s. Modern dance training spread throughout Asia, implemented by other American and local institutions, and international festivals gave increased visibility to performing companies.

These and other global encounters have resulted in highly regarded fusion companies like Batsheva of Israel and Cloudgate of Taiwan. Modern dance also leaves its philosophical traces—its independence from classical ballet's regimentation and its commitment to personal expression—in the work of soloists and groups abroad. Notable for their blending of traditional dance and ritual, their theatricality, their imaginative use of the body, and their search for identity are artists like Vincent Mantsoe from South Africa, Sardono (Indonesia), Tero Saarinen (Finland), Akram Khan (an Anglo-Bangladeshi), and Nora Chipaumire (from Zimbabwe).

What keeps this art form in a state of timely evolution continues to be the creative imagination of individual artists. Modern dancers, eclectic, diverse, whether driving toward the mainstream or content to remain on the borders, still believe in their own bodies as the medium for singular expression, and still work to realize that expression through the bodies of other dancers.

Notes

1. Arnold Genthe, *The Book of the Dance* (© 1916 by Arnold Genthe); Boston: International Publishers, 1920.
2. Ann Daly, *Done into Dance - Isadora Duncan in America*; Bloomington & Indianapolis: Indiana University Press, 1995. p.128.
3. Ted Shawn, *Every Little Movement* (1954). New York: Dance Horizons, 1963.
4. Genevieve Stebbins, *Delsarte System of Expression* (1902); New York: Dance Horizons, 1977. p.113.
5. Franklin Rosemont, ed., *Isadora Speaks*; San Francisco: City Lights Books, 1981. p.33.
6. Robert Henri, "My People" (1915) in *The Art Spirit* (1923); New York: Harper & Row, 1984. p.144.
7. Emile Jaques-Dalcroze, preface to "Exercises de Plastique Animée" - Méthode Jaques-Dalcroze; Lausanne: Jobin & Cie., 1917. pp.5-6. (my translation)
8. Irma Duncan, *The Technique of Isadora Duncan* (1937); New York: Dance Horizons, 1970. p.x.
9. Elizabeth Selden, *Elements of the Free Dance*; New York: A.S.Barnes and Company, 1930. p.vii.
10. Merle Armitage, ed., *Martha Graham* (1937). Reprinted by Dance Horizons, 1966. p.97.
11. Sali Ann Kriegsman, *Modern Dance in America: The Bennington Years*. Boston: G.K. Hall & Co., 1981. p.232.
12. Quoted in "Nik: A Documentary," ed., Marcia B. Siegel. *Dance Perspectives* No.48, winter 1971. p.11.
13. "Space, Time and Dance," originally published in Trans/Formation I/3, 1952. Reprinted in *Merce Cunningham—Dancing in Space and Time*. Ed. Richard Kostelanetz. New York: Da Capo Press, 1998.
14. For example, see extended discussions of dance postmodernism a decade and a half apart in: *TDR* T65, Vol.19 No. 1, March 1975, "Postmodern Dance Issue" ed. Michael Kirby. pp.3-52; and *TDR* T133, Vol.36 No.1, spring 1992, "What Has Become of Postmodern Dance?" ed., Ann Daly. pp.48-69.
15. "Some retrospective notes on a dance for 10 people and 12 mattresses called Parts of Some Sextets, performed at the Wadsworth Atheneum, Hartford, Connecticut, and Judson Memorial Church, New York, in March, 1965," in *TDR*, Vol. 10, No. 2, Winter, 1965.
16. *Movement Research* #19, fall-winter, 1999. p.11.

References

Banes, Sally, *Terpsichore in Sneakers—Post-Modern Dance*. Boston: HoughtonMifflin Company, 1980.
Bremser, Martha, ed., *Fifty Contemporary Choreographers*. London and New York: Routledge, 1999.

Foster Susan Leigh, *Dances That Describe Themselves — The Improvised Choreography of Richard Bull*. Middletown, CT: Wesleyan University Press, 2002.

Franko, Mark, *Dancing Modernism/Performing Politics*. Bloomington and Indianapolis: Indiana University Press, 1995.

Graff, Ellen, *Stepping Left—Dance and Politics in New York City, 1928-1942*. Durham and London: Duke University Press, 1997.

Horst, Louis and Carroll Russell, *Modern Dance Forms*. San Francisco: Impulse Publications, 1961.

Humphrey, Doris, *The Art of Making Dances* (1959). New York: Rinehart & Company/Grove Press, 1962.

Jackson, Naomi M., *Converging Movements—Modern Dance and Jewish Culture at the 92nd Street Y*. Hanover, N.H.: Wesleyan University Press/University Press of New England, 2000.

Kendall, Elizabeth, *Where She Danced*. New York: Alfred A. Knopf, 1979.

Kriegsman, Sali Ann, *Modern Dance in America—The Bennington Years*. Boston: G.K. Hall & Co., 1981.

Lloyd, Margaret, *The Borzoi Book of Modern Dance* (1949). New York: Dance Horizons, 1974.

Martin, John, *The Modern Dance* (1933). New York: Dance Horizons, 1963.

Mazo, Joseph H., *Prime Movers—The Makers of Modern Dance in America*. New York: William Morrow, 1977.

Morris, Gay, *A Game for Dancers—Performing Modernism in the Postwar Years, 1945-1960*. Middletown Connecticut: Wesleyan University Press, 2006.

Nietzsche, Friedrich, *The Birth of Tragedy* (1870–71). New York: Doubleday/Anchor Books, 1956.

Novack, Cynthia J., *Sharing the Dance—Contact Improvisation and American Culture*. Madison: University of Wisconsin Press, 1990.

Perpener, John O., III, *African-American Concert Dance—The Harlem Renaissance and Beyond*. Urbana and Chicago: University of Illinois Press, 2001.

Prevots, Naima, *Dance for Export—Cultural Diplomacy and the Cold War*. Hanover, N.H.: Wesleyan University Press/University Press of New England, 1998.

Ruyter, Nancy Lee, *Reformers and Visionaries—The Americanization of the Art of Dance*. New York: Dance Horizons, 1979.

Siegel, Marcia B., *The Shapes of Change - Images of American Dance* (1979). Berkeley: University of California Press, 1985.

Stebbins, Genevieve, *Delsarte System of Expression* (1902). New York: Dance Horizons, 1977.

Toepfer, Karl, *Empire of Ecstasy—Nudity and Movement in German Body Culture, 1910-1933*. Berkeley: University of California Press, 1997.

Chapter 5

Ballet

Ballet: Reinvention and Continuity Over Five Centuries

Lynn Garafola

People have always danced, and throughout history there have always been entertainments that involved some form of dance. However, it was in the Renaissance, and specifically in the courts of Renaissance Italy, that ballet had its beginnings. Not that it was recognizable as ballet, or what we understand today as ballet; for that we must wait until the early nineteenth century. But the Renaissance brought together a group of ideas that laid the foundation for ballet and its development as an art form.

The Renaissance began earlier in Italy than elsewhere and, by the mid-fifteenth century, was at its apogee. It was an intensely urban phenomenon. Italy was a patchwork of city states, and every city had its court. Those of Florence, Rome, Milan, and Naples were especially brilliant, ruled by princes, dukes, or popes who were among the country's greatest patrons. The Renaissance brought a revival of learning and a flowering of the arts and literature. There were marvelous artists, like Michelangelo, who celebrated the beauty of the naked human body in his sculpture, and Leonardo da Vinci, who painted the Mona Lisa with her still tantalizing smile. Poets and composers abounded. The revival of trade produced great wealth, which was used to beautify cities like Florence and Rome. Public spectacle was very much a part of this program. In the huge public spaces was pageantry galore—processions and parades, carnival masquerades and equestrian displays. And inside the banquet halls and ballrooms there was also dancing.

The first known treatises on the art of dance were written in fifteenth-century Italy. They were written in Latin, the lingua franca of the educated, and described dances for both public and private occasions, in addition to giving their music. The authors were dancing masters, men (as yet there were no women) hired to teach members of the court to dance, to compose dances for weddings, betrothals, and other important occasions, and also to perform. The position of the dancing master within the aristocratic court was far from elevated, a reflection of the status of dance relative to music, painting, or literature. Still, for the Renaissance courtier, "a lithe and airy grace of movement" was added to the list of necessary accomplishments.[1]

The word "ballo" was the generic term for dance. It could indicate any kind of dance or an entertainment devoted to dancing. (The diminutive "balletto"—literally "little ballo"—became the word ballet when it passed into French.) According to scholar Barbara Sparti, there were three types of dancing at Renaissance banquets and festivities—dances performed by the host and his guests; dances in which everybody took part; and "moresche," which were interludes performed as entertainment.[2] These interludes could portray heroic, exotic, or pastoral scenes; they were danced by courtiers, dancing masters, and dancers called "ballerini" (the origin of the word ballerina). The performers wore costumes and masks, and there could be special effects like fire. No expense was spared. The allegorical themes and symbolism flattered and idealized the prince, dramatizing his power through the conspicuous display of his wealth.

Although presented within a theatrical context, the dances performed in these moreschi were identical to fifteenth-century social dances. These included the bassadanza (or "low dance"), the slowest of the era's dances, which was performed with the feet close to the ground (hence the name). Another was the piva (the word for pipe or bagpipe), a lively dance of rustic origin. "The most merry dance of all" was the saltarello, a sprightly couple dance performed in villages and towns as well as at court, often for hours on end.[3] Not until the eighteenth century would the line dividing social and theatrical dance become clear.

Ballet was born within the context of Renaissance magnificence. Although individual dances, as well as some of the dancers, might have a popular origin, the ballo itself was an elite practice, dependent on the court. Thus, very early on, ideas of aristocracy and patronage, spectacle and display, performance and self-presentation became associated with ballet. This association grew even closer when Catherine de Medici brought the tradition of Italian dance spectacle to France in the sixteenth century. Although the Italian contribution continued until the late nineteenth century, in France ballet would acquire a national identity.

Le Ballet Comique de la Reine
(The Ballet of the Queen)

Born in 1519 into the celebrated Florentine family of Medicis, Catherine was well-educated in literature, philosophy, music, and dance. While still a teenager, she was married to the future Henry II and in 1547 became queen of France. When Henry died and the first of their three sons came to the throne, she became the country's dominant political personality, a position she retained for decades.

Like her Italian forebears, she understood the political value of theatre. In 1573, a year after the Massacre of St. Bartholomew's, when thousands of Protestants were killed in a single night, she organized a splendid fête to celebrate the election of her second son as King of Poland. The climax was *Le Ballet des Polonais* (The Ballet of the Poles) in which sixteen ladies, representing the sixteen provinces of France, were presented to the King, Queen, and "other lords of France and Poland"[4]—a vision of political unity that was far from real.

This was followed in 1581 by *Le Ballet Comique de la Reine* (The Ballet of the Queen), sometimes called the first ballet. Conceived as a unified dramatic spectacle, a synthesis of music, poetry, and dance, *Le Ballet Comique* marked the advent of a new form of dance entertainment, the "ballet du cour" or "court ballet." Conceived by Balthasar de Beaujoyeulx, a musician and dancing master who had come to France from Italy some thirty years before, it pitted the mythological enchantress Circe against a knightly hero whom she has ensnared and who seeks to be released from her spell.

Le Ballet Comique was staged in a vast hall of the Louvre. The royal party sat beneath a canopy at one end; other spectators were ranged along the adjacent sides, so the playing space was three-quarters in the round. Scenery was distributed around the floor, and the splendidly costumed characters entered on floats. There was sung and spoken dialogue. All the performers, save the instrumentalists, were noble amateurs.

Dance appeared in several of the tableaux. In one, a corps of Naiads, led by strings and a dozen pages, performed a dance with a dozen geometric figures. There was a processional led by the Queen, and as the finale, a grand ballet, danced by sixteen "princesses and ladies," with no fewer than forty geometric figures, including squares, circles, ovals, and triangles, many with symbolic meaning.

Le Ballet Comique laid out fundamental principles about the use of space in ballet—the emphasis on symmetry, geometry, abstract patterns, and complex configurations. It also showed that these patterns could have meaning, that movement could be a form of symbolic action, an expression of cosmic harmony, of the noble, heroic, and ideal.

Court Ballet

Le Ballet Comique de la Reine initiated the vogue for court ballet. Despite its name, this was a hybrid form, consisting of sung and spoken dialogue, as well as dance. The theme could be drawn from classical mythology or heroic literature. The structure, however, was episodic, consisting of numerous individual scenes called *entrées*, or entrances, in which it was often difficult to find a coherent narrative thread.

Court ballets were immensely popular. The wealthy staged them in their homes and the Jesuits in their schools. But the grandest were presented in court, carrying on the tradition of royal and aristocratic display. In some instances these ballets were first performed at the Louvre, then in the early hours of the morning repeated at the Hôtel de Ville, another vast structure that was the seat of the municipal Paris government.

By the 1620s and 1630s the taste for comic or "burlesque" spectacles had overshadowed the older geometric or symbolic dance, with its implications of cosmic harmony, idealism, and nobility. Audiences applauded devils and monkeys, clowns and exotic Tartars, fools and astrologers, Incas and headhunters, even Ghengis Khan, who made his entrance on a camel (not a real one). Lobsters sprouted from hats, coral from elbows; musicians dressed as soldiers, and bonneted bottles turned into ladies who were really men. It was a topsy-turvy world—the court at play—and it marked the triumph of the "grotesque" dance.

The era of the court ballet witnessed rapid development of dance technique. In 1588 Thoinot Arbeau published *L'Orchésographie* (Orchésography), a treatise about dancing (as well as fencing, piping, and drumming) that defined in a rudimentary way three of the five basic positions of the feet. These positions remain the foundation of all ballet training. Another basic principle evident in *L'Orchesographie* and other early treatises was turnout, the outward rotation of the hips that allows the legs greater freedom of movement than if they were in parallel. Although the degree of turnout was extremely modest, its presence underscored the role both of physical control and visual display in the development of ballet technique. No detail was too small to be ignored—not the touch of a hand, the position of the feet, the carriage of the head, and the elegance of a gesture. Through the discipline of technique, the body was remade, its rough edges smoothed, its natural movements refined. Here was the essence of the "danse noble" or noble dance, the aristocratic ideal in movement.

The introduction of the proscenium or "picture box" stage in the 1640s (it had been invented earlier in Italy) gave a new visual focus to the court ballet. The audience now sat in front of the stage, rather than on three sides of the playing area. A curtain gave a beginning and an end to the action, while painted backdrops and elaborate backstage machinery created dramatic changes in scenery. On the new stage, unlike the banquet hall, the dancer could not turn his back on the audience. With all eyes trained on him, he had to command the stage by moving grandly and attending to intricate foot movements. Spurred in large measure by the acrobatic displays of the "grotesque" dance, technique grew by leaps and bounds. By the 1640s an ever growing number of professionals was dancing side-by-side with noble amateurs.

Louis XIV and Pierre Beauchamps

No monarch was more closely identified with ballet than the "Sun King," Louis XIV. Born in 1638, he had a passion for dancing and loved to perform. He appeared several times a year in ballets presented at one of several royal palaces, dancing for ambassadors and visiting dignitaries as well as members of his glittering court. He played all kinds of roles, including "grotesque" and women's roles, but his favorite was Apollo, the Greek god of music and the Sun King, whose emblem he adopted as his own. His performances were state occasions and often had political overtones. He made his debut as the Rising Sun, for instance, in a ballet that celebrated his coming of age and assumption of royal power.

With Louis XIV, the court ballet reached its glittering apogee. He himself was the last and greatest of the form's noble amateurs, the ultimate embodiment of its aristocratic ideal of manliness. But, increasingly, even at court, technically expert professionals were crowding the field. Among them was Pierre Beauchamps, the most illustrious of seventeenth-century choreographers.

Born in Paris in 1631, Beauchamps came from a large family of violinists. He probably began his training at eight or nine with one of his father's colleagues. What did he study? According to scholar Régine Astier, "the aspiring dancer would be made to practise his *entrechats, cabrioles, demi-coupés* and minuet steps in all direction. Some early engravings show gentlemen practising capers and entrechats holding on to the backs of two chairs, an indication that dance technique was moving toward more daring feats of virtuosity."[5]

Beauchamps made his debut when he was about fifteen. He mainly played "grotesque" or character roles—drunkards, jealous husbands, witches, tramps, exotic Moors and Egyptians. He was endowed with great suppleness and elevation, and his technique was prodigious. He danced in all the major ballets at court, winning Louis' heart and unstinting support. In 1661, when he made his debut as a choreographer, it was in *Les Fâcheux* (The Bores), a comedy-ballet written by the great French playwright Molière to celebrate the king's name day.

The comedy-ballet was another of the hybrid forms that dominate the history of ballet before the mid-eighteenth century. The idea, Molière explained,

> was to give a ballet with the play, but as there were but a small number of excellent dancers, one was forced to separate the "entrées" . . . and it was thought fit to insert them between the acts of the comedy. . . . But in order not to break the thread of the comedy by these sorts of intermèdes [interludes], it was thought judicious to tack them on to the subject and to make one thing of the ballet and the play.[6]

The comedy-ballet, in other words, made its dancing plausible. If the hero fell asleep and dreamed of Scotland or Naples, this would provide the pretext for national dances. Scenes with dancing masters abounded. The dancers were required to mime, and the distinctions between the noble, grotesque, and figured dance were largely eliminated. For the choreographer, *Les Fâcheux* marked the start of a long and fruitful collaboration with Molière.

Founding of the Paris Opéra

In 1661 Louis founded the Académie Royale de Danse, or Royal Academy of Dance. Its purpose, he wrote, was "to restore the art of dancing to its original perfection and to improve it as much as possible."[7] The Academy consisted of a dozen dancing masters, who offered classes to aspiring teachers, conferred teaching credentials, maintained a list of Paris dancing masters, and elected new members. For the first time, the study of dance had a legal structure of its own.

Beauchamps was not among the Academy's twelve original masters although he would later become its director. But he was closely associated with another of Louis' institutions— the Académie Royale de Musique (Royal Academy of Music), better known as the Paris Opera. Founded in 1669, around the time that Louis himself stopped dancing, the Opera is the oldest dance institution in continuous existence (although it has occupied several different buildings over the centuries).

The Opera enjoyed a unique place in the French cultural world. Its license limited the use of dancers and musicians by other French theatres, which meant that the Opera enjoyed a virtual monopoly on opera and ballet. Generously funded by the royal purse, the Opera brought the entertainment and sumptuary display once reserved for the court within reach of a paying public of commoners. Now, instead of courtiers, the children of theatre people, fairground entertainers, and the poorer classes would embody the aristocratic ideal of nobility. Even if ballet had left the court, it remained closely identified with the French state.

In 1672 Jean-Baptiste Lully purchased the royal performance license. Italian-born, Lully came to the French court as a dancer and violinist, appeared in several ballets (for which he also composed instrumental music), and became a great favorite of Louis XIV. As director of the Paris Opera, Lully joined forces with Beauchamps and the designer Carlo Vigarani (another Italian!) to create the "tragédie lyrique," or lyric tragedy.

Yet another hybrid or composite genre, the "tragédie lyrique" was basically a form of opera, a sung tragedy, with dance interludes interspersed throughout. Used chiefly as a divertissement, dance served a decorative or ornamental function, underscored by the magnificence of the costumes. Most of the dances were social dances, and included the relatively new menuet, along with older chaconnes, gigues, and sarabandes. Carrying on the tradition of public display associated with the court ballet, the tragédie lyrique was big on spectacle, and magic scenes, pastoral scenes, and battle scenes were especially popular. For the next hundred years the history of dance at the Opera would remain closely linked to that of opera.

Beauchamps worked closely with Lully at the Opera. "These two great men," wrote François Raguenet in 1702, "brought [ballet] to a high degree of perfection which no one in Italy or any other part of the world has ever exceeded."[8] From 1672 until 1687, when he retired from the Opera, Beauchamps choreographed scores of dances, winning praise for his skill and refinement, and the variety of his groupings and floor patterns. He was an outstanding teacher, training a generation of dancers who would make French ballet the envy of Europe. His success as a pedagogue reflected his analytic understanding of technique. According to Pierre Rameau in his 1725 treatise *The Dancing Master*, it was Beauchamps who codified the five positions of the feet and insisted on them being used to "to give a definite foundation to the art."[9]

Around 1680 Beauchamps developed a system of notation in which he recorded some of his dances. Among them is a virtuoso solo with many unusual changes of direction, balances on one foot, and a great variety of jumps, including early versions of steps that form the basis of today's ballet vocabulary. This suggests the rapid advance in technique that accompanied professionalization.

For reasons that are unclear, Beauchamps was denied credit for the invention of his notation system. Instead, it was Raoul Auger Feuillet who secured the right "to engrave . . . publish, sell and distribute all new dances either composed by him and by others."[10] Thus, Feuillet notation became the first comprehensive method of recording dance movement, and beginning in 1700, when Feuillet published his first collection of dances, the lingua franca of the European ballroom. For the most part, the dances published by Feuillet and the many other dancing masters who adopted his system were ballroom dances—the courants, minuets, and (later) contredanses danced in polite society. These dances were also performed in the theatre, suggesting that in the early eighteenth century the relationship between stage and ballroom continued to be fluid.

The Appearance of the Ballerina

Women of the nobility had taken part in *Le Ballet Comique de la Reine*. However, for the most part French court ballet was a male practice, with women's roles danced by men in masks. This was also true of the Paris Opera, which opened the ballet troupe to women only in 1681. Although men may have appeared "in drag" (to use a contemporary phrase), ballet was not, as Régine Astier points out, a "feminine concept" in the seventeenth century, when "[d]ance was still considered a martial art, prominently featured in the education of young aristocrats traditionally destined to the army. . . . The five basic positions of classical ballet were borrowed from fencing, as were many baroque dance terms."[11]

Françoise Prevost made her official debut at the Opera in 1699 and remained the Opera's foremost ballerina for the next thirty years. She combined technical brilliance with expressiveness. "All the advice which . . . we can offer in regard to our art," enthused Rameau, "is contained in a single one of her dances." She moved with "grace, lightness and precision," and was also a marvelous actress, "enchant[ing] the eager eyes that watch her and . . . conquer[ing] all hearts."[12]

Her pupil Marie Anne de Cupis, better known as La Camargo, was even more famous. Born in Brussels, she made her debut at the Opera in 1726. From the outset she was a star, a virtuoso who excelled at the beaten steps and sparkling footwork considered the prerogative of the male dancer. "Her *cabrioles* and *entrechats* were effortless," wrote a critic.[13] "Ah! Camargo," sighed the philosopher Voltaire. "How brilliant you are!"[14] "Her dancing," observed the choreographer Jean-Georges Noverre, "was quick, light, full of gaiety and brilliancy."[15] Given what she was wearing, this was all the more remarkable.

Camargo, it is said, was the first ballerina to shorten her skirts—to a few inches above the ankles. Conservatives were incensed at the sight of so much flesh. But those few inches gave the ballerina greater physical freedom than she had ever known. Still, with her corset and the panniers or hoop skirts that remained standard until the 1770s, she was anything but unencumbered. Male dancers, for their part, wore a stiff bouffant skirt called a *tonnelet* and tight breeches. Still, their legs were free, and almost without exception the great dancers of the age were men.

With women, the theme of sexual impropriety entered the history of ballet. The Paris Opera, someone once remarked was "a passport to a life of evil and immorality."[16] Once a dancer was "on the list" of the Opera, she was no longer subject to the authority of her parents but only that of the king—a situation that rakes were quick to exploit. Camargo's own life was far from exemplary. She lived openly as the mistress of the Comte de Clermont, and both she and her rival Marie Sallé were painted in pastoral settings known as "fêtes galantes" that depicted amorous play in an atmosphere of rococo charm.

Opera-Ballet

"Opera-ballet" was the last of the hybrid forms pairing music and dance. It dominated the first half of the eighteenth century, and its divertissements were a repository of the era's most popular stage dances. For the most part, they were unrelated to the dramatic action, an ornament to the story, "divertissements," as Louis de Cahusac remarked, "in which one dances just to dance."[17]

The composer most closely identified with eighteenth-century opera-ballet was Jean-Philippe Rameau. Dance melodies had an important place in his works, and he included several in each act or entrée. He was endlessly inventive, a man, in Noverre's words, "of . . . vast genius," in whose works all was "beautiful, grand and harmonious."[18] Among his best works was *Les Indes Galantes* (The Gallant Indies), which premiered in 1735 and catered to the eighteenth-century taste for exoticism, with acts set in Persia and Peru as well as North America.

By then the "baroque" dance was at its height. Among the steps and step-units that appear in reconstructed dances of the period are assemblé, coupé, glissade, jeté, cabriole, entrechat, gargouillade, chassé, tombé, pas de bourrée, and pirouettes—all in many varieties. Beats, pliés, élevés, walks on demi-pointe, and low circular leg gestures called "tour de jambe" were other typical movements. Although turnout did not approach 180 degrees until 1800, the "tourne hanche" or "hip turner" was in use well before that, indicating that by the mid-eighteenth century turnout had grown significantly. Feet were stretched, but not fully pointed, because of the heeled shoes that men as well as women continued to wear until the end of the century.

The danse noble was the heart of French ballet as it had evolved since the late sixteenth century. By the mid-1700s, however, it began to seem like an anachronism and its practitioners a little ridiculous. Far more popular in the early decades of the century were the Italian Players. These were dancers bred in the commedia dell'arte traditions of Italy, and their dancing had the robust physicality of popular fairground performers. Where the French favored elegance, the Italians preferred energetic jumps and acrobatics. In Gregorio Lambranzi's *New and Curious School of Theatrical Dancing*, published in 1716, the dancers leap and jump, perform splits and a host of other acrobatic stunts that offered a seductive alternative to the conventions of French opera-ballet. Many dancers, including Marie Salle, cut their teeth in the fairgrounds.

The Italian influence would continue to be felt in technique, in the emphasis, above all in male dancing, on virtuosity. Such dancing, performed by so-called "grotesque" dancers, presaged the "demi-caractère" virtuosos of the early nineteenth century.

Jean-Georges Noverre and the "Ballet d'Action"

The "opera-ballet" was the last of the hybrid genres that preceded the emergence of ballet as an independent art. Beginning with the "ballet d'action" or "action ballet," ballet acquired a narrative dimension: it began to tell stories in movement. Nature, drama, poetry, verisimilitude, expression—all became rallying cries of a movement that changed the face of ballet. Although a number of choreographers were experimenting along similar lines, the ballet d'action is most closely identified with Jean-Georges Noverre.

Born in 1727, Noverre studied with Dupré and made his debut in Paris at the Opéra-Comique in 1743. For the next thirty years he worked extensively abroad—in London (where the celebrated actor David Garrick called him "the Shakespeare of the dance"), Dresden, Stuttgart, Strasburg, Vienna, Milan. In 1760 he published *Letters on Dancing and Ballets*, which brought him instant fame and lasting renown.

Noverre pressed for a thorough-going reform of ballet as it then existed. Ballet, he wrote, had to be expressive. "A well-composed ballet is a living picture of the passions, . . . it must be expressive in all its details and speak to the soul through the eyes."[19] A man of the Enlightenment, he held nature dear, arguing that in the "action" or mime scenes, "symmetry should give place to nature."[20] He had a horror of tonnelets and panniers, and pleaded for "light and simple draperies" that would "reveal the dancer's figure" and allow greater freedom of movement.[21] Finally, he urged dancers to throw away their masks "and gain a soul."[22]

Even if Noverre's own ballets have disappeared, his legacy survives. Quite simply, he believed that ballet could stand on its own. That it could persuade as well as entertain, tell a story and depict the emotions. Although ballet remained linked to opera in the sense of sharing venues and even bills, it was no longer a part of opera. It was finally independent.

The French Revolution and Its Aftermath

The French Revolution, which began in 1789, transformed all of French life. Inspired by the country's outmoded social and economic system, by the success of the American Revolution, and by Enlightenment ideas such as rationalism and liberalism, it began as a movement for reform and ended in the Reign of Terror, when hundreds of nobles, including Louis XVI and his queen, Marie Antoinette, were sent to the guillotine. Along the way the monarchy was abolished, and "Liberty, Equality, Fraternity" became the rallying cry of the dispossessed all over Europe.

Because ballet had close ties to the court (Noverre, for instance, staged festivities for members of the royal family during his tenure at the Opera), these events reverberated throughout the dance world. Dancers and choreographers (along with much of the nobility) left the country to seek work abroad. At the Opera, huge changes were underway. The system of "privilèges" was abolished, encouraging scores of new theatres to open, while ballets, operas, and choral dramas celebrated the glorious events of the Revolution. There was a resurgence of interest in antiquity, and this produced a revolution in stage dress. Panniers, tonnelets, and corsets vanished. Men as well as women donned tunics or togas, and instead of heeled slippers, they wore flat Grecian sandals or glove-fitting slippers, the ancestor of the modern ballet shoe.

The change in dress spurred equally dramatic changes in technique. By 1830, when Carlo Blasis published *The Code of Terpsichore*, dancers wore now familiar soft ballet slippers. Blasis laid out the elements of the ballet class, with its structured sequence of exercises. He insisted on the need for daily "practice," full turnout, and extensions to ninety degrees. He listed many virtuosic steps, including different kinds of multiple pirouettes.

Blasis distinguished among three types of dancer. The first was the "serious" dancer, who had to be "of a noble, elegant, elevated carriage, replete with dignity and gracefulness."[23] Far more popular was the "demi-caractère" dancer, fleet and lively, who excelled at roles such as Mercury and Zephyrus, the Greek god of the West Wind. Finally, there was the "comic" dancer, a dancer of middle stature and "athletic" proportions. This system of typecasting by physique remains a characteristic of ballet, especially in companies with a traditional repertory.

Although Blasis did not neglect the female dancer, his typology was based upon the attributes of the male dancer. For Blasis, writing on the eve of the Romantic ballet, ballet was still a male-identified form of expression. Romanticism would significantly alter this.

The Romantic Ballet

On March 12, 1832, the curtain of the Paris Opera rose on *La Sylphide*. The ballet was choreographed by Filippo Taglioni, an itinerant Italian ballet master, for his daughter Marie, who danced the title role of the mysterious, ethereal Sylphide. She wore a white diaphanous skirt and a bodice with little wings that was the prototype of the tutu. On her feet were satin slippers darned at the tip and sides that enabled her to linger momentarily on the very tips of her toes and were the homemade ancestor of today's boxed pointe shoe. Taglioni was an aerial dancer. She jumped with lightness and was blessed with suppleness and fluidity. With her modest demeanor, Taglioni was a new kind of ballerina. She inspired a generation of dancers to "taglionize," and made the tutu and the pointe shoe badges of ballerina identity.

La Sylphide, for its part, represented a new kind of ballet. The setting was Scotland, dear to the Romantic imagination and novelists such as Sir Walter Scott. The hero, an impetuous young man named James, dreams on his wedding day of a mysterious sylph. Enraptured, he abandons his flesh-and-blood fiancée, Effie, and follows the Sylphide, as she flies (literally, thanks to wires) to a sylvan abode. The witch Madge gives him a magic scarf, but when he uses it to capture the Sylphide, she dies, surrounded by grieving sylphs. The ballet was thus set in two worlds—an everyday one of the familiar, and another conjured from dream and desire. In the first, "realistic" act, the dancers wore Scottish plaids and performed Scottish reels and step dances, while in the second, they wore tutus and danced in classical style. With its mixture of dramatic action and pure dancing, *La Sylphide* and the ballet-pantomimes that followed in the 1830s and 1840s made good on Noverre's dream of a self-contained dance narrative.

Taglioni was not the first ballerina to dance on pointe. However, it was only in *La Sylphide* that this relatively new technique acquired a metaphysical dimension and became uniquely an expression of the eternal feminine. "When a dancer rises on her points," critic André Levinson wrote many years later, "she breaks away from the exigencies of everyday life and enters into an enchanted country—that she may thereby lose herself in the ideal."[24]

One glimpses that "enchanted country" in lithographs of the era. Romantic prints could be varied in subject matter, but they belonged above all to the ballerina. Often she was shown in flight, eluding the arms of a lover. Or she might stand demurely on a scallop shell, tantalizing in her nearness. She was a creature of the air and a daughter of nature, who made her home in secluded valleys, misty lakesides, secret glades, and wild heaths that extolled a Romantic idea of nature.

Of course, there was more to the Romantic ballet than tutus and pointe shoes, even if these were the most obvious of the ballerina's new attributes. National dances, sometimes referred to as "character" dances, were a key part of the Romantic ballet. Although France did not lack for folk traditions, the overwhelming majority of national dances on the French stage came from Europe's underdeveloped periphery—southern Italy, Spain, Scotland, the Tyrol, eastern and central Europe. Dances like the mazurka, fandango, and tarantella provided local color as well as visceral excitement. Influential critics such as Théophile Gautier praised the "suppleness, vivacity, and Andalusian passion" of the Spanish dance, comparing it unfavorably to the "geometrical poses" and academic traditions of the French school.[25]

More than anyone else, it was the Austrian ballerina Fanny Elssler who epitomized the exotic aspect of the Romantic ballet. In 1836, in *Le Diable Boiteux* (The Devil on Two Sticks), she introduced her celebrated rendering of the Spanish cachucha. Wrote Gautier: "How charming she is with her big comb, the rose behind her ear, her lustrous eyes and her sparkling smile. At the tips of her rosy fingers quiver ebony castanets. Now she darts forward; the castanets begin their sonorous chatter. With her hand she shakes down great clusters of rhythm. How she twists, how she bends! What fire! What voluptuousness!"[26] Nothing could be further from the "ballet blanc."

Like the Romantic ballerina, the ballet blanc was new. The "white act" of a multi-act Romantic ballet, this was the classical interlude when the hero glimpsed his

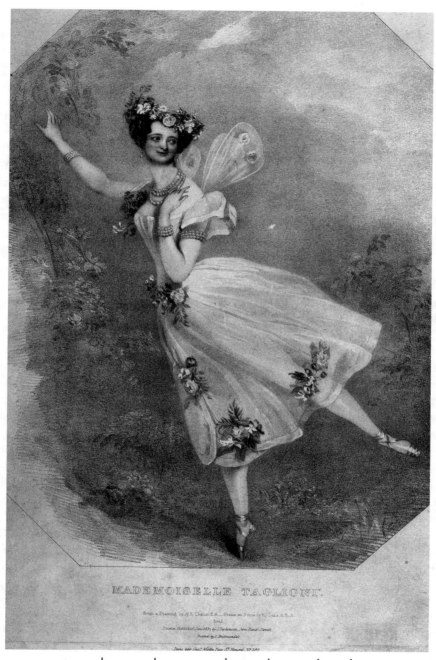

MADEMOISELLE TAGLIONI.

Marie Taglioni in Flore et Zéphire (Flora and Zephyrus).
Courtesy of The Performing Arts Collection, New York Public Library.

unattainable love among white or pastel-skirted sylphs, Wilis, naiads, and other night creatures. The ballet blanc belonged to the corps de ballet; it was a group dance, performed solely by women, a vision of enchanted sisterhood and ethereal femininity. Unmoored in time and space, the ballet blanc stood outside the story; it was a pure dance sequence, couched in the universal language of classicism. The craze for national dances notwithstanding, it was during the Romantic period that the Spanish bolero school, the Italian grotteschi tradition, and the French baroque dance—vital eighteenth-century idioms—fell into abeyance. When they survived, it was as an exotic or antiquarian taste.

There were two kinds of dancers, Gautier famously said: "Christians," like Taglioni, who evoked Romanticism's spiritual yearnings, and "pagans," like Elssler, who expressed its obsession with the carnal and the exotic.[27] Finally, there was the "danseuse en travesti" or travesty dancer—women who donned breeches to play shipboys and sailors, hussars and toreadors. By 1840 the travesty dancer had all but displaced men from the vast majority of male roles on the French ballet stage. Critics applauded. "There is nothing more disagreeable," wrote Gautier in 1838, "than a man showing his red neck, great muscular arms, parish beadle legs, and the whole of his heavy frame shuddering with leaps and pirouettes."[28] Added his critical colleague Jules Janin two years later: "Today, the dancing man is tolerated only as a useful accessory."[29] Ballet was rapidly becoming a female ghetto.

La Sylphide was an overnight sensation. Taglioni herself danced it in London, Berlin, and St. Petersburg; her brother and sister-in-law brought it to New York. But like most ballets staged in the heyday of French romanticism, it did not survive the nineteenth century. Giselle, which premiered in 1841, proved a happy exception. Danced by companies all over the world, Giselle is both an enduring love story and a defining work of the classical repertory. The idea for the ballet was Gautier's, inspired by a German legend of the Wilis, the spirits of women betrayed in love who performed their ghostly dances at midnight and danced to death any man who wandered into their glen. Giselle had all the trappings of a Romantic ballet. There was a realistic first act, set in a Rhineland village during the grape harvest, and a second act ballet blanc, full of romantic yearning, in which Giselle, now transformed into a Wili, is reunited with her unfaithful lover, Albrecht, beyond the grave. The choreography of the group dances was by Jean Coralli, although this was significantly revised in the 1880s, when Marius Petipa restaged the ballet in Russia. However, the dances for Giselle and the magnificent pas de deux in Act II, were by the greatest of Romantic choreographers, Jules Perrot. The title role, which was created by the Italian ballerina Carlotta Grisi, posed numerous challenges, from the acting required in the mad scene (when Giselle discovers Albrecht's duplicity) that brings Act I to a dramatic close, to the almost unearthly lightness of her moonlit dances in Act II. Critics fell over one another in praising the ballet. Wrote Jules Janin in Le Journal des Débats:

> In order to complete this beautiful dream, this feast for the eyes, . . . this danced drama that so little resembles the faded compositions that we have described for ten

years, in order to describe this new Sylphide, you need to slip, if you can, into the midst of these sweet landscapes, overflowing with pastoral poetry. . . . Nothing is missing from this charming work: there is invention, poetry, music, newly arranged dances, lots of pretty danseuses, lively harmony, grace, energy . . . and, especially la Carlotta Grisi. This, for sure, is what a ballet should be![30]

From the Romantic Ballet to "Spectacle" Ballet

By the 1850s the Romantic ballet was played out. Sylphs had vanished, leaving only a memory of their ethereal lightness. A new generation of ballerinas came to the fore, but for the most part they were neither light nor French. Beginning with Carolina Rosati, who first danced at the Paris Opera in 1853, Italian-trained "étoiles"—or stars (the highest category in the French dance hierarchy)—displaced native-born ballerinas at the cradle of French ballet. Most of the early Italian stars were students of Carlo Blasis, who taught the "class of perfection"— or advanced class—at the ballet school affiliated with Milan's La Scala Theatre. His classes were rigorous, and his students were celebrated for their precision, speed, and strength. Over the next several decades La Scala produced nearly all the virtuoso ballerinas appearing in Europe and the Americas. They toured everywhere and made "Italian" virtually a synonym for ballet, just as "French" had been in the eighteenth century and "Russian" would become in the twentieth.

By the 1850s audiences had tired of the conventions of the Romantic ballet; they wanted dancing, not storytelling, spectacle, not poetry. Benjamin Lumley, the director of Her Majesty's Theatre, the London home of the Romantic ballet, had nothing but scorn for the new trend: "The majority of the male supporters of the ballet (as a mere display of dancing) had long decided upon eschewing all pantomime. They disliked the trouble of understanding a story. . . . They wanted only dancing, not acting, they said. . . . And so it was the the mere *divertissement* obtained an undue position on the great choreographic stage of London."[31]

The ballets of the 1850s grew ever more splendid, with gorgeous costumes and scenery, and transformation scenes that left audiences gasping for more. *Le Corsaire*, a tale of pirates, pashas, and slave girls choreographed by Joseph Mazilier at the Paris Opera in 1856, opened with a spectacular shipwreck and ended with an equally spectacular rescue of the hero and heroine. *Marco Spada, ou La Fille du Bandit* (Marco Spada, or The Bandit's Daughter), staged by Mazilier the following year, featured a split stage, with a forest on the upper level and a bandits' cave on the lower.

Another hallmark of post-Romantic ballet was the divertissement—a group of dances unrelated to the plot that made individual dancers shine. Mazilier's works celebrated the technical virtuosity of their ballerinas, above all in the realm of pointe-work. This had grown by leaps and bounds since Taglioni's lingering balances in *La Sylphide*. "Mme. [Amalia] Ferraris does not dance," wrote a critic of the former Blasis pupil who became an étoile at the Paris Opera in 1856: "[S]he runs, she flies, she bounds, she darts, hardly does her foot skim the ground, scarcely does she glide over the boards. . . . [S]he rises with . . . *ballon* and elasticity; [and] thanks to her supple and sinewy foot, she raises herself with an incomparable strength *sur les pointes*, without apparent effort."[32]

The earliest pointe shoes were darned at the front and sides, allowing the dancer to hover almost imperceptibly on the tips of her toes. Gradually, the darning grew heavier, the sole shortened and was reinforced, and in the 1860s Italian shoemakers began adding a "box" or reinforced base that enabled the dancer to turn and perform more complicated steps on pointe. With the invention of the "blocked" shoe, pointe technique entered a period of rapid development. Multiple turns and extended balances became commonplace, and many steps were reworked for pointe. By the 1880s ballerinas were jumping, running, and hopping on pointe, performing complicated feats of balance and in Italy, at least, beginning to master the fouetté turns that remain a yardstick of female virtuoso technique.

Divertissements were the strength (or weakness, depending on your point of view) of Arthur Saint-Léon's many works. The most important figure of the 1850s and 1860s, he packed his ballets with dances. He was in great demand as a choreographer and revived many of his ballets as well as established favorites in cities throughout Europe. He played and composed for the violin and devised a system of dance notation, called *Sténochorégraphie*, in which he recorded some of his ballets. In Moscow he choreographed *The Little Humpbacked Horse* (1864), the first ballet on a Russian subject. *La Source*, which he choreographed in 1866 for the Paris Opera, was lavish and picturesque. But in Paris, as in London, audiences were bored with stories.

Although the Paris Opera retained its prestige throughout the second half of the nineteenth century, the number of productions fell precipitously. Virtually the entire repertory was jettisoned in 1873, when a fire destroyed not only the existing Opera but virtually the entire stock of ballet sets and costumes as well. In 1875, when the sumptuous Palais Garnier opened, they were not replaced. Thus, the Romantic repertory disappeared from the stage that had witnessed its finest hours. Those few ballets that survived did so in versions handed down elsewhere—*La Sylphide*, in the version staged by August Bournonville for the Royal Danish Ballet; *Giselle*, in Marius Petipa's revival for the Imperial Ballet, St. Petersburg. Between 1870 and 1900 fewer than twenty ballets were created at the Paris Opera, and of those only Saint-Léon's *Coppélia*, with its spunky heroine and hero enamoured of a doll, has survived. By then, as Edgar Dégas revealed in his many paintings of dancers, French ballet was a world made up largely of women. Although real men continued to play character roles, women (as in *Coppélia*) now took over the hero's role, revealing the shapely legs that identified ballet with sexual license. The number of boys at the Opera school could be counted on one hand.

Music-Hall and "Spectacle" Ballet

During this period, however, ballet became popular entertainment. There were troupes at the Folies-Bergère and other Paris music halls, as well as variety theatres all over Europe. At the Alhambra "Palace of Varieties" in London's West End, not one but two ballets were standard fare in the 1880s, while at the Empire Theatre, ballets were a regular part of the weekly program until 1915. Contemporary themes were sometimes featured in these ballets. In 1893, at the Alhambra, a ballet called *Chicago*, complete with dancing "redskins," Buffalo Bill, and the Statue of Liberty, coincided with the Columbian Exposition in that city. Exotic themes were popular, as well as military parades and character dances. And everywhere there were girls, girls galore, and many, many girls in tights—pretending to be boys. For the Victorian "gent" it was very exciting.

The top dancers, however, were nearly always Italian and graduates of La Scala, artists who made their living shuttling between the best of the music halls and the best of the Opera houses. Pierina Legnani was one such globe-trotter. An Alhambra star of the late 1880s and early 1890s, she danced throughout the 1890s at La Scala and St. Petersburg's Maryinsky Theatre. Ballet masters were also globe-trotters. Belgian-born Joseph Hansen, for instance, wedged his work at the Alhambra in the mid-1880s between engagements at Moscow's Bolshoi Theatre and at the Paris Opera.

Spectacle ballet was not solely a phenomenon of the popular stage. On the opera house stage no choreographer was more identified with the genre than Luigi Manzotti. Born in Milan in 1835, he came to ballet after studying mime. In 1881 at La Scala he choreographed his masterpiece, *Excelsior*. In six parts and eleven scenes it was a huge production, a hymn to modernity and scientific progress, ideas that galvanized the Italian public in the aftermath of the country's unification. Scenes were set in New York and Washington, Lake Como and the Suez Canal, and celebrated inventions such as the steamboat, electricity, and the telegraph. The sets were sumptuous; there were numerous transformation scenes, and more than five hundred people in the first act alone. The ballet was a triumph, and 100 performances were given in Milan before the year was out. Performances followed in Paris, London, the United States, and elsewhere; everywhere the ballet met with success.

Other grand-scale productions followed, including *Sport* (1897), inspired by the new fad for athletics. Like other forms of spectacle ballet, Manzotti's productions emphasized the colossal, both in scenic display and in the sheer concentration of human bodies on stage. But in their championing of science and progress, so dear to the heart of Italy's northern elite, they also belonged to the opera house. Only a fine line separated Western opera house ballet of the late nineteenth century from ballet on the popular stage.

Marius Petipa and the Imperial Russian Ballet

It was during this same era that ballet in Russia reached a creative zenith unmatched— and unknown—in the West. Ballet in Russia was an imported art. The first school was founded in St. Petersburg in 1738, and the earliest ballet masters came from abroad. Ballet in Russia was also preeminently a court art, patronized by the country's rulers, the tsars, and performed in theatres open only to the elite. The Imperial court was generous to foreigners, especially artists, and many settled in the Russian capital.

Dance personalities of the first rank found their way to St. Petersburg, either as visitors or as long-term residents. Filippo Taglioni revived most of his ballets for the Imperial Ballet, including *La Sylphide*, with his daughter, Marie, the most celebrated of Romantic ballerinas, in the title role. Balletomanes—a term coined in Russia for fanatical enthusiasts of ballet—mobbed her performances and even, it is said, sipped champagne from her ballet slipper.

In 1847 Marius Petipa, then twenty-nine years old, landed in St. Petersburg. Like so many other dancers and choreographers, he was drawn to Russia because of the decreasing opportunities for male dancers in the West and the generous terms of an Imperial contract. He remained in Russia until his death in 1910, marrying there (both times to Russian ballerinas), raising a family, and ruling the Imperial Ballet from 1869, when he became chief ballet master, to 1904, when he retired. His long stewardship of the company had an incalculable effect on Russian ballet. Indeed, what we call "Russian ballet"—in terms of repertory and style—is virtually synonymous with Petipa, his colleagues and descendants. Petipa choreographed scores of ballets and innumerable dances. He also revived many older ballets, including *Giselle*, which had disappeared elsewhere but survived in Russia (and later returned to the West) because of the stability of the Imperial system. Many of his own works fell into oblivion, but those that continued to be performed, often in much altered or "modernized" versions, became the so-called "classics" of twentieth-century ballet.

Although Petipa headed the Imperial Ballet, he was not his own boss. He reported to the Director of the Imperial Theatres, who was himself an appointee of the Minister of the Imperial Court, who was appointed by the Tsar. Of all the directors under whom Petipa served, he had the highest regard for Prince Ivan Vsevolojsky. Director from 1881 to 1899, Vsevolojsky contributed costumes and libretti to many ballets, including *The Sleeping Beauty*. With music by Tchaikovsky, *Beauty* premiered in 1890. From the first it was recognized as Petipa's masterpiece.

The story of a princess, Aurora, who pricks her finger on a spindle, goes to sleep for a hundred years, and is awakened by Prince Charming's kiss, *Beauty* was the apogee of nineteenth-century ballet, a summation of the conventions elaborated over the course of the century. It was a grand spectacle, four hours long, with a prologue, three acts, and an apotheosis. Like all ballets of the time it drew on a multiplicity of movement idioms. There were long mime scenes, "character" or national dances to give local color to "realistic" scenes, ballroom dances, as well as classical dancing. As always, there was a splendid role for the ballerina, in this case Carlotta Brianza, an Italian visitor, that called for virtuoso balances, brilliant pointework, lightness, and stamina. And in the Vision Scene, where Desiré (as Prince Charming is sometimes known) searches for Aurora among a corps of sea nymphs, Petipa created a ballet blanc that embodied the idealism identified with the ballerina. Scenes such as this had their origins in the Romantic era. But in Petipa's hands they became brilliant examples of the mass dance, with a huge corps of women, garbed identically in tutus, who moved through a seemingly endless array of symmetrical figures.

Petipa never threw anything away; on the contrary, he reiterated movement phrases and steps to imprint themselves on the spectator's imagination. A phrase would be done to one side, then the other; beaten steps would be repeated, perhaps four times, often as many as eight or even sixteen times; in *Swan Lake* Odile does thirty-two fouetté turns. In the Shades scene in *La Bayadère* a simple phrase is reiterated until the entire corps (twenty-four or thirty-two today, forty-eight originally) entered.

It is impossible today even to imagine the human density on the Imperial stage of the late nineteenth century. In 1903–1904 the Imperial Ballet consisted of 122 female and 92 male dancers—plus ballet masters and régisseurs, and dozens of children and advanced students of the ballet school. The Imperial stage teemed with life. But it was also a representation of the hierarchy that governed all aspects of Russian life. Rank determined the minimum and maximum number of dancers who could appear in a group. Coryphées could dance in groups of no more than eight; second soloists in groups of no more than four; first dancers in groups of no more than two. The ballerina danced alone, surrounded by the static frame of the corps de ballet.

Another major focus was the pas de deux. Each act climaxed in a grand pas de deux for the ballerina and her partner. Petipa did not invent the classical pas de deux, but he significantly transformed it, codifying it as a multi-part number that opened with a supported adagio, in which the ballerina, assisted by her partner, offered a display of harmonious poses and extensions. This was followed by one or two pairs of solos or variations—the first for the cavalier, the second for the ballerina—that segued into a triumphant coda. Petipa choreographed hundreds of variations; even in old age his imagination never failed him, and he delighted in showing off the personality of a favorite dancer. His variations in *The Sleeping Beauty* comprise a virtual encyclopedia of the female bravura technique as it existed in 1890. In fusing the virtuoso technique associated with the Italian school with the elegance of the French school, Petipa created the foundation of modern Russian ballet.

For much of his career Petipa worked with what musicologist Roland John Wiley has called "specialist composers." These were in-house conductors and instrumentalists who specialized in producing ballet music tailored to the needs of the choreographer. Ballet music had to be tuneful and rhythmic. It had to evoke mood and character, heighten the drama, and follow the ballet master's instructions closely. Petipa was fully aware of the importance of his collaboration with Tchaikovsky, even if meeting the composer halfway was not always easy. With Tchaikovsky, ballet music entered a new era.

Following the triumph of *The Sleeping Beauty*, the Imperial Ballet mounted two other works by Tchaikovsky—*The Nutcracker* (1892) and *Swan Lake* (1895). Incredible as it may seem, given its staying power, *The Nutcracker* was not a success. Petipa's libretto was weak; the heroine was a child, and the only pas de deux came at the end of the second act. Very different was the reception of *Swan Lake*. The ballet had actually premiered eighteen years earlier in Moscow. But it had quickly lapsed, and was thus pretty much a novelty when it was reborn in St. Petersburg after Tchaikovsky's death.

Perhaps the most beloved of ballets, *Swan Lake* represented the final flowering of the nineteenth-century Romantic myth. The ballet was set in Germany, where Siegfried, a prince, is told by his mother to choose a bride at the ball celebrating his birthday. He goes off to hunt and by a lake discovers a flock of enchanted swans led by Odette, to whom he swears eternal love. However, at the ball, he is tricked into forgetting his vow by Odile, who looks just like Odette (they are played by the same ballerina), except that she wears a black rather than a white tutu. When he chooses Odile as his bride, havoc erupts. Siegfried flees to beg Odette's forgiveness, but the sorcerer Rothbart claims her, and the lovers throw themselves to death in the nearby lake.

Petipa choreographed Acts I and III, including the famous "Black Swan" pas de deux, which, with its thirty-two fouetté turns for the ballerina, remains a virtuoso showpiece. His assistant Lev Ivanov, with his more lyrical temperament, choreographed the lakeside scenes, including the memorable encounter of the lovers in Act II, with its haunting pas de deux and images of ethereal sisterhood. The double role of Odette-Odile was a tour de force for the ballerina, not only technically but also artistically. As the swan, as critic Deborah Jowitt reminds us, Odette was "a traditional Russian symbol of purity and redemption,"[33] a descendant of Romantic heroines, a singer of female loss. But as Odile, she was a temptress, closer in her projection of sexual power to the Salomés of the European fin de siècle than to the female idealism of her "White Swan" counterpart. Probably no ballet, with the exception of *Giselle*, has proved so enduring as *Swan Lake*.

For the most part Petipa rejected developments in ballet outside Russia. "I consider the Saint Petersburg ballet company the best in the world," he told an interviewer in 1896, "precisely because it has fully preserved the kind of serious art that the rest of the world has lost."[34] The reasons for this were many—the company's hothouse environment; the fact that it was entirely subsidized by the state, physically isolated from the West, artistically isolated from contemporary developments in Russia, and ever more tightly circumscribed in terms of subject matter. Ballet may have been an exemplary art on the Russian imperial stage, but it was also an art in which change was limited to details of technique and execution.

Michel Fokine

In 1904 the American interpretative dancer Isadora Duncan made her first tour of Russia. In the audience of her first St. Petersburg concert was Michel Fokine, a handsome young "first dancer" and a teacher at the Imperial Ballet School. He was thrilled by what he saw. "Duncan," he wrote many years later in *Memoirs of a Ballet Master*, "reminds us of the beauty of simple movements. . . . She . . . proved that all the primitive, plain, natural movements—a simple step, run, turn on both feet, small jump on one foot—are far better than all the richness of the ballet technique, if to this technique must be sacrificed grace, expressiveness, and beauty."[35]

Fokine choreographed his first dances in the aftermath of Duncan's concerts. Like her, he found his music in the concert hall—in composers like Chopin and Schumann, who had never written for the ballet stage. He created ballets on Greek themes, took his women out of pointe shoes and tutus, freed the torso and the arms, and emphasized both expressiveness and subjectivity. By 1908 he had choreographed *Chopiniana* or *Les Sylphides*, as it is known in the West, a one-act ballet that was plotless. Hailed by his supporters as the "new ballet" (as opposed to Petipa's "old ballet"), Fokine's work was a source of controversy within the Imperial Ballet and its audience.

Petipa may have built up the finest ballet company in the world, but only those who had seen it dance in Russia knew that it existed. The Imperial Ballet did not tour, and its soloists seldom danced abroad. It was Europe's best-kept secret until 1909, when Serge Diaghilev presented the first of his Russian dance "seasons" in Paris. The troupe, made up of Imperial dancers from both the St. Petersburg and Moscow companies, was a sensation. So, too, was the repertory, composed chiefly of ballets by Fokine. The following summer Diaghilev returned with yet more new works, and the following year—1911—he formed the Ballets Russes (or "Russian Ballet"). With this company, ballet entered the twentieth century.

Serge Diaghilev and the Ballets Russes

Founder and director of the Ballets Russes, Diaghilev had a profound and far-reaching influence on twentieth-century ballet. Under his aegis, the first of the century's classics came into being—works such as *The Firebird, Les Sylphides, Petrouchka, Les Noces, Les Biches, Apollo,* and *The Prodigal Son* that transformed ballet into a vital, modern art. He nurtured several outstanding choreographers, including Fokine, Vaslav Nijinsky, Léonide Massine, Bronislava Nijinska, and George Balanchine, and through them influenced ballet choreography until the 1970s. He brokered remarkable marriages between dance and the other arts. From the numerous dancers who passed through the Ballets Russes during its twenty-year history came the teachers, choreographers, and company directors who carried on its work throughout the West. A man of ferocious will and discerning taste, encyclopedic knowledge and passionate curiosity, Diaghilev was both a Napoleon of the arts and a Renaissance man.

Born in Russia in 1872, Diaghilev grew up in Perm. Music was his first love, and when he moved to St. Petersburg in 1890 to study law, his ambition was to be a composer. But his talent was unequal to his ambition, and he turned to the visual arts, writing criticism, mounting exhibitions, and founding Russia's first modern art journal. He also spent a few years working as a special assistant to the director of the Imperial Theatres, a post that whetted his appetite for ballet. His discontent with Russia grew, and after the Revolution of 1905, which promised but did not deliver arts reform, he turned his sights abroad. In 1906 he organized the first of his Russian enterprises for export, a huge exhibition of Russian art at the Salon d'Automne in Paris. The following year he returned with a concert series of Russian music, and in 1908, at the Paris Opera, he made his debut as a theatre producer with the opera *Boris Godunov*, seen for the first time outside Russia. The following year his "Russian Season" at the Théâtre du

Châtelet included opera as well as ballet. The operas were greeted appreciatively, but the impact of the ballets was overwhelming. This triumphant season launched Diaghilev's career as a ballet impresario.

In the next twenty years Diaghilev would selectively revive the "old" repertory. He presented *Giselle* in 1910, *The Sleeping Beauty* in 1921, and at various times (and in various incarnations) *Swan Lake*. What interested him above all, however, was the new—contemporary art in all its manifestations. He viewed ballet as a collaborative art, one in which choreographer, composer, and designer contributed equally to the whole. He dreamed of fusion, of creating a "total" art work—or Gesamtkunstwerk—the term coined by composer Richard Wagner. Diaghilev hired easel painters to design both the scenery and costumes of his ballets, making artistic coherence a Ballets Russes trademark. His earliest designers were the St. Petersburg artists Alexandre Benois and Léon Bakst, the virtuoso colorist of fin-de-siècle orientalist fantasies. But by the end of World War I he had embraced former fauvists like Matisse and cubists like Picasso, as well as Russian neoprimitivists and Italian futurists, allying the Ballets Russes with international modernism. With Diaghilev the stage became a total visual environment, set off from everyday life even as it resonated with the forms and colors of contemporary art.

"It is not an exaggeration," composer William Schumann once remarked, "to claim that the great patron of twentieth-century music has been the art of dance."[36] With Diaghilev, ballet acquired a remarkable body of new music, equally at home in the concert hall as in the theatre. Among the composers who owed their careers to Diaghilev, none was greater, or more closely identified with the Ballets Russes, than Igor Stravinsky. Plucked from obscurity, he was the first of Diaghilev's first great "discoveries." His first ballet for the company was *Firebird* (1910), and it catapulted the young composer to international fame. Diaghilev called Stravinsky his "first son," and together, over the next two decades, despite ruptures and financial bickering, they sired nearly a dozen works, including several masterpieces— *Petrouchka* (1911), *The Rite of Spring* (1913), *Les Noces* (1923), and *Apollo* (1928). These works underscored not only the "Russianness" of the Diaghilev enterprise but also its commitment to modernism. On the other hand, the presence of Debussy, Ravel, Falla, Satie, and Poulenc among the roster of Ballets Russes composers, emphasized the company's international identity. The use of preromantic French and Italian music—a new repertory for ballet—underscored this as well. By 1914, Fokine could write, "The new ballet accepts music of every kind, provided only that it is good and expressive."[37]

Although Fokine's earliest ballets predated the Ballets Russes, the company refined his thinking, while offering a framework for his most sophisticated choreography. In a letter to the London *Times*, written in 1914, he spelled out his aesthetic. The emphasis was on expression—of the group, the crowd, the movement, the body. He argued for the elimination of nineteenth-century choreographic conventions, ready-made step combinations, forms like the grand pas de deux, ornamental groupings, mime, conventional ballet dress, and "ballet music."[38] What he advocated came alive in his works—exotic ballets such as *Schéhérazade* (1910) and *Cléopâtre* (1909), with their fatal temptresses, exotic settings, and atmosphere of sexual promise; neoromantic reveries such as *Les Sylphides* (1909), *Carnaval* (1910), and *Le Spectre de la Rose* (1911); Russian works like *Firebird* (1910) and above all *Petrouchka* (1911). In this, probably his greatest work for the Ballets Russes, Fokine depicted a St. Petersburg street carnival of the 1830s, with the richness of detail and fidelity to nature of Stanislavsky's Moscow Art Theatre.

By the time Fokine laid out his principles in the *Times*, he was at the end of his career with the Ballets Russes. Nevertheless, they formed the cornerstone of Ballets Russes practice. Not only were they embodied in the many Fokine works that remained in active repertory until the company's demise, but they provided the basis for the radical break that marked the company's passage to modernism. The catalyst for that seismic shift was Vaslav Nijinsky. A graduate of the Imperial Ballet School, he was the company's great star, the lover on whom Diaghilev lavished his knowledge, passion, and resources. Numerous works were created for him, with roles tailored to his virtuoso technique and charismatic personality.

Nijinsky the choreographer was Diaghilev's second great discovery—proof, again, of his gift for developing raw talent. In *L'Après-midi d'un Faune* (or "The Afternoon of a Faun," 1912), Nijinsky abandoned the aesthetics of Fokine's "new ballet," while treating sexuality with an explicitness many found shocking. (At the end of the ballet, Nijinsky, as the Faun, seemed to spill his seed into the scarf abandoned by a fleeing nymph.) The following year, with *The Rite of Spring* (1913), he crossed the threshold of choreographic modernism with a vision of ancient Slavic rites and human barbarism that gave rise to one of the century's legendary art scandals, when the audience rioted on opening night. In both these works Nijinsky abandoned formal ballet technique, including such basic elements as turnout and the rounded, harmonious arm movements of the traditional port de bras. In *Faune* the dancers wore sandals; they held their limbs and heads in profile, like the figures of an antique frieze; their feet were flexed, their movement slow and ritual-like. *Rite* ventured even further afield. Unlike Debussy's shimmering music for *Faune*, Stravinsky's score for *Rite* was hammering, violent, and terrible. Set in ancient Russia, the ballet was a vision of primal man and the ritual sacrifice of a girl—the Chosen Maiden—to appease the sun god Yarilo. The dancers trembled, shook, shivered, stamped; they jumped crudely and ferociously; circled the stage in wild khorovods; crowded, like animals in heat, around the hapless victim. Nijinsky "takes his dancers," wrote the critic Jacques Rivière, "rearranges their arms, twisting them; he would break them if he dared; he belabors these bodies with a pitiless brutality, as though they were lifeless objects; he forces from them impossible movements, attitudes that make them seem deformed."[39] What a distance ballet had traveled since the days of Petipa.

In 1913 Nijinsky left the company. His ballets were dropped (although *Faune* was later revived), and his path abandoned. In the years to come, Diaghilev would ally the Ballets Russes with artists whose roots lay in the West. Accompanying him on the initial phase of this journey was Leonide Massine, a young Bolshoi dancer who joined the

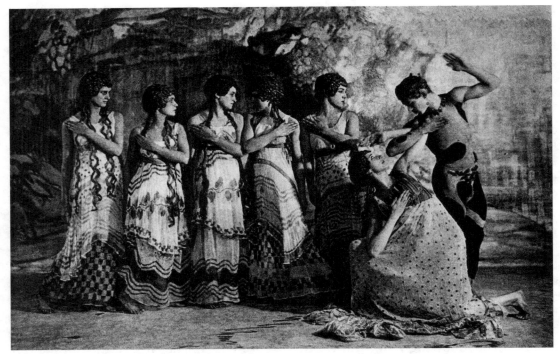

Vaslav Nijinsky and Nymphs in L'Après Midi d'un Faune, 1912.

Courtesy of The Performing Arts Collection, New York Public Library.

Ballets Russes in 1914, and the Russian painters Natalia Goncharova and Mikhail Larionov. Under their aegis Massine began to choreograph, revealing the angularity, simplification, and stylization that were markers of modernism in the visual arts. These characteristics, along with an emphasis on speed and rhythm, appeared in all of Massine's early works, including those on period themes, such as *The Good-Humoured Ladies* (1917), or inspired by folk material, such as the Spanish-themed *Le Tricorne* (1919). "I believe," he wrote in 1919, "that in the art of ballet we must strive to reach a synthesis of movement and form, of choreography and plastic art, a blend in which the two essentials would be balanced, but with a certan inclination, perhaps, towards the plastic element."[40]

Beginning with *Parade* (1917), Diaghilev began to shift his sights to Paris and its international community of artists. *Parade* was conceived by the poet Jean Cocteau as a homage to French popular culture; it had music by Erik Satie and designs by Picasso, by now a hero of the French avant-garde. Picasso created sets, costumes, and curtains for no fewer than five Ballets Russes productions, while also contributing numerous drawings to company souvenir programs. Although Diaghilev initially failed to follow up on *Parade*'s contemporary subject matter, by the mid-1920s the repertory included any number of ballets set in the here-and-now of movie stars and tennis champions, gigolos and aviators, fancy house parties, flapper dresses, and Chanel sportswear. In numerous ballets, including those produced by the rival Ballets Suédois (or Swedish Ballet), the modern was conveyed as much by the decors and costumes as by the choreography.

When Massine left the company in 1921, his place was taken by a woman, Bronislava Nijinska, Nijinsky's younger sister. Nijinska worshipped at her brother's shrine and viewed his work as a prelude to her own, even if she rejected the overt sexuality and male-centered stories of his ballets. She began to choreograph in Russia during World War I. Isolated from her brother, she presented her first independent choreography, a program of solos that recalled the performances of early twentieth-century interpretative artists like Isadora Duncan. In 1919 she opened a studio in Kiev. She called it the School of Movement—not dance, not ballet, but movement. Working with a group of teenage students, Nijinska created her first plotless ballets.

By then, Nijinsky had succumbed to mental illness. In 1921 Nijinska left Russia, rejoining the Ballets Russes, where Diaghilev, now bereft of Massine, hired her as a choreographer. Two years later she created *Les Noces*. The music was by Stravinsky, but the story of a peasant wedding in Old Russia touched a personal chord. She saw the bride as an innocent, her soul in disarray as she "bid[s] good-bye to her carefree youth and to her loving mother." With *Les Noces*, she later wrote, she resumed her "new path." There were no leading parts; rather it was the corps de ballet, raised "to the highest artistic level" that expressed the "whole ballet-action."[41] The choreography itself had many elements of abstraction. It was detached and impersonal, a form of symbolic gesture, a story, a form reduced to the barest essentials. For all its modernism *Les Noces* marked a partial return to the past. All the women were on pointe. The last scene was a great mass dance, worthy of Petipa, albeit totally different in style. However distorted, the choreography was rooted in the traditional ballet lexicon.

This encounter of the modern and the traditional also appeared in the works of Nijinska's successor. Born in Russia in 1904, George Balanchine joined the Ballets Russes in 1924. Trained at the Imperial Ballet School in St. Petersburg, he emerged as a choreographer during the experimentalist moment that followed the 1917 Russian Revolution. Balanchine made his first dances when he was sixteen, and in the years before he left the Soviet Union (as Russia had become), he choreographed concert pieces, theatre movement, cabaret entertainments, and ballets. He discovered modern composers such as Stravinsky and, with the dancers of his Young Ballet company, took part in Fedor Lopukhov's path-breaking *Dance Symphony: The Magnificence of the Universe* (1923), which was plotless. Conservatives criticized both the modernism of Balanchine's work and also what they perceived as its eroticism; some of his earliest and most radical experiments were in the realm of partnering. In 1924 Balanchine and the Young Ballet left Russia for a German tour. They never returned. Instead, they auditioned for Diaghilev and joined the Ballets Russes.

Balanchine's early choreography for the Ballets Russes is difficult to categorize. Critics spoke of the acrobatic character of his work—the high extensions, innovative lifts, and unusual promenades that seemed to parody the traditional pas de deux but at the same time extended its form. In *The Prodigal Son* (1929) the Siren wrapped herself around the Son and slithered down his back in a display of female sexual power that left Petipa's chaste partnering far behind. Another modern note was Balanchine's extensive use of parallel; still another the Art Deco sleekness of the female body, elongated by pointework and ultra-short tutus that revealed the full length of the leg. From the first he could choreograph anything—classical divertissements, ballroom dances, character dances, expressive movement for actors, even a "fairy" ballet that recalled the snowflakes scene in the original *Nutcracker*.

Of all Balanchine's works for the Ballets Russes, *Apollo* (1928) was the most important. "The events with which *Apollo* deals," Balanchine's biographer, Bernard Taper, has written, "are simple, compressed, evocative: Apollo is born, discovers and displays his creative powers, instructs three of the Muses in their arts, and then ascends with them to Parnassus. The theme is creativity itself—Apollonian creativity, vigorous but lucid, untortured, civilizing."[42] *Apollo* was both an homage to Petipa and an early example of what later came to be called neoclassicism. The roots of the ballet lay in the nineteenth century, but the forms belonged to the twentieth: it viewed the past through the lens of a modernist present. Balanchine himself considered the ballet a turning point—the first time, as he later put it, that he dared "not to use all my ideas." It was Stravinsky's score that showed him the way, that suggested "that he, too, could clarify his art by reducing all the multitudinous possibilities to the one possibility that was inevitable."[43]

By 1929, when Diaghilev died, ballet had changed dramatically, above all in the West. Thanks to the Ballets Russes it had become a vital, creative, and respected art. Although it continued to have a popular following and be performed on popular stages, it reestablished its identity as an elite art—both in terms of its artistic character and the select nature of its core audience. Diaghilev brought ballet into the twentieth century. He all but abandoned the multi-act ballet. A typical ballet performance now consisted of three one-act ballets. He transformed ballet subject matter and nineteenth-century ballet conventions. He used outstanding composers and visual artists, and through his commissions made the Ballets Russes both a concert hall and an art gallery. Although he remained loyal to classical technique, he urged his choreographers to experiment with other kinds of movement. Last but not least, he returned real men to the Western ballet stage and, for the first time, made ballet an expression of homosexual desire.

Nationalism in Ballet

Beginning in the 1920s, nationalism became a potent idea in ballet. In part, this was a reaction against the success of Diaghilev's Ballets Russes; in part an attempt to capitalize on the model it represented. People talked about the company as a uniquely Russian phenomenon, even if the technique was based on the universal idiom of the ballet studio. Now companies as well as movements were likely to be identified by nationality. Nowhere was the issue of nationalism more pressing than in England. Here the influence of the Ballets Russes ran deepest, and by the 1920s Marie Rambert and Ninette de Valois were making "British ballet" a reality. Rambert was the more quixotic of the two. She had an eye for talent and a passion for nurturing it, and from her classes came both Frederick Ashton and Antony Tudor, choreographers who defined a British sensibility in ballet. De Valois was an empire builder, the founding mother of the Vic-Wells, later Sadler's Wells company that in 1956 became the Royal Ballet. She dreamed of an all-British company that would combine both the creative spirit of the Diaghilev enterprise and the repertory and institutional stability of the Maryinsky. Under her aegis, Ashton choreographed his greatest works, and *Swan Lake*, *The Sleeping Beauty*, and *The Nutcracker* were staged in their entirety. They became the cornerstone of the company's repertory, at the same time acquiring the status of "classics."[44] By the 1950s, the company had become a pillar of ballet tradition and Britain's artistic establishment.

Americana Ballet and the Founding of American Ballet Theatre

What was American dance? In the 1930s this was a question that was asked time and again. For modern dancers, it was what *they* did, something so unique to America that it was sometimes referred to as "the American dance." It was American because of the nationality of the dancers and choreographers, because of the idiom they used, and because of the subject matter and themes of their dances.

For American ballet dancers the issue was more complicated. Ballet, according to the moderns, was not American. It had arisen in the courts of Italy and France and reached a zenith in tsarist Russia; it was an art of foreign stars, foreign teachers, foreign companies, and foreign works. So what was nationalism in ballet, and how did it apply to America? Was it expressed in technique? In the nationality of the dancers? The nationality of the choreographer? The place of production? Or the subject matter?

Lincoln Kirstein's Ballet Caravan offered a solution to the nationality conundrum that many found congenial. Kirstein, a Boston brahmin and impassioned balletomane who had brought Balanchine to the United States in 1933, founded Ballet Caravan three years later. Just about everything, except the technique, was American. The dancers were American, as were the mostly young choreographers, composers, and painters. With titles like *Pocahontas* (1936), *Yankee Clipper* (1937), *Filling Station* (1938), and *Billy the Kid* (1938), the subject matter was also American, drawn from the national folklore. *Billy* was the most important Caravan work. Choreographed by Eugene Loring to a commissioned score by Aaron Copland, it was American but with a modernist thrust that recalled Diaghilev's approach to "ethnic" and popular subject matter.

In 1939 World War II broke out in Europe. The conflagration brought the leading "international" companies to the U.S. The De Basil Ballet Russe went on to spend most of the war years touring in South America. The Ballet Russe de Monte Carlo, on the other hand, criss-crossed the U.S., becoming in the process an American enterprise. Not only were more and more dancers American-born and trained, but so, increasingly, were the designers, choreographers, and composers. *Rodeo*, which the company premiered in 1942, catered to a public hungry for native subject matter.

Choreographed by Agnes de Mille, the ballet was an instant hit—pure Americana, with a feminist twist. The score was by Copland, the set design by Oliver Smith, and the costumes by Kermit Love. De Mille herself played the spunky, high-spirited Cowgirl, a tomboy who has to put on a skirt to get her man. Set in the West, the ballet makes use of riding movements and includes such vernacular forms as a square dance and a tap dance cadenza.

Rodeo led de Mille to Broadway. In 1943 she choreographed the Rodgers and Hammerstein musical *Oklahoma!* Her dances were unique in two respects: they were the first to be fully integrated with the dramatic action, and they required dancers with training in both ballet and modern dance. Overnight hoofers crowded ballet studios, while a generation of choreographers came to the fore with roots in ballet and modern dance. The golden age of the Broadway musical had opened.

The founding of Ballet Theatre in 1940 marked the coming of age of American ballet. Founded as a choreographers' collective, the new company had three wings—a Russian one headed by Fokine; a British one headed by Antony Tudor, and an American one headed by Loring and de Mille. Although most of the dancers were American trained, if not always American born, the company's artistic outlook was cosmopolitan. The repertory embraced "international" classics such as *Giselle* and *Les Sylphides*, along with "modern" ballets such as Tudor's *Pillar of Fire* (1942), whose theme of repressed sexuality spoke directly to a generation reared on Freud.

It also included that enduring Americana favorite, *Fancy Free* (1944), a ballet about three sailors on shore leave during World War II. Choreographed by Jerome Robbins, *Fancy Free* was set in a bar on the far West Side of Manhattan. With New York a major point of embarkation, the city teemed with G.I.s enroute to the battlefields of Europe. They wanted to have fun, pick up girls, go dancing. *Fancy Free* caught the mood brilliantly. The score by Leonard Bernstein has a jazz-cum-Latin undercurrent, like the social dances of the time that Robbins made part of the choreography. "What has happened," Robbins told readers of *The New York Times Magazine*, "is that ballet, that orchidacious pet of the Czars, has come out of the hothouse and become a people's entertainment in our energetic land."[45] Ballet was booming.

New York City Ballet

In 1946 a recently demobilized Lincoln Kirstein teamed up with George Balanchine to form Ballet Society. Subsidized by Kirstein family money, the new enterprise was organized on a subscription basis. Its goal, according to the prospectus, was the "presentation of new theatre pieces, including ballet, ballet-opera, and chamber opera, either commissioned by Ballet Society or unfamiliar to the American public." Most of the dance works were choreographed by Balanchine, and they had a strong experimentalist edge.

Thirteen years had passed since Balanchine had arrived in New York to form the professional American company that was Kirstein's dream. In 1934 they founded the School of American Ballet, and Balanchine choreographed his first American ballet, *Serenade*, for its students. The following year the American Ballet—the first of several ill-fated Kirstein-Balanchine companies—made its debut. During the next ten years Balanchine discovered America. He choreographed a dozen Broadway and Hollywood musicals, working with dancers as different as Katherine Dunham, José Limón, Ray Bolger, and Vera Zorina. He also created the first of several ballets that paid homage to Petipa and the Imperial tradition. Among these were *Theme and Variations* and *Symphony in C*, both choreographed in 1947, abstract neoclassical works that distilled the pristine beauty and architectural grandeur of Petipa's greatest ballets.

Balanchine's "re-remembering" of Petipa in this decade coincided with the first of his overtly "modern" works, *The Four Temperaments* (1946). Produced by Ballet Society, it had music by Paul Hindemith and choreography that was not only modern in design and contemporary in energy, but also plotless. Kirstein, who viewed ballet as a composite art, had commissioned sets and costumes from the surrealist Kurt Seligmann. Balanchine hated them. He snipped away at the costumes, until in 1951, he got rid of them entirely. He put the dancers in practice clothes, and bared the stage, except for a blue "cyc." The "leotard" ballet was born, and it quickly became a signature of the New York City Ballet, which succeeded Ballet Society in 1948.

With the founding of the new company, Balanchine went into high gear. He was amazingly prolific, his works amazingly diverse. He choreographed "leotard" ballets to twelve-tone music, but also the first *Nutcracker* (1954) to become a Christmas classic. He choreographed ballets poignant with romance and pure-dance works that offered a classical vision of the sublime. He invoked styles past and continued to experiment with narrative, while also celebrating high-stepping showgirls and razzamatazz Americana. And even apart from *The Nutcracker*, he choreographed original full-length works, including one, *Jewels* (1967), that was totally plotless.

An exceptionally gifted musician, Balanchine defined the essential nature of ballet as movement to music. "The music is always first," he once said. "I cannot move, unless I hear the music first. I couldn't move without a reason, and the reason is music."[46] His taste in music was catholic. He loved Tchaikovsky and Delibes, Bach and Mozart, but from his earliest years he also choreographed to contemporary music. He had a long and inspired collaboration with Stravinsky that began with *Apollo* and culminated in the New York City Ballet's 1972 Stravinsky Festival. With twenty-two new works presented in a single week, along with performances of Stravinsky ballets already in the company's repertory, the festival was a magnificent tribute to the recently deceased composer.

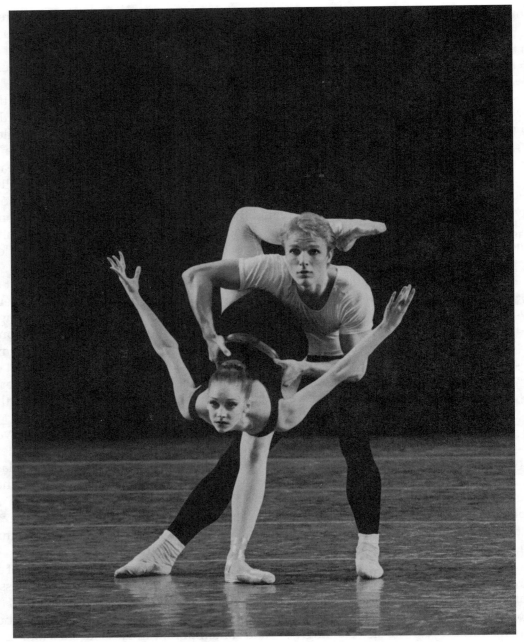

María Kowroski and Nilas Martins in George Balanchine's Agon.
Courtesy of photographer Paul Kolnik.

Through the New York City Ballet and its affiliated School of American Ballet, Balanchine transformed the landscape of professional dance in the United States. He was instrumental in creating a style of classical dancing that came to be regarded as distinctly "American." This had to do with attack, speed, clarity, energy, and an absence of manner. He reemphasized the classical basis of ballet and extended the classical language beyond anything Petipa or any other nineteenth-century choreographer could ever have imagined. Through his teaching and his choreography he brought about a profound rethinking of the *danse d'école*. Had Balanchine not lived, the history of ballet would have been very different, above all in the United States.

"Crossing-over": Ballet and Postmodern Dance

By the 1970s ballet choreography in the West had reached its own impasse. The masters of the 1940s, 1950s, and 1960s—Balanchine, Ashton, Tudor, Robbins, de Mille—were at the end of their careers, and no immediate successors were in sight. All had honed their craft on companies with little money but a strong creative bent, some of which grew into major institutions. Ballet needs institutions to survive, because they provide continuity, conserving the past and passing it on. But institutions do not foster originality. The choreographers who emerge from them tend to create within the limits of a "house" style. The ballet "boom" of the late 1960s and 1970s created a huge need for choreography. Companies multiplied, above all in the United States, where foundations and the newly established National Endowment for the Arts were pumping money into the regional ballet movement. Unlike Ballet Theatre (or American Ballet Theatre, as it was now known) in its early years or the New York City Ballet, few of these young companies had a choreographic identity; most grew out of a school or a "civic" (i.e., non-professional) company. The emphasis was on training, not creativity.

In 1973 Robert Joffrey, the founder and artistic director of the Joffrey Ballet, commissioned *Deuce Coupe* from Twyla Tharp, the most exciting choreographer to emerge from the postmodern ferment of the 1960s. Performed by members of her own company as well as Joffrey dancers, *Deuce Coupe* made history. The music was by the Beach Boys, a popular rock-and-roll group. The choreography was in Tharp's rapidly developing signature style—"loose-limbed, seemingly spontaneous but totally controlled . . . with off-centered ease, torquing bodies, unusual lifts and turns, big, breathtaking physicality as well as throwaway squiggles."[47] *Push Comes to Shove*, which followed in 1976, teamed Tharp with the Russian defector and ABT superstar Mikhail Baryshnikov in a work that wittily juxtaposed classical virtuosity with her idiosyncratic movement style.

The "cross-over" phenomenon, as the pairing of young postmodern choreographers with ballet companies was soon called, was a funder's delight. It filled two pressing needs: providing commissions for the choreographers and choreography for the companies. However, unlike Tharp's experience with Joffrey or ABT, few of the pairings were successful. Most choreographers had no experience working with ballet dancers and little understanding of ballet vocabulary and technique. They did not come away from the experience untouched, however. A perceptible shift could be discerned in the style of many choreographers, a concern for line and technical detail that enriched their vocabulary and complemented their interest in structure. Many postmoderns returned to ballet class and hired dancers who were proficient in both ballet and modern techniques. Meanwhile, in upscale quarters of the U.S. modern dance world and especially on the contemporary fringe of the European ballet world, ballet technique was appropriated as a means of giving a virtuoso edge to non-balletic or even anti-balletic choreography. In companies as different as the Alvin Ailey American Dance Company and William Forsythe's Frankfurt Ballet, ballet-trained bodies have created a bravura form of modern dance, a form enhanced by the dancers because of their training. Exploited as a system of physical gymnastics, ballet is the means to an end, not an end in itself.

Return of the Multi-Act Ballet

The one-act ballet introduced by the Ballets Russes dominated Western repertories well into the 1960s. In the United States, apart from *Giselle*, few multi-act ballets were performed in their entirety. Even when Balanchine staged *Raymonda* for the Ballet Russe de Monte Carlo in 1946, the version was truncated, as if audiences needed more variety than a single work could provide. Amazing as it may seem, no U.S. company danced the full Petipa-Ivanov *Swan Lake* until 1967, when it was staged by American Ballet Theatre. In Britain, however, Ninette de Valois had acquired full versions of the Tchaikovsky classics and other nineteenth-century ballets for Sadlers Wells in the 1930s. With the move to the Royal Opera House, Covent Garden, in 1946, de Valois began downplaying the company's modernist identity, emphasizing instead its Maryinsky lineage. In 1948, at her behest, Frederick Ashton choreographed his first full-length ballet, *Cinderella*, followed in 1952 by *Sylvia*.

The Bolshoi Ballet's 1956 tour gave a tremendous boost to the full-length ballet, especially in England. The Royal Ballet added several to its repertory, including Ashton's *La Fille Mal Gardée* (1960), John Cranko's *The Prince of the Pagodas* (1957), and Kenneth MacMillan's *Romeo and Juliet* (1965). Even Balanchine choreographed no fewer than three original full-lengths in the 1960s—*A Midsummer Night's Dream* (1962), *Don Quixote* (1965), and *Jewels* (1967). In the decades that followed, multi-act ballets occupied a growing place in the repertory of Western ballet companies. Some were newly minted; others were remakes of older ballet subjects; still others, including *Le Corsaire* and *La Bayadère*, were Russian imports. No matter what their origin, these works embraced a neotraditional aesthetic. They were story ballets with big casts, big stars, and lush production values that appealed to the upscale, conservative audiences that increasingly patronized ballet.

Apart from the choreography, what distinguishes a neotraditional full-length from real nineteenth-century ballet is the augmented male presence. In Petipa's day, ballet was dominated by women. Today, they are increasingly overshadowed by men. Even in ballets as traditional as *Swan Lake*, male roles have been added and existing ones rechoreographed to display the dazzling virtuosity of a new generation of men, many of them trained in Spain, Argentina, and especially Cuba. Today, multi-act works account for almost the entire repertory of American Ballet Theatre's lengthy spring season in New York. They also occupy a growing place in the repertory of the New York City Ballet, which in an effort to expand audiences, has added productions of *The Sleeping Beauty, Swan Lake, & Romeo & Juliet* all choreographed by the company's artistic director Péter Martins.

Ballet, its opponents argue, is a hothouse bloom. Yet in recent decades it has grown exponentially, setting deep roots in Japan and in many parts of the United States, where regional companies are now redrawing the national ballet landscape. Critics sometimes say that ballet is dying, because no choreographer of the stature of Balanchine, Ashton, or Jerome Robbins has appeared on the horizon. While that is certainly the case, it is also true that ballet is thriving. Companies have multiplied; technical standards have risen; training is excellent. In fact, in many parts of the U.S., the only dance training available is ballet training. Although older companies may find themselves in the artistic doldrums, new ones have emerged, often associated with a choreographer, while in cities like New York, chamber groups are flourishing. Ballet is yet again reinventing itself.

Notes

1. Quoted in Lincoln Kirstein, *Dance: A Short History of Classic Theatrical Dancing* (New York, 1935; rpt. New York: Dance Horizons, 1974), p. 138.
2. *Guglielmo Ebreo of Pesaro: De Pratica seu arte tripudii (On the Practice or Art of Dancing)*, ed., trans., and introd. Barbara Sparti (Oxford: Oxford University Press, 1993), pp. 47–48.
3. Ibid., pp. 218, 223, 225. These definitions come from Sparti's very useful glossary.
4. Pierre Brantôme, quoted in Kirstein, *Dance*, p. 149.
5. Régine Kunzle [Astier], "Piérre Beauchamp: The Illustrious Unknown Choreographer," Part 1, *Dance Scope*, 8, no. 2 (Spring/Summer 1974), p. 40.
6. Quoted in Régine Kunzle [Astier], "Pierre Beauchamp: The Illustrious Unknown Choreographer," Part 2, *Dance Scope*, 9, no. 1 (Fall/Winter 1974–1975), p. 36.
7. Quoted in Regine Astier, "Académie Royale de Danse," *International Encyclopedia of Dance* (hereafter *IED*).
8. Quoted in Régine Astier, "Beauchamps, Pierre," *IED*.
9. P[ierre] Rameau, *The Dancing Master*, trans. Cyril W. Beaumont (London, 1931; rpt. New York: Dance Horizons, [1970]), p. 5.
10. Quoted in Kunzle, "Pierre Beauchamp," Part 2, p. 41.
11. Régine Astier, "Review—Dance and the Jesuit Theatre of the Ancien Régime," *Dance Chronicle*, 21, no. 2 (1998), p. 301.

12. Rameau, *The Dancing Master*, pp. xiv–xv.
13. Quoted in Kirstein, *Dance*, p. 207.
14. Quoted ibid., p. 208.
15. Quoted in Régine Astier, "Camargo, Marie," *IED*.
16. Parmenia Migel, *The Ballerinas: From the Court of Louis XIV to Pavlova* (New York: Macmillan, 1972), p. 51.
17. Quoted in James R. Anthony, "Opera Ballet and Tragédie Lyrique," *IED*.
18. Noverre, *Letters on Dancing and Ballets*, trans. Cyril W. Beaumont (London: C.W. Beaumont, 1951), p. 59.
19. Noverre, *Letters*, p. 16.
20. Ibid., p. 12.
21. Ibid., p. 73.
22. Ibid., p. 98.
23. Carlo Blasis, *The Code of Terpsichore*, trans. R. Barton (London, 1828; rpt. New York: Dance Horizons, [1976]), p. 88.
24. André Levinson, "The Spirit of the Classic Dance," in *André Levinson on Dance: Writings from Paris in the Twenties*, ed. Joan Acocella and Lynn Garafola (Hanover, N.H.: Wesleyan University Press/UPNE, 1991), p. 47.
25. Théophile Gautier, "Las seguidillas de Andalucía and Las boleras de Cádiz at the Opéra," trans. Ivor Guest, *Dance Chronicle*, 10, no. 1 (1987), p. 31.
26. Quoted in Cyril W. Beaumont, *Complete Book of Ballets* (London: Putnam, 1937), p. 147.
27. Théophile Gautier, "Opera: Return of Fanny Elssler in *La Tempête*," in *Gautier on Dance*, trans. and ed. Ivor Guest (London: Dance Books, 1986), pp. 15–16.
28. Gautier, "Opera: Benefit of Mlles Elssler," ibid., p. 35.
29. Quoted in John V. Chapman, "Jules Janin: Romantic Critic," in *Rethinking the Sylph: New Perspectives on the Romantic Ballet*, ed. Lynn Garafola (Hanover: UPNE/Wesleyan University Press, 1997), p. 232.
30. Ibid., p. 241.
31. Quoted in Beaumont, *Complete Book of Ballets*, pp. 262–263.
32. Quoted ibid., p. 273.
33. Deborah Jowitt, *Time and the Dancing Image* (New York: Morrow, 1988), p. 243.
34. Quoted in Vera M. Krasovskaya, "Petipa, Marius," *IED*.
35. Michel Fokine, *Memoirs of a Ballet Master*, trans. Vitale Fokine, ed. Anatole Chujoy (Boston: Little, Brown, 1961), p. 256.
36. Quoted in Andrea Olmstead, *Juilliard: A History* (Urbana: University of Illinois Press, 1999), p. 203.
37. Michel Fokine, "The New Russian Ballet," *The Times*, 6 July 1914, p. 6.
38. Ibid.
39. Quoted in Lincoln Kirstein, *Nijinsky Dancing* (New York: Knopf, 1975), p. 166. The translation is by Miriam Lassman.

40. Leonid [*sic*] Massine, "On Choreography and a New School of Dancing," *Drama*, 1, no. 3 (Dec. 1919), p. 69.

41. Bronislava Nijinska, "Creation of 'Les Noces,'" trans. and introd. Jean M. Serafetinides and Irina Nijinska, *Dance Magazine*, Dec. 1974, p. 59.

42. Bernard Taper, *Balanchine: A Biography*, rev. ed. (Berkeley: University of California Press, 1996), p. 99.

43. Ibid., p. 100.

44. For a discussion of how this happened, see Beth Genné's "Creating a Canon, Creating the 'Classics,'" *Dance Research*, 18, no. 2 (Winter 2000), pp. 132–162.

45. Jerome Robbins, "The Ballet Puts On Dungarees," *The New York Times Magazine*, 14 Oct. 1945, p. 9.

46. George Balanchine, *By George* (New York: San Marco Press, 1984), p. 8.

47. Nena Couch, "Tharp, Twyla," *IED*.

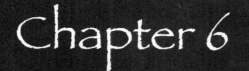

Chapter 6

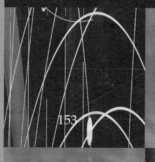

African American Influences on Dance

Social Dances of African Americans

Sally Sommer

One of the most notable aspects of the evolution of American social dance from the late seventeenth century to the end of the twentieth century is the emerging dominance of African American dance styles. During the first two hundred years the development of a recognizable American dance style progressed slowly through a blending of African and European movement and music forms. By the end of the 1890s, however, a distinct pattern unfolded in which dances created in African American communities spread out to the American mainstream, moving from the United States to Europe and eventually to other parts of the world, such as the Charleston in the 1920s and the hiphop/freestyle in the 1970s and '80s. During the twentieth century the process accelerated. Propelled by the aggressive exportation of American movies, television, records, and videos, African American dances spread quickly. And since the early 1980s, with worldwide satellite television broadcasting and the consequent expansion of the music-video industry, a world youth culture has developed. Linked together through CDs and music videos and tuned to the latest move, an adolescent in Paris or Tokyo dances to the same beat as a New York hip-hopper. The styles they are trying to master are decidedly African American, and the teenagers dance more like each other than like their parents.

Although American dance has been fused from many different cultural sources over hundreds of years, the two main traditions of movement and music that shaped the way we move and those of Western Europe and West Africa. In constant flux, American dance encompasses older traditional dances as well as the newest fads, stage dance and street forms, classical African dances, ballet, square dancing, and the most recent club inventions.

Because popular dances are created democratically by thousands of people over a long period of time and are learned through observation and imitation, traditional movements pass and are recycled from one generation to the next. For example, some of the steps used in hip-hop/RAP/freestyle look like updated versions of the fast, slipping footwork of the Charleston, which, in turn, echoes the rapid grinding and crisscrossing steps basic to some of the traditional dances of West Africa. The cycle works the other way as well, and contemporary African social dances recycle and retranslate modes of popular American dances.

Because it is nonverbal, dance information can cross temporal and geographic borders. It slips ethnic boundaries, and it blurs the imaginary lines that separate folk art from fine art, popular dance from classical dance. As a result of this flexibility, original functions and forms get altered, movements get reshaped to fit new situations and contexts. Paradoxically—because body language is learned early and strongly and is a fundamental cultural identifier—dance, the most fugitive of artistic expressions, remains one of the most persistent of all cultural retentions.

Carried in the kinetic memories of African slaves and European immigrants, dances arrived whole or in fragmented forms. Subjected in North America to radically different environmental and cultural mixes as well as the harsh conditions of slavery, dances adapted. Circumventing verbal communication, dance (like music) provided a way for Africans from disparate geographic areas to come together, to move together, to bond together in a strange land. Gradually, over time, an African American style evolved as dances got recreated by those who recalled their dance inheritances whole, those who recalled them only partially, and those of other cultural origins for whom it was not a legacy.

In colonial America the majority of African slaves resided in the middle and southern colonies. The rapid establishment of religious circular dances (grouped under the generic name of "ring shouts") and secular circular dances (called "juba" dances) indicates a probable legacy of compatible movement characteristics shared by the various African groups. These early African Americans also practiced seasonal dances that marked seasonal changes and harvesting and planting times, or dances that celebrated rites of passage such as marriage dances. In addition there seemed to have been a variety of animal dances (probably a fusion of hunting dances and mask-cult or religious dances), and processional dances, used during funeral celebrations.

In the late 1730s slaves were forbidden use of their drums in several colonies, in part because of the 1739 Cato Conspiracy of STONO REBELLION in South Carolina, which led to the subsequent passage of a series of laws forbidding slaves to congregate or to play their big *gombe* drums. Deprived of their larger percussion instruments, the slaves turned to smaller means of percussion. They used their bodies as musical instruments. Previously used in complementary rhythmic accompaniment, these now became dominant: hand clapping and body slapping (also known as "patting" or hamboneing), and rhythmic footwork. Small percussive instruments, such as tambourines and "bones" (the legbones, ribs, or jawbones of animals played with pieces of wood or metal rasps) became widespread. (At times the bones could be fashioned into two fine, thin, long pieces that were held in the hand and played like castanets.) In both the religious ring shout and the secular juba, the feet slid, tapped, chugged, and stamped in rhythmic harmony with antiphonal singing and clapping as the dancers moved around the circle. The juba and the ring shout shared other characteristics, such as moving counterclockwise, with the dancers in the surrounding circle providing musical, movement, and percussive motifs in a call-and-response pattern with a changing leader. In the juba, individual improvisations occurred in the middle of the circle; in the ring shout, individual ecstatic possession occurred among some of the participants. In the juba especially there was a fluid relationship between the improvisers and the surrounding circle of watchers and music makers. Those in the center would dance until exhausted; then others from the circle would move in to take their places.

Colonial slave masters rarely allowed religious dances to be performed openly, so religious dances continued to be practiced clandestinely. At times they merged with other, more secular dances and continued to exist syncretically. Although these new dances retained many characteristics of those from the Old World, they had become their own distinctive dance forms.

Certainly the most powerful changes were caused by the mixing of African and European dance styles. European dance featured an upright posture with head held high and a still torso with no hip rotations. Arms framed the body and—because European dance was usually performed inside, on floors, in shoes—there was careful placement and articulation of the feet. Men and women danced in couples, and in this partnership, body line and placement, as well as couple cooperation, were emphasized over individual movement. In European "figure" dances, floor patterns were valued above personal invention (in "figure" or "set" dances many couples will move together as a group in specific designs, similar to a modem-day Virginia reel or square dance). Music and dance tempos were organized around simple rhythms with regularly stressed beats and syncopations, and musical compositions emphasized melody. The pervasive dynamics of European dancing were control and erectness.

By contrast, African dance "gets down" in a gently crouched position, with bent knees and flexible spine. Traditional African dance tends to be performed in same-sex groups. Danced in bare feet on the bare earth, it favored dragging, sliding, and stamping steps. The supple upper body, with its flexible relationship to the lower limbs, could physically carry many rhythms simultaneously, mirroring the polyrhythms of the music. A polyrhythmic, multi-metered, and highly syncopated percussive dynamic propelled movement and music. Movement often initiated from the pelvis, and pelvis rotations caused a sympathetic undulation in the spine and torso. Animal motions were imitated and quite realistically portrayed on the entire body. Improvisations were appreciated as an integral part of the performance ethos.

These last two qualities would make especially important contributions to the development of African American dance. First, when the dancer imitates the animal's motions fully, habitual patterns of locomotion and gestures are bypassed. Timing and tempos get altered, usual choices are supplanted by fresh movements, fueling the dance vocabulary with new material, expanding the lexicon of motion. For example, "peckin'" (the head thrusts forward and backward like a bird feeding) and "wings" (the arms are flapped like the wings of a great bird, or sharply bent elbows beat quickly) spiced the larger body movements of the Charleston in the 1920s. The monkey and the pony were popular dances of the 1960s, and break dancers of the 1980s did the crab and the spider (see BREAKDANCING). In the early 1990s, the butterfly (the legs open and close like butterfly wings) became a popular dance in REGGAE and dance hall styles.

The emphasis on improvisation advanced the evolution of dance styles. The improviser accomplishes two things simultaneously. While staying within the known stylistic parameters (reinforcing traditional patterns), the improviser is an inventor whose responsibility is to add individual flavor to the movement or timing that updates and personalizes the dance. This keeps social dance perpetually on the edge of change and also helps explain why social dance fads come and go so quickly.

The inevitable exchange between European and African styles led to incorporation and synthesis, and what evolved was neither wholly African nor European but something in between. As they served at the masters' balls, slaves observed the cotillions, square dances, and other "set" or "figure" dances. In turn, European American dances were altered by observation and contact with African American music and dance. Sometimes black musicians played for the white masters' balls. It was also not uncommon on southern plantations for the children of the slaves to play with the masters' children. It was common practice for the masters to go down to the slave quarters to watch slave dances or to have their slaves dance for them on special occasions. At times, slaves engaged in jig dance competitions, where one plantation would pit its best dancers against the best dancers from another. At first, "jig dance" was a generic term that European Americans gave to different types of African American step dances where the feet rhythmically played against the floor, because this fancy footwork resembled the jigs of the British Isles. Informal jig dance contests occurred in northern cities on market days, when freedmen and slaves congregated to dance after the market closed (in Manhattan this happened in the Five Points Catherine Square area), and along the banks of the great transportation river highways, where slaves hired out by their masters worked as stevedores alongside indentured or immigrant workers. In New Orleans, "Congo Square" was designated as the place where slaves could congregate and celebrate in song and dance on Sunday.

The majority of the earlier European colonists came from the British Isles, and within that group were large numbers of poor Irish settlers and Irish indentured servants. More than any other ethnic group, the Irish mixed with African slaves doing heavy labor—the Irish as indentured servants, the Africans as slaves—for the master. Later they lived alongside each other in slums of poverty, so that the mutual influence of Irish step dances like the jig and hornpipe and African step dances was early and strong.

General patterns of fusions suggest the following progression. Between the late 1600s and early 1800s, Africans and African Americans adopted aspects of European dance for their use. For example, they began early to move in male/female couples (mixed couples and body contact in traditional African dance is extremely rare) in

European figure dances, such as quadrilles and reels. However, they retained their own shuffling steps and syncopated movements of feet, limbs, and hips. After the 1820s that trend reversed, as Europeans and European Americans began to copy African American dance styles—a trend still in effect. In general, as the African elements became more formal and diluted, the European elements got looser and more rhythmic. Religious dancing became secular; group dancing gave way to individual couples on the dance floor; and following the rise of urbanization and industrialization and the consequent migration of black workers, rural dances moved to the towns. Since the late 1930s, in reverse, urban dances that became dance crazes spread back to rural communities and out to the world.

The 1890s was the decade that marked the beginning of the *international* influence of African American dance. The cakewalk had been developing since the late 1850s, and by the 1890s was well established as an extremely popular dance in both theatrical and nontheatrical contexts. According to ex-slaves, the cakewalk, with its characteristic highkneed strut walk, probably originated shortly after the mid-1850s. The dance had begun as a parody of the formal comportment and upright posture of the white ballroom dancers as they paraded down the center of the floor, two by two, in the opening figures of a promenade that would have begun the formal balls. The simplicity of this walk made it easy to mimic and exaggerate, it fit easily into the African tradition of satiric song and dance, and the formality of the walk resonated with African processional dances. Apparently the dance had been a "chalkline" dance, where the dancers had to walk a line while balancing containers of water on their heads.

By the 1890s the cakewalk had been adapted as a ballroom dance by the whites, who grafted the high-kneed walking steps with a simple 2/4 or 4/4 rhythm of early RAGTIME jazz and blended it with the promenading steps that were already a central motif in many of the schottisches and gallops popular in the ballrooms of the time. The cakewalk quickly translated to the stage and had been regularly performed in the big African American touring shows since the beginning of the decade, by such troupes as *Black Patti's Troubadours* and in shows like *The South Before the War* and *A Trip to Coontown*, among others. The cakewalk was danced on Broadway by excellent black performers in *Clorindy: The Origin of the Cakewalk* (1898). As well, there were numerous cakewalk competitions done regularly by whites (one of the largest annual events took place at Madison Square Garden in Manhattan). The enormous popularity of the dance is clear from even the most cursory perusal of sheet music from 1890 to 1907. A few exhibition dance teams of African American performers traveled to Europe to perform the dance (the most famous was the husband-and-wife team of Charles JOHNSON and Dora Dean), and in 1904 the cakewalk received the validation of aristocratic society when the Prince of Wales learned the dance from the comedy-and-dance team of African American performers Bert WILLIAMS and George WALKER. The structural framework of the cakewalk had open sections for improvisation that shifted emphasis to the individual's role, changing the focus from the group to the couple and the person. It was the turn of the century, and as the incubator of individual invention, the cakewalk was the perfect artistic catalyst to launch dance into the modernist sensibility of the twentieth century.

A rash of rollicking animal dances gained ascendancy between 1907 and 1914, overlapping the cakewalk and replacing it in the public's favor. The turkey trot, kangaroo hop, and the grizzly bear (three among many) incorporated eccentric animal gestures into the couple-dance format, a blend that had long been practiced by African American dancers—elbows flapped, heads pecked, dancers hopped—in bits of motion that were derived from such African American animal dances as the buzzard lope. The rising popularity of these dances paralleled the rise in sheet music publication. For a small investment, people got music *and* dance instructions, since the song lyrics told how the dance should be done.

A typical example of the instructional song is the well-known ragtime dance ballin' the jack, which developed in about 1910. (The meaning of the title is obscure, but it probably originated from railroad slang, with the general meaning of enjoyable, rollicking good times.) As described in 1913 in its published form by two African American songwriters, Chris Smith and Jim Burris, the dance had the following steps:

First You put your two knees close up tight,
then you sway 'em to the left, then you sway 'em to the right.
Step around the floor kind of nice and light,
then you twis' around and twis' around with all your might.
Stretch your lovin' arms straight out in space,
then you do the eagle rock with style and grace,
swing your foot way 'round, then bring it back,
now that's what I call ballin' the jack.

Between 1900 and 1920 a dance fever gripped America. Since the early 1900s couples had been moving closer together, and with the evolution of the slower, more bluesy early JAZZ styles, close-clutching dances like the slow drag, which had always been done at private parties, began to surface in public places. The hip motions and languid gliding feet in such African American dances as the grind and mooch (both a couple or solo dance) indicate that body contact and postures were already racially shifting. Certainly this prepared the way for the arrival of the tango and its immediate acceptance as a dance craze in 1913. (The tango originated in Argentina. Although its precise origins are quite complex, it was also a likely synthesis of European and African influences.) The tango is a difficult dance to do, necessitating dance lessons, a reality happily exploited by the numerous exhibition tango teams who demonstrated the dance to the eager public, then taught it to them in their studios, or at the local dance hall or tango teas. If few could afford this luxury, thousands of people nevertheless danced what they believed to be the tango. In reality, the frank sensuality of thigh and pelvic contact coincided more readily with familiar close-couple

African American dances of the juke joints, small dance halls, and white- and-tan clubs that peppered mixed neighborhoods of every American city.

By the late 1910s a flood of migrating workers moved northward, seeking jobs in urban industries built for the war effort of WORLD WAR I. As great numbers of African Americans moved into cities, they formed a critical mass of talent that erupted in a variety of artistic expressions. Their energy gave birth to the HARLEM RENAISSANCE of the 1920s and turned Harlem—and black neighborhoods in other industrial cities—into crucibles of creativity in the popular and fine arts. The golden years of black Broadway (1921–1929) began with the hugely successful *Shuffle Along* (1921), written, directed, composed, and choreographed by African Americans (its four major creators were Noble SISSLE, Eubie BLAKE, Flournoy Miller, and Aubrey Lyles). This production, and subsequent road shows, brought African American jazz music and jazz dances to a wide audience. There was little distinction between social dances and stage adaptions, and current popular dances were simply put onstage with few changes. As a result of *Shuffle Along's* popularity, Broadway dance began to re-shape itself, shifting to a jazz mode, as Florenz Ziegfeld and other producer-directors began to copy *Shuffle Along's* choreography. A spate of new studios opened in the Broadway area to teach this African American vernacular jazz dance to professional actors and to an eager public (one important instructor was Buddy BRADLEY, who taught the Astaires and a host of other Broadway and film actors, then went on to choreograph English revues).

Then, with the 1923 Broadway show *Runnin' Wild*, the Charleston burst onstage and into the hearts of the American public, especially through the eponymous song James P. JOHNSON composed for the show. However, the Charleston had been a pop-ular dance among African Americans long before the 1920s. Although its origins are unclear, it probably originated in the South, as its name suggests, then was brought north with the migrating workers. Jazz historian Marshall Stearns reports its existence in about 1904, and the late tap dancer Charles "Honi" COLES said that in about 1916 as a young child he learned a complete version of the dance, which had long been pop-ular in his hometown of Philadelphia.

The Charleston is remarkable for the powerful resurgence of Africanisms in its movements and performance and for shattering the conventions of European partner-ing. The Charleston could be performed as a solo, a couple dance, partners could dance together side by side or in the closed-couple position. For women in particular, its wild movements and devil-may-care attitude broke codes of correct deportment and pro-priety. It was quick and decidedly angular, and the slightly crouched position of the body imparted a quality of alert wildness. The steps (and the early jazz music it was performed to) are syncopated, the knees turn in and out, the feet flick to the side, and a rapid forward-and-backward prancing step alternated with pigeon-toed shuffles and high kicks. As the arms and legs fling in oppositional balance, elbows angled and pumping, the head and hands shake in counterpoint. Knock-kneed, then with legs akimbo, body slightly squatted, this beautiful awkwardness signaled the aesthetic demise of European ideals of symmetry and grace in social dance. The fast-driving rhythms of the music smoothed the flow of broken motions into a witty dance punctuated with shimmies, rubber-legging, sudden stops, and dance elements such as the black bottom, spank the baby, or truckin'. Although these new dances often caused alarm because of their seeming anarchy of motion, and the uncontrolled freedom that that implies, the Charleston in particular roused the ire of the guardians of public morality. Warning that the Charleston would lead to sexual and political dissolution, the dance was condemned by several clerics and was banned in several cities.

Although the Charleston was immediately introduced to Europe by American jazz artists touring there, it was Josephine BAKER (she had been a chorus girl in *Shuffle Along*) who personalized the dance. She went to Paris in 1924 and became the darling of the French, and it was Josephine's charming, humorous, and slightly naughty version of the Charleston that caused such a sensation in Europe. The Charleston, and all the bold young women who performed it, came to symbolize the liberated woman of the twenties, and the rubber-legging "flapper" became an icon of the era.

Then, in 1926, the SAVOY BALLROOM opened in New York City's Harlem. Nicknamed "The Track" or "Home of Happy Feet," the Savoy could accommodate up to four thousand people. Because it had the reputation of being the place to go and hear good music and dance, all the best bands wanted to play there. It was the practice to feature two different bands on the same night, playing one after another on two different bandstands placed at opposite ends of the ballroom. This subsequent "battle of the bands" energized dancers to new heights of daring and improvisation. For thirty years the Savoy would be the center of dance in New York City, and there dances were brought to such a level of excellence that the name "the Savoy" was synonymous with the best in dancing. As its reputation grew, the Savoy also became a showplace, a kind of informal stage arena where people could go to watch the finest Savoy dancers as each tried to outdance the other.

Great dancing is inspired by great music, and the history of African American social dance parallels the history of African American jazz music. In truth these social dances are most accurately described as "vernacular jazz dance" (from the title and subtitle of Marshall and Jean Stearns's magnificent historical study of tap and popular dance, *Jazz Dance: The Story of American Vernacular Dance*). The juke joints of the South and the dance halls of the North served as forums where musicians and dancers worked together. The sharing of ideas, rhythms, and the heated excitement of music and movement feeding each other produced an environment of experimentation where the spirit moved and dances got created on the spot. Certainly the arrival of big-band swing music, fathered by the great jazzmen and their groups, all of whom played the Savoy, parented the next great African American dance as well.

Existing concurrently with the Charleston and evolving from it, a kind of Savoy "hop" was getting formulated on the floor of the Savoy Ballroom. Then, in 1928, the dance was christened "the lindy hop" by a well-known Savoy dancer, Shorty Snowden, in honor of Charles Lindbergh's 1927 solo flight across the Atlantic. The dance, which would become an international craze and an American classic, contained many ingredients of the Charleston—the oppositional flinging of the limbs, the wild, unfettered quality of the movement, the upbeat tempos, the side-by-side dancing of partners. But the two most outstanding characteristics were the "breakaway," when two partners split apart completely or barely held on to each other with one hand, while each cut individual variations on basic steps (a syncopated box step with an accent on the offbeat) and the spectacular aerial lifts and throws that appeared in the mid-1930s. The tradition of individual improvisation was, of course, well entrenched. However, with the lindy hop, it was the climactic moment of dance, and the aerial work set social dance flying. The lindy hop contained ingredients distilled during the evolution of social dance since the 1890s. It had a wide range of expressive qualities, yet it was grounded in steps and rhythms that were simple enough to be picked up readily *and* were capable of infinite variations. It would, in fact, become one of the longest lasting of all African American social dances. Commonly known as the jitterbug in white communities, the dance adapted to any kind of music: There was the mambo lindy, the bebop lindy, and during the 1950s, the lindy/jitterbug changed tempos and syncopations and became known as rock 'n' roll; when looked at carefully, the 1970s' "disco hustle" reveals itself as a highly ornamented lindy hop cut down to half time. In the 1980s and '90s, "country-western swing" looked like the lindy hop framed by fancy armwork, and in the South, "the shag" was another regional variation of the lindy hop theme.

On the floor of Harlem's Savoy Ballroom the lindy hop was brought to its highest level of performance, fueled by the big-band swing played by brilliant musicians in orchestras led by such men as Fletcher HENDERSON, Chick WEBB, Al Cooper, Duke ELLINGTON, Earl HINES, Cab CALLOWAY, Count BASIE, Billy ECKSTINE, Benny Goodman, and many more. As the dynamics of swing music heated up to its full musical sound and fast, driving, propulsive "swing" beat, the dancers matched it with ever more athletic prowess. In the mid-1930s the lindy took to the air, and using steps with names such as the hip to hip, the side flip, the snatch, over the back, and over the top, the men tossed the women, throwing them around their bodies, over their heads, and pulling them through their legs until the women seemed to fly, skid-land, then rebound again.

The Savoy lindy hop was renowned for its spectacular speed and aerials. An entrepreneurial bouncer at the club, Herbert White, decided to capitalize on this dancing talent, and he formed "Whitey's Lindy Hoppers." Choosing a large group of lindy hop dancers, the best from the ballroom, White split them into smaller troupes or teams that toured the country, appearing in movies, vaudeville, on Broadway, at the 1939 World's Fair in New York City, and in many other venues. The lindy spread out to the world, first through newsreels and films, and then the dance was carried personally to Europe and Asia by American GIs during the 1940s.

As the language of jazz moved from swing to be-bop, rhythmically more complex and harmonically daring, so did the nature of jazz dance. With the passing of the great dance halls, the smaller venues that featured the five- or six-piece jazz combo that was the basic form of bebop became the main site for jazz performance, and though many of these clubs had no space for dancing, bebop-influenced jazz dance nonetheless flourished.

Bebop jazz often sounded barely in control with its fast pace and solo improvisations, and bebop dancers mirrored the music. The at times private, introverted quality of musical performance was reflected by the bebop dancer's performance, which appeared disassociated and inward. Rather than having the movement scattering outward, as in the Charleston and the lindy, the bebop dancers used footwork that slipped and slid but basically stayed in place, the dynamic of the dance was introverted and personal, and the dancer appeared to gather energy into the center of the body.

Like the music, the dance was dominated by males. And if the bebopper used many of the same steps as the lindy hopper, there were enormous stylistic differences in the focus and body language. Bebop was almost the reverse of the lindy: partners broke away for longer periods of time than they spent together. Bebop dance could be done as a solo, in a couple, or in a small group of three or four. This open relationship was perfect for a dance that placed the strongest significance on individual improvisation and devalued group cooperation. The body rode cool and laid-back on top of busy feet that kept switching dynamics, tempo, flow, timing, direction, impulse, and emphasis. Off-balance and asymmetrical, the dance wobbled at the edge of stability. The dance was filled with slips and rapid splits that broke down to the floor and rebounded right back up, and the bebopper was fond of quick skating-hopping steps that appear to be running very fast while remaining in the same place. Elbows pulled into the body, shoulders hitched up, hands lightly paddled the air. Balanced on a small base—the feet remained rather close together—with swiveling body and hips, the dancer seemed made of rubber. Partners rarely touched each other or looked directly at each other. Bebop dancing influenced the dance styles of rhythm and blues and other black popular music of the 1940s. It is also known as "scat" dancing (the comparison is to the vocal freeflights of the scat singer). James BROWN is perhaps the best-known entertainer who dances in bebop mode. Watered down and simplified to rapidly rocking heel-and-toe steps that alternated with pigeon-toed motions in and out, with the occasional splits, bebop lost most of its glittering individualism when translated to the mainstream. Yet the effect of bebop dance was to give the social dancer a new "cool" persona, that of the "hipster," whose sensual slipperiness provided a rest, a contrast, to the heat and speed of the jitterbug lindy. This hip attitude had an enormous effect on Broadway jazz. Bob Fosse, Jerome Robbins, and Jack Cole, three powerful Broadway and film choreographers, would convert the physical language of bebop dance into a style of laid-back, cool jazz that would be viewed as epitomizing the best of Broadway jazz dance.

During the 1950s, with the explosion of a "teen culture" and a "teen market," an entertainment industry, led by the record companies, was established to service this market. Bepop dance influenced the dance styles of rock 'n' roll. The record industry, ever quick to seize an opportunity, made the crossover, renaming RHYTHM AND

BLUES rock 'n' roll. The jitterbug got renamed as well, now called by the music's name of rock 'n' roll dance. Partners continued to split apart. With the infusion of the bebop mentality, a slippery smoothness in the footwork calmed down some of the flinging of the older forms of jitterbug, while the twisting hips were beginning to even out the sharp bouncing of the fast-paced Savoy style. Toward the end off the 1950s, gyrating hips (the trademark of Elvis Presley), previously only one movement phrase in the midst of many, would be singled out and made into an individual dance. "The twist," which became another worldwide dance fad, structured an entire dance around a single movement. Its simplicity made it easy to do, and its virtues were promoted in Chubby Checker's beguiling rock 'n' roll song "The Twist" (1960, a close copy of Hank Ballard's 1958 original). Also in the 1950s there was a resurgence of close-clutching couple dances, similar to the older mooch and grind (now known as "dirty dancing"), danced to sweet harmonics of five-part *a cappella* singing groups who were developing a singing style that became known as doo-wop. It is notable and interesting that in the 1950s, during a period when there was a strong sense of conformity, group line dances such as the stroll and the madison became popular.

During the 1960s, the civil rights movement was reflected in a re-Africanization of dance forms in such dances as the Watusi, the monkey, the bugaloo, and a series of spinewhipping, African-inspired dances such as the frug and the jerk. Animal gestures and steps reentered dances with a vengeance, formulated into dances such as the pony, the chicken, and the fish (also known as the swim). Partners did not touch. Instead, they danced face-to-face, but apart, reflecting each other's movements, using a dialogue of movement that was essentially a call-and-response mode of performance.

MOTOWN singing groups whose carefully tailored and tasty dance routines were choreographed by Cholly ATKINs had an inestimable effect on dance styles. The teenagers who admired these groups and bought their records now watched them perform on television. Then they copied the Motown style, whose choreography was made to underline the message of the song. A variety of pantomimic dances was created in which the words, or story line, of the song were enacted by the dancers. For example, one of the most popular and beautiful of these tunes was Marvin GAYE's "Hitchhiker" (Atkins worked with Gaye on this tune). The major gesture-motif of this dance recurred as the dancer—feet doing little prancing steps, hips swiveling, head bobbing—circled the hand in front of the torso, then swung it off to the side, thumb stuck up, as if he or she were trying to hitch a ride on the road, watching the cars go by.

The 1970s disco explosion featured the hustle (if one strips away the ornamentation of multiple turns and sharply pointing arms and poses as the man swings out his partner, the lindy hop becomes visible). The line dance made popular by the movie *Saturday Night Fever* (1976) is actually the old madison, retooled for the 1970s (the same is true for the 1980s' bus stop and the 1990s' electric slide). However, with the explosion of breaking and electric boogie in the Bronx during the late 1970s, and popping in Sacramento and Los Angeles, dance styles underwent a radical change in the United

States, then in Europe, Asia, and Africa as the styles spread to the world on television and music videos.

Breakdancing was part of a larger cultural movement known as hip-hop, which got established in the South Bronx neighborhood of New York City. Hip-hop had a variety of artistic expressions—graphic arts (graffiti or "writing"), spoken poetry (rapping), music (scratchin', which developed into the rap music of the 1980s and '90s), religion and philosophy (Zulu Nation and the politics put forth in the lyrics of the rap), and dance (breaking, electric boogie, and popping and/or locking). Breakdancing took the structural principle of the breakaway and expanded it into a solo dance form. Accompanying the breakdancers musically were street DJs who were using the techniques of scratchin' (holding the record by its edge, the DJ moves it back and forth on the same groove) and mixing (shifting back and forth between turntables, the DJ replays the same sound bits of a couple of records over and over) to create new syncopations and "breaks" in the old records, thereby improvisationally composing new musical scores. Then, using one or more microphones, rappers would talk rhythmically over the music.

Intensely competitive, breaking was primarily a solo, male dance form that re-Africanized the aesthetics of African American dance. Visually it retains powerful reverberations of gestures and phrases derived from capoeria, the martial-art dance that came to the New World with the slaves captured in the Angola region of southwestern Africa.

Breaking stressed acrobatic fluency in the spins and in the dancer's buoyancy. In fact, bouncing is one of its most obvious characteristics. Performers effortlessly spring from dancing on their feet in an "up-rock" style to "breaking" down to twirl on the floor; then they rebound to an upright position. There is little distinction between up and down, and because the breaker moves within a circle, the focus is multidirectional, as a consequence of its bounding-rebounding quality. Breaking seems to defy gravity, to exist almost at the edge of flight.

Popping and locking are other hip-hop dance styles that were performed along with breaking and were developed first on the West Coast. In these styles the body seems to be broken into segments. As motion moved from the fingers of the left arm through the chest and out the fingers of the right arm, the joints "locked" or "popped" into sharp millisecond freezes. The movement looks as if it were a living rendition of a video game, and popping and locking did evolve from an earlier dance known as the robot. A related but more undulating version of popping and locking, called the electric boogie, developed on the East Coast; in this dance the body seemed to move in fluid, increasingly complex minifreezes.

Breaking was the dance of the young and tough hip-hop subcultures of the ghettos, and the rawness of the sounds and the movements made breaking the dance of protest that rallied against the mainstream disco styles of music and movement. Because of its brilliance, its technical display, its physical virtuosity, and its machismo, and because breaking got immediate and near-hysterical media coverage, it became popular worldwide. Breakers sprung up in Tokyo, Rome, Calcutta, Rio de Janeiro, and Paris, and long after it had faded in popularity in the United States (in about 1984), it was still flourishing in the 1990s in other parts of the world. Breaking was the most powerful and early expression of the hip-hop culture, and because of its worldwide success, it prepared the way for the eventual ascendancy of rap, which deemphasized the dancer for the rapper and was the centerpiece of the hip-hop movement of the 1980s and early 1990s.

In the late 1980s and '90s, the young adults who are creating the current social dances do little that is reminiscent of traditional European dance and much that is re-flective of the ancient African legacy. On the dance floor they gather in casual circles that randomly arise, then disintegrate. Male/female partnerships, if they exist at all, change and shift throughout the night, and a partner is simply another dancer who is focused upon for a while. Dancers move in loose groupings that may or may not mix genders (males often dance together, or there will be a group of females dancing). Though they move in stylistic harmony, improvisation is highly prized, and each par-ticipant brings individual flavor to the movements.

There are many reverberations with traditional African motion. The body is slightly crouched with bent knees, feet flat on the floor. The footwork favors sliding, stamping, or digging steps. When the music is hard-hitting and fast, dancers burst out in vigorous jumps and athletic maneuvers; a phrase may consist of diving down to the floor ("breaking" down) in belly slides or shoulder rolls, then smoothly pulling the body up-right, swinging back into the beat with fast, sliding steps. Digitalized and engineered, the African drum has been transformed into a sonic bass boom that blasts through the speakers. With volume turned up to the "red zone," the bass power pops the body, vi-brating bones, internalizing the beat. The dancers use their torsos as as multiunit in-strument with an undulating spine, shimmying shoulders, and swiveling hips. Movement is poly-rhythmic, and ripples through the body in waves, or it can lead to very briefly held positions known as freezes. Heads circle and bob, arms do not frame the body so much as help it balance. Dances are named for the style of music that is played, such as house, rap, hip-hop or dance hall, or they are called "freestyle" because each dancer improvisationally combines well-known steps as the fancy strikes.

A prime example of an Africanized dance was one performed to Chuck Brown's "The Butt," which hit the top of the commercial pop charts in 1988 and was notable for its bold call-and-response structure. As the title suggests, movement concentrated on shaking buttocks. Dancers "get down" in a deep squat. Placing hands on butts or thighs, they arch their spines, nod their heads, and swivel the pelvis in figure eights. In the early 1990s, this same dance remained popular. It was now called "winding," performed by young, urban, black, and white club goers to reggae or go-go (a Washington, D.C., musical style influenced by Jamaican reggae). "Winding" alludes to the circular winding motion of the hips. In 1901 the same moves were called "the funky butt," and in the 1930s they were known as "grinding."

African American underground club dancers continue to create new dances that will be picked up by the mainstream tomorrow, disseminated through music videos. All musicvideo dance styles originate in the clubs and on the streets, so one must look at the places of origination to get a glimpse into the dance styles of tomorrow.

Club dancers, mostly African American and Latino youth, are the most active, influential, and democratic of the social dance choreographers. The club community is a specialized one, which has coalesced around an action rather than a neighborhood or through bloodlines. Relationships are made because of a shared obsession with dancing. Perhaps the distinguishing characteristic of a real "clubhead" is that dance is passion and possession, and through movement, they experience "going off," a kind of secular spirituality that echoes the spiritual possession of the older African circle dances brought to this country four hundred years ago.

Music is provided by DJs mixing at their consoles with a couple of turntables, merging the sounds of one record into another in a seamless musical flow, composing on the spot. They are musicians of consoles and amplifiers; they are today's bands and orchestras and conductors. Using raw recorded "cuts" that have not been engineered into their final form (this is not the stuff of commercial radio), DJs are the high priests of the clubs who regulate the emotional and physical heat of the dancing. A good DJ knows how to play the songs that inspire movement. He shifts the mood and pace through musical combinations, acting and reacting to what he sees on the floor. Reading ephemeral signals of movement and energy, breath and beat, a constant flow of information is exchanged between dancer and DJ.

In the early 1990s, dance styles fall into rough generational divisions. Hip-hop *tends* to be done by the younger generation of early through late teens, while lofting (this style of dance is called different names in different parts of the country) and house tend to be done by a slightly older group in their late teens and twenties. Lofting is a softer assimilation of the "old school" breaking, whose immediate predecessors are the lindy hop, and whose older progenitors are the capoeria and other African acrobatic dances. The "New Jack" style of hip-hop uses footwork reminiscent of the Charleston and earlier West African step dances. The pose and punch and stylized gestures of voguing exaggerate the syncopated isolations of jazz, and like the cakewalk, voguing makes satiric commentaries on the mannered postures of the monied classes, as represented in the images of models of high-fashion magazines.

Social dance is a structure of movement that is always open to modification. Propelled by improvisational innovation, dancers can transform a recreational participatory event into a performance within a circle. Perhaps the greatest African aesthetic gift was the reverence for improvisation. It keeps social dance democratic, it is not tied to any one institution or controlled by a small elite group who determine who shall perform and who shall observe. Improvisation and individuals keep dance a celebration of imagination, while the flexibility and power of movement itself is what links the past to the present and the community to the person.

References

Brandman, Russella. *The Evolution of Jazz Dance from Folk Origins to Concert Stage.* Ph.D. diss., Florida State University, 1977.

Emery, Lynne F. *Black Dance in the United States from 1619 to 1970.* 1972. Reprint. Brooklyn, N.Y., 1980.

Frank, Arthur H. *Social Dance.* London, 1963.

Gorer, Geoffrey. *Africa Dances.* London, 1949.

"Jazz Dance, Mambo Dance." *Jazz Review* (November 1958).

"New Orleans Marching Bands: Choreographer's Delight." *Dance* (January 1958).

"Popular Dance in Black America." *Dance Research journal* 15, no. 2 (Spring 1983). Special issue.

Stearns, Marshall, and Jean. *Jazz Dance: The Story of American Vernacular Dance.* New York, 1968.

Wittke, Carl. *Tambo and Bones.* Durham, N.C., 1930.

Yarborough, Camille. "Black Dance in America: The Deep Root and the Strong Branch." *Black Collegian* (April–May 1981): 10–24.

_____. "Black Dance in America: The Old Seed." *Black Collegian* (October–November 1980): 46–53.

The Home-Grown American Dance Forms— Jazz and Tap Dancing

Katita Milazzo

Jazz dance is the most visible of dance forms in the United States, yet most Americans would be hard pressed to accurately describe it. Moreover, it does not seem to have much in common with present-day jazz music. Jazz music is usually syncopated and improvisational. Jazz musicians take a set melody line and play with it in endless imaginative ways. Conversely, most jazz dance we see now on the stage and especially on television is very set and rigid in its choreography and usually emphasizes the downbeat of the music. Another problem with identifying jazz dance is that it is constantly changing. About every twenty years, it has an entirely new look. During its history it has covered a range of dance fashions and throughout its existence has garnered vague descriptions such as a "feeling"[1] or it "is likely to call up a mental snapshot of the jitterbug."[2] Further complicating the identification issue is that there are different styles of jazz dance, such as lyrical jazz, Broadway style, funk, and modern jazz. Each era has reinvented jazz dancing, dating from the time of the Charleston in the 1920s through modern jazz in the 1950s, up to the newer forms such as hip-hop. In truth, it is these continually shifting trends that make it current, accessible, and so popular. But what exactly is it?

It is known that jazz dance evolved from tap dance. Although they were not called jazz then, early jazz steps were the movements between the audible tap steps or they were the same steps as tap without the sound. One would think, therefore, that tap dance would be easier to identify because of the metal plates on the bottoms of the shoes that amplify the percussive sounds, but even those are not a given. One of the greatest tappers of all time, Bill "Bojangles" Robinson, danced in shoes with wooden soles. Tap does seem to have more in common with jazz music than jazz dance because of its musicality, syncopation, and improvisation, but yet it is called tap dance. Furthermore, tap, like jazz, is diversified and cannot be pinned down to one style. There are different schools such as jazz tap, Broadway tap, and rhythm tap. However, both jazz and tap, in whatever reembodiment, are driven by a percussive, rhythmic force. Rhythm is integral, essential—whether it is self-induced with sounds made by tapping feet or slapping, clapping hands, or propelled by the pulsating beats played by musicians. Indeed, these are the attributes that make tap and jazz very accessible and easy to enjoy. It does not take long before the pounding of drums and percussive reverberations become irresistible and contagious, compelling us to join the beat with our bodies and with our souls.

Jazz and tap dancing were born in the Americas. They are the only two theatrical dance forms that people of the United States can truly claim as their own. Furthermore, these rhythmic, exciting styles of dancing have since spread throughout the entire world. Although the family tree of tap and jazz can be traced to multiple roots, it must be mentioned that if it were not for the contributions of Africans with their rhythms, style, attitudes, and aesthetics, the only indigenous dances in the Americas would belong to the Native Americans.

For Africans[3], dance is not entertainment, nor is it art. It is life. It may celebrate life and its cycles or it might ask for protection and prosperity. It might be educational, teaching social norms, or it might be in honor of the ancestors, asking for their intervention or their blessing. For the Africans torn asunder from all of their possessions, their ancestors, and their homes, dance and music were the two things they carried with them. The entire slave trade—from the capture, through the horrific Middle Passage, through the humiliation of the sale—is one of the lowest points in American history. That the Africans held on to some vestiges of their heritage through all of this heartache is astounding. That their American legacy evidenced in music and dance would one day become the most imitated on the planet is perhaps some sort of poetic justice.

The African aesthetic has become the keystone of American vernacular dance, and several identifiable attributes encapsulate this dance form. One of the first and foremost scholars to delineate these characteristics was Robert Farris Thompson in his 1974 book, *African Art in Motion*. Brenda Dixon Gottschild has distilled them into several points. Some of these are:

1. Ephebism or the youthful power, vitality, and attack that is apparent not only in dance, but can be identified in music, clothing, and lifestyle.
2. The simultaneous suspension and preservation of the beat that can be observed in syncopation. The dominance of percussion is integral in African as well as African American music and dance and cannot be overemphasized.
3. The get-down quality. Gottschild describes this as the "descending direction in melody, sculpture, gesture, and dance. 'Getting down' is a metaphorical, honorific attribute and is not to be interpreted solely as the physical stance of groundedness."[4]
4. Multiple meter or polyrhythms—more than one rhythm occurring simultaneously. Musicians can create tension and excitement by playing several rhythms at the same time. Dancers can articulate some of these rhythms in different

parts of the body, especially by isolating body parts, but it is very important that the beat is visually clear.

5. Looking smart refers to the brilliance, flair, virtuosity, or even showing off displayed in clothing, hairstyles, and movements.
6. Correctness in entrance and exit or being aware that the beat does not dissipate either in the beginning or the end of a dance.
7. Call and response. This attribute can also be thought of as question and answer. One dancer makes a statement rhythmically, and a second dancer takes that same phrase and either repeats it or embellishes it. This same sort of "conversation" can occur between dancers and musicians or one dancer and a group of participants.
8. Coolness. Thompson considers this to be "an all-embracing, positive attribute which combines notions of composure, silence, vitality, healing and social purification."[5]

As such, these selected attributes are in actuality basic components of American culture not only in dance, but also in styles of dress, modes of flirtation, hairstyles, speech patterns, and in other aspects of our lifestyles. Yet, as Gottschild notes, these enriching gifts are frequently the object of defamation in our ongoing process of homogeneity and segregation. Time and time again, African American choreographers have not been credited for their work. Jazz and tap dancing have, in their history, frequently been denigrated as lesser types of dance compared to concert dance forms. Yet as mentioned, these characteristics have been widely copied and distilled not only in those concert forms, but in popular culture throughout the world.

The History

One of the first African American dances to gain worldwide notoriety was invented during the slave era. The cakewalk, as mentioned in the Sally Sommer chapter, was one of the early dances to come from southern plantations and become a staple in most black variety shows. Curiously, it also was broadly imitated by white dancers. This dance was originally a parody of pretentious white manners. The dancers, costumed in Sunday dress clothes, executed such steps as strutting in parade-like patterns that generally mocked white masters. Apparently, whoever danced the best won a cake.

Competition was encouraged by plantation owners and was accompanied by percussive elements as simple as clapping when the drums were banned. Winning dancers would subsequently compete against those from other plantations. Besides the cakewalk, another popular challenge dance was the jig. This dance was essentially an early form of tap dance in that it incorporated audible footwork, but the legwork seems to have been more frenzied. Evidently, a slave by the name of Tom in Palestine,

Texas, was an expert jigger. His master was so sure of Tom's abilities that he built a platform and invited slaves from all around to compete. An eyewitness recounts the event:

> I must tell you 'bout the best contest we ever had. One nigger on our place was de jigginest fellow ever was. Everyone round tries to git some body to best him. He could put de glass of water on his head make his feet go like trip hammers and sound like de snaredrum. He could whirl round and sich, all de movement from his hips down. Now it gits noised round a fellow been found to beat Tom and a contest arm 'ranged for Saturday evening'. There was a big crowd and money am bet, but master bets on Tom, of course.
>
> So dey start jiggin'. Tom starts easy and little faster and faster. The other fellow doin' de same. Dey gits faster and faster and dat crowd am a-yellin'. Gosh! There am 'citement. Dey jus' keep a gwine. It look like Tome done found his match, but there am one thing yet he ain't done—he ain't made the whirl. Now he does it. Everyone holds he breath, and de other fellow starts to make de whirl and he makes it, but jus' a spoonful of water sloughs out his cup, so Tom am de winner.[6]

The term *jig* comes from the Irish folk dance. Today modern tap dancers consider the use of the word "jigging" to be old-fashioned and humiliating.[7] Nonetheless, some steps used then are recognizable today in tap, such as the shuffle (a slapping movement made with the ball of the foot) and the buck and wing (flat-footed heelwork with waving arms). During the slave era these dances were primarily only seen on an amateur level.

Minstrelsy

Blacks had been ridiculed in the legitimate theater both here and in Europe, or if they did perform, it was under the guise of nonsensical comedy. In 1794 when the Revolutionary War was over and Mexico still owned most of the southwestern United States, one of the first black performers, by the name of William Nesbet, appeared in Balltimore. There was no mention in the newspapers if Mr. Nesbet was a slave or a free man. His specialty was "while dancing a slackwise hornpipe, 'he will fold his arms on his breast, and clap one of his legs on his knee.' Another Nesbet specialty was his 'SPANISH FANDANGO, BLIND-FOLDED, over FIFTEEN EGGS, and break none.'"[8] Like the cakewalk, this farcical version of a Spanish dance was not left to the black performer for long. By August 20, 1796, there was a listing in the *New Hampshire Gazette* announcing that one Don Pedro Cloris, the principal performer in Donegan's Company, who exhibited some years previously to great applause, would, on the Monday next August 22, be dancing "the Spanish Fandango, blindfolded, over thirteen eggs, placed in different situations, and imitating the drunkard, stagger amongst them, without breaking."[9]

Such was the attitude toward the Afro-American performer when T. D. Rice came on the scene. Thomas Dartmouth Rice, a white man, created the character of Jim Crow

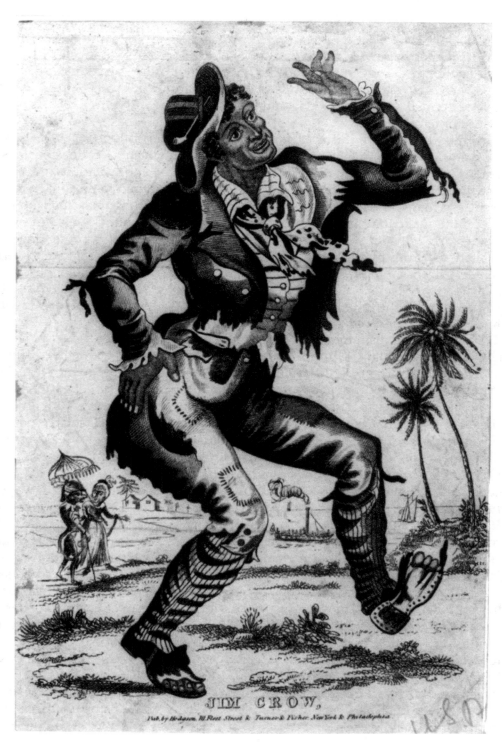

T.D. Rice as Jim Crow.

around 1820 after he saw a lame black man singing and dancing. Rice presented his characterization by exaggerating and distorting the postures and dance of the old, crippled Mr. Crow, making it ludicrous in order to capture audience appeal. Furthermore, Rice donned a curly black wig and painted his face with burnt cork, becoming the first actor in minstrelsy.

Minstrelsy began with this mocking, derisive characterization. T. D. Rice was the first of many white actors who imitated the African American. Certain scholars such as Brenda Gottschild question whether these actors were doing imitations or were creating their own biased interpretations of what they considered to be a black person. Nevertheless, many followed, blackening their faces and circling their lips with red or white paint to make their mouths twice the normal size. From the 1820s through the Civil War, early minstrel shows traveled all over the United States, presenting white interpretations of this hybrid African American dancing. But at the same time, certain African Americans were raising the bar on this new American vernacular dance.

William Henry Lane was born a free man. He took the stage name of Master Juba from a dance called the Juba, which came from Africa to the West Indies and involved rhythmic stamping and clapping. In 1845 Master Juba was recognized as the greatest of all dancers[10] and was famous for his "jigging." He was challenged to a "jigging" duel by Master Diamond, a white minstrel performer. Master Juba won the distinctive title of "King of All Dancers" after an arduous contest. He subsequently headlined white minstrel shows touring in the States and in Europe, finishing in London in 1848, where he died a few years later. A critic in London was much impressed with Lane's dancing and noted that he had never witnessed such mobility, elasticity, footwork, grace, vigor, and endurance.[11] Juba's feet twinkled and he could tie his legs into knots and fling them about recklessly. Master Juba's dancing contained new elements not readily apparent in other Afro-American dances at his time.

Lane grew up in an area of New York that was divided almost equally between Irish and African Americans in the mid-nineteenth century. He was described as a "jig" dancer at a time when the word was changing in meaning—from an Irish folk dance to a term used to describe the general style of black dancing. Lane's popularity and abilities probably hastened this change and, as such, he has been identified as the originator of tap dance. The Irish influence on the development of tap can be seen in the leg movements; the African inspiration can be found in the rhythmic syncopation of the feet and the body movements. Other influences identified in tap dancing include the reel, clogging, and the hornpipe. William Henry Lane has been recognized as the most influential single performer of nineteenth-century American dance, and the repertoire of any current tap dancer today contains elements that he established theatrically.[12]

After the Civil War, freed black slaves took to the stage to perform theAfrican American dances that had been mostly performed by white actors in the minstrel shows. Unfortunately, in order to continue to be marketable in the American capitalistic society, they, too, had to don the blackface and assume the ridiculous characters that had been codified by their white predecessors. They had to play black men imitating white men who were imitating (or doing their biased interpretations) of black men. Many stereotypes were developed on the minstrel stage: the happy, funny, shuffling, lazy Jim Crow character; the childish and irresponsible but loyal and contented singing and dancing slave; and the freed Negro whose prototype was a character by the name of Zip Coon. This third character was the town Negro: the gaudily dressed, shifty, smart-talking dandy of the streets, with ruffled shirt, gold watch chain, and patent leather shoes.[13] Minstrelsy was to maintain a solid presence on the stage into the twentieth century. Sadly, vestiges of the caricaturizing of the black performer in demeaning roles can still be seen today. Fortunately, most black actors today are more respectable and continue to put out remarkable work.

Vaudeville to Broadway

Many black performers continued to find work in show business throughout the latter part of the nineteenth century. They performed a style of dancing that was based on a patchwork of folk material, such as shuffles, struts, hops, twists, grinds, and buck and wing, and became the new vernacular dancing of America. By the early twentieth century, the range of performing opportunities for the black performer expanded with medicine shows, gillies, carnivals, and circuses, as minstrelsy began to wane. Black vaudeville even had its own chain of theaters. By the middle 1910s an organization called the Theatre Owners' Booking Association (TOBA) was formed, which organized venues open to black performers. The TOBA circuit was prevalent throughout the South and penetrated several northern cities as well. Typically three shows were given nightly, each about forty-five minutes long. They featured jazz bands, actors in blackface, and set. It was a hotbed for the development of home-grown dancing. Two characteristics inherent in African dance and music were carried on: continual improvisation and propulsive rhythms. These qualities became the hallmarks of American jazz and tap.

One of the most important incubators of dancing talent for black shows on the TOBA circuit was the Whitman Sisters troupe. This group began performing around 1900 and continued until 1943. Beginning at their father's church in Kentucky, the sisters would raise money for benefits by singing and dancing. One of the two older siblings, Mabel, began managing the family and booking them throughout the South. For a while, white shows had been hiring young, black children who sang and danced, thus adding a "cute" factor to increase sales. These children were known as *picks* or *pickaninnies*. This is where this derogatory term originated. Taking a cue from the white acts, the Whitman Sisters began to book youngsters to fill out their roster. Even though they publicity stated that these children were homeless or orphans to create sympathy and build audiences, the Whitmans were a class act and parents knew their children would be safe touring with them. While on the road, the children were educated in religion, academics, and show business. The size of the troupe would fluctuate between twenty and thirty performers,[14] so many future dancers moved through the company. In their day the Whitman Sisters were the highest-paid act on the TOBA circuit; they were royalty of black vaudeville. They also were strong believers in quality dancing, which would pave the way for what was coming on Broadway.

TOBA outlasted white vaudeville, maintaining vigor until the 1930s. New dances created by the stars of these shows included the Black Bottom, in which the dancer spun on his rear end on the floor; the soft shoe, in which a dancer scraped his/her feet rhythmically in sand strewn on the stage, thus creating a "sshh" sound; and a lot of what was called *eccentric* dancing. "The term 'eccentric' is a catchall for dancers who have their own non-standard movements and sell themselves on their individual styles."[15] This covered a large range of dances, such as Buzzin' Barton's Buzz dance, where he executed long, sliding steps forward, knees bent and arms flung out to the sides with hands turned down and fingers vibrating in an imitation of a bee's wings.[16] Rubberlegs Williams combined "legomania" with high kicks, wiggles, and shimmies, and with steps such as the Boogie Woogie and the Camel Walk. Flash dancers offered their audiences acrobatic and other tricks. The Shake dance was a mixture of belly dance and the Afro-American Grind and has since risen in popularity several times since its creation in the early 1900s.

One of the most renowned eccentric dancers was Earl "Snake Hips" Tucker, who arrived in New York in the 1920s. His act was mesmerizing, and for its sheer theatricality would probably be popular today.

> When Snake Hips slithered on stage, the audience quieted down immediately. Nobody snickered at him, in spite of the mounting tension, no matter how nervous or embarrassed one might be. The glaring eyes burning in the pock-marked face looked directly at and through the audience, with dreamy and impartial hostility. Snake Hips seemed to be coiled, ready to strike.
>
> . . . He came slipping on with a sliding, forward step and just a hint of hip movement. . . . Using shock tactics, he then went directly into the basic Snake Hips movements, which he paced superbly, staring out innocently enough, . . .
>
> Gradually, however, as the shining buckle threw rays in larger circles, the fact that the pelvis and the whole torso were becoming increasingly involved in the movement was unavoidably clear. As he progressed, Tucker's footwork became flatter, rooted more firmly to the floor, while his hips described wider and wider circles, until he seemed to be throwing his hips alternately out of joint to the melodic accents of the music. . . .
>
> The next movement was known among dancers as the Belly Roll, and consisted of a series of waves rolling from pelvis to chest—a standard part of a Shake dancer's routine, which Tucker varied by coming to a stop, transfixing the audience with a baleful, hypnotic stare, and twirling his long tassel in time with the music.[17]

Tucker staggered and shocked his Broadway audience when he appeared in the production of *Blackbirds of 1928*. Another dancer who leapt to fame doing a riveting dance tapping on a set of stairs in this show was fifty-year-old Bill Robinson, better known as Mr. Bojangles. Robinson, like William Henry Lane, did much to expand and popularize tap dance. Although Robinson was "discovered" in the 1928 Broadway show, he had been performing for a long time. He was born in 1878 in Richmond, Virginia, and began his career as a pick for fifty cents a night. Robinson moved to New York in 1898 and worked in the Bowery and at various restaurants in Coney Island. He then became one of the few black performers on the white vaudeville circuit and, at his peak, was making $6,500 a week. After *Blackbirds* he moved to Hollywood, where he starred in several films including the 1935 movie *The Little Colonel* with Shirley Temple, in which he re-created his famous stair dance. Cholly Atkins, who will be discussed later in this chapter, knew Bojangles well. Atkins had this to say:

> Uncle Bo really knew how to mesmerize people with his feet. Being on stage with him was like going to school every night, because he had so much style and finesse. And you just can't imagine how many different ways he could engage an audience. That was one of the greatest experiences of my career. In fact, I often think about how much I learned from watching the master work. Years later, when I was choreographing a dance in honor of him with some of the buck dancers, I could contribute a lot because I knew exactly how he moved.[18]

Tap, up to this point, had been danced flatfooted with the weight primarily over the heels. Robinson's contribution to tap was that he brought it up on the toes, dancing upright and swinging. Clogging and jigging had also been danced on the balls of the feet, but they did not swing. Robinson made tap light and fleetfooted. He was the epitome of the African aesthetic of cool. Bill "Bojangles" Robinson's act and persona exuded nothing if not class. His favorite phrase was "Everything is copasetic," and he did much to further the dignity of the African American performer.

Blackbirds of 1928 was not the first show to feature black acts on Broadway. *Shuffle Along* premiered in 1921 and was a huge box office success. It pioneered theatrical jazz dancing and it introduced a chorus girl who would soon bring Afro-American jazz dance to Paris—Josephine Baker. *Runnin' Wild* in 1923 brought extensive exposure to the Charleston. The Charleston, as Sally Sommer stated, was a social dance that probably originated in Charleston in the early 1900s, but it took over twenty years to be discovered by white dancers.

After the Civil War blacks expanded the social dances enjoyed in the honky-tonks and juke joints in black communities. These venues were social clubs frequented by the newly free African Americans, places where they could relax with their music and dance. Without the constraints of white masters or theatrical entrepreneurs, the African American vernacular dance exploded with innovative movements that were to leave a profound mark on American theatre. Furthermore, these clubs became the training ground for dancers in minstrel, carnival, and other early theatrical venues.

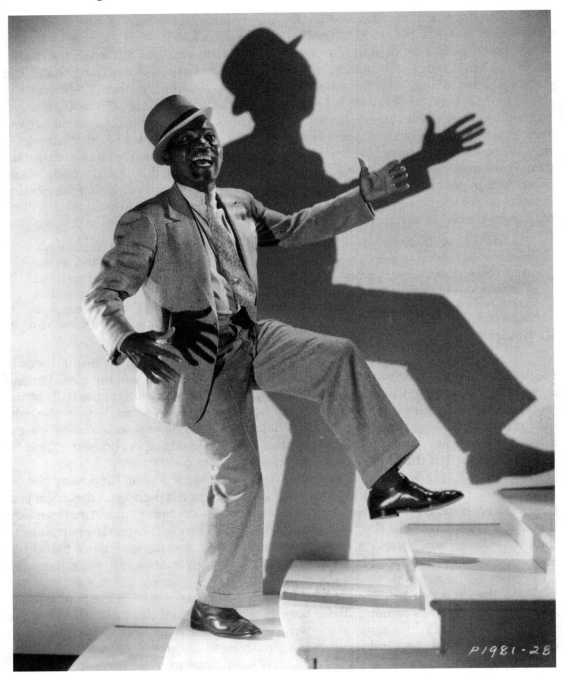

Bill "Bojangles" Robinson.

These dancers were talented at picking up steps and knew how to hold their audiences, but usually they had no formal training as we know it. It was out of this milieu that theatrical tap and jazz dance were born. Jazz and tap began as the expressions of everyday people. To this day, social dance (and by extension, street dance) feeds the concert stage.

The early dance steps in both tap and jazz were inherently the same. Hoofers, the name given to these dancers who picked up steps as they went along, incorporated steps from both styles in their routines. The jazzy movements were evident in the flashy and acrobatic movements. The tap steps incorporated more footwork and sound. As chorus lines became more popular in nightclubs and on the Broadway stage, metal taps were added to dance shoes so the audiences could hear the feet of the dancers over the orchestras. The sound of dozens of pounding feet became positively thrilling. This early vernacular dance was performed to the popular music of the time. At the turn of the last century, ragtime—with its very square, danceable meter—was all the rage. The term "jazz" was first applied to this type of music.

Up to this point, the focus of this dance history has been on the contributions made by Africans and their descendents. As mentioned before, dances of other countries such as Ireland also made their mark in this country. European dances such as the polka had long been popular in the western dancehalls. The waltz had been in the United States since the 1820s, scandalizing puritanical Americans with the close embrace of the dancing couples. But social dance had not been widely accepted on the East Coast. That was to change in 1910, when all of America went mad for dance. Early ballroom dance, after the waltz, polka, and cakewalk, went through an animal dance phase with such dances as the Turkey Trot and the Buzzard Lope. Although the steps were inspired by black vernacular, couple dancing had never been inherent in African dance. This hybridic ballroom dancing acquired its first stars when Vernon and Irene Castle burst on the scene in 1913, performing the Turkey Trot in the show *The Sunshine Girl*. The Castles became very popular, giving exhibitions for society and formulating printed instructions for anyone to follow. Dancing, especially ballroom dance, soon spread like wildfire.

One of the most famous dancers of all time who executed the most elegant combination of ballroom, tap, and ballet was Fred Astaire. Like Robinson, Astaire, a white dancer, exuded a sense of "coolness," but he smoothed and polished his cool pose of polite unconcern into a mature and engaging style of carefree sophistication.[19] He looked "smart." Astaire danced in vaudeville with his sister Adele for many years, and then achieved his greatest success in Hollywood musicals starring with Ginger Rogers. He considered himself a musical comedy performer, and wrote that even he did not know how it all started for him, nor did he want to know.[20] Astaire raised understatement to a fine art, but he was classically trained. His use of arms and hands, as well the entire body, was his greatest contribution to American dance. He did, however, consider himself to have an "outlaw" streak, which added to his devil-may-care attitude. This was to pave the way for the James Brown generation to come.

Another early theatrical contributor to the jazz/tap/ballet/ballroom dance style was Gower Champion. Champion also studied ballroom dance prodigiously and worked primarily as one half of a ballroom couple performing in nightclubs and restaurants throughout the country. He brought a youthfulness and enthusiasm to American dance and choreographed with a keen eye for theatrics. "When asked once what his choreographic impulse was, however, he replied that he was simply looking for applause."[21] He was a master at the Broadway extravaganza, creating memorable shows such as *Hello Dolly!*, *Bye, Bye, Birdie*, and *42nd Street*. Champion's sense of theatrical timing in knowing just how to perfectly pull off an entrance or a kick line was legendary.

This era in the 1950s marked a change in the development of American vernacular. Dancers more highly trained in classical ballet, modern dance, and ballroom became the material for choreographers by the 1940s. Jazz dancing began to be presented with an eye towards calculated, set, theatrical effect rather than relying on improvisation and swing. Gene Kelly became a master of this sort of theatrical presentation. He was a dancer turned actor turned choreographer turned director. In his heyday in the 1950s he invented new ways of filming, combining animation and special effects with dance. His work changed camera angles and editing techniques, which created new spaces for dancers in film. Kelly's most famous movies were *American in Paris* in 1951 and *Singin' in the Rain* in 1952. His goal was to increase the popularity of the American male dancer with his athletic and gymnastic qualities.

It must be mentioned that, as in the vaudeville era, there was a split between black and white performers and black and white shows. This is still the case today. Astaire, Champion, and Kelly were white performers who made the black vernacular palatable to white audiences by toning down overly suggestive elements. Black shows tended to be less constrained. That is not to say there was or is no cross over, but Broadway still tends to present shows that feature one ethnicity or another.

The Hoofers Club and Its Antecedents

Meanwhile, black social dance was at its apogee in the 1930s and 1940s with the Harlem Renaissance and the lure of the Savoy Ballroom. For pure tap and jazz dancing, the unacknowledged headquarters and incubator of black talent was a small cellar room on 131st Street in New York City's Harlem. This back room was known as the Hoofers Club, and from the 1920s through the 1940s, this was the place where great dancers went to see others and to be seen. The 15-square-foot room contained benches, maybe one chair, and a battered upright piano. The tradition was that anybody could practice any step he wanted for as long as he pleased. But the cardinal rule was: "Thou Shalt Not Copy Another's Steps—Exactly."[22] A young dancer could learn a lot by having time and a place to practice, but

> the code decreed that a fledgling dancer was not to bother the great ones, even with
> a question. If you were lucky enough to be inside when one of the kings arrived, you

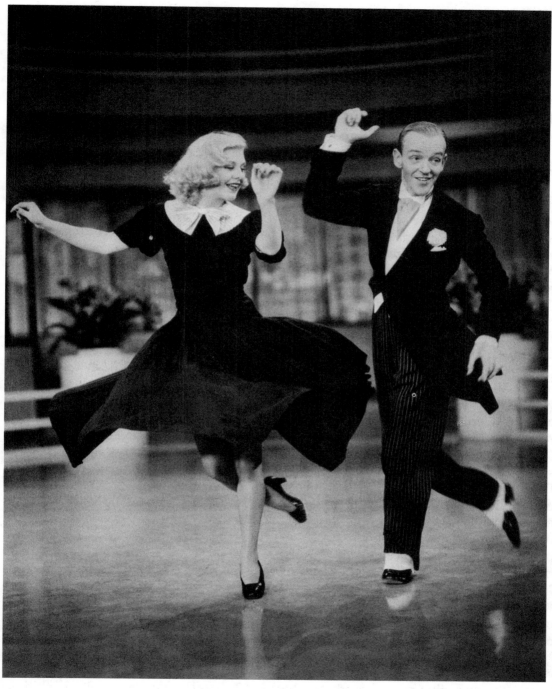

Fred Astaire and Ginger Rogers.

remained seated on the bench utterly motionless and "cool," although, curled up beneath you, your feet maybe moved as you watched, imitating a step. But your face was expressionless, and when the great man stopped dancing and sat down, you stayed glued to the bench, no matter how great the strain, until he left.[23]

Some dancers, such as King Rastus Brown, enjoyed showing the youngsters a few steps. Although he was an outstanding Buck dancer and has been credited with the development of the time step, he did not fare well theatrically. He lacked a gift for comedy and so fame eluded him.

In 1920, one cocky eighteen-year-old named John "Bubber" Sublett could not control himself. After he jumped up and did a few steps he was laughed out of the Hoofers Club and told "You're hurting the floor."[24] He stayed away for over a year practicing his tap, multiplying and changing steps so fast that each step was mounting the next. When he returned, he was a success and was crowned a new king. Newly anointed John "Bubbles" teamed up with Ford Lee "Buck" Washington and created a highly successful act called "Buck and Bubbles." The new style that Bubbles created soon became known as rhythm tap. He would mentally cut the tempo in half, thereby giving himself twice as much time to add new inventions.

Harold and Fayard Nicholas, better known as the Nicholas Brothers, were one of the best flash tap acts of all time. They opened at the Cotton Club in Harlem in the 1930s when Harold was eight and Fayard fourteen. Their acrobatic act, their abundant charm, and their undeniable talent made them an overwhelming success. From the Cotton Club they went to Hollywood and made *Kid Millions* in 1934. They toured England with a revival of *Blackbirds* and then returned to New York to dance in the Broadway musical *Babes in Arms*. Throughout their career they alternated between night clubs, concerts, Broadway shows, Hollywood, and a series of tours to South America, Africa, and Europe. There is a great clip of their outstanding dancing in the movie *Stormy Weather*, where, after tapping up and down stairs, on drums, and all over the stage, they catapult off the steps and over each other, landing from flying splits. Evidently they executed these splits in a correct ballet style of one leg in front and the other in back so as to prevent injury and not with one leg doubled up underneath on one side. Flash dancers such as the Nicholas Brothers "*compress* acrobatics and jazz dance together, creating a shock effect. By so doing, they communicate a feeling of desperate sophistication, a calculated impulse of *carpe diem*, reflecting a hot defiance that makes the rebellious movements of the Charleston seem low-key. This style of dancing evolved with the Depression and perhaps mirrors something of its mood."[25]

Unlike the simplified routines performed in unison set on chorus lines for the big commercial Broadway shows, these tap dancers were dancing with the great big bands of the time, blending their syncopated rhythmic feet with the music and creating highly intricate patterns. Today great tappers such as Savion Glover continue this tradition. Glover describes the process as having a conversation. His rhythms can be converted to words that are nuanced and shaded. "Trained as a drummer, Glover thinks of his tap shoe as a drum; the inside toe of the metal tap is the hi hat, the outside toe of the tap is the snare; the inside ball of the foot is the top tom-tom, the outside rim of the

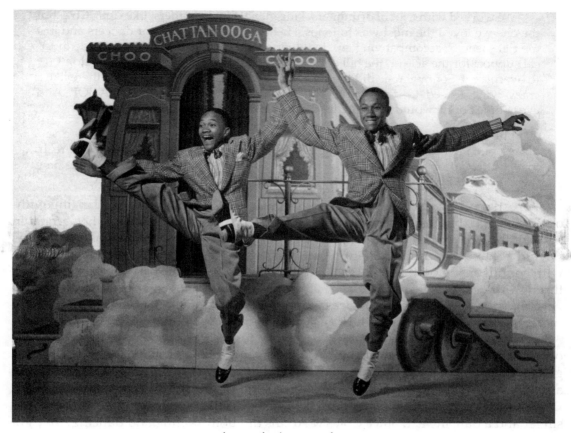

The Nicholas Brothers.

Image © Bettmann/CORBIS

ball is the cymbals, his left heel is the bass drum, and the right heel, the floor tom-tom-tom."[26] Music and dance are highly intertwined with each player inspiring the other. Jazz drummers learned much from the rhythms of the dancers and vice versa. And again, the intricate rhythms were improvisational. Tap dancers were essentially jazz musicians. This symbiotic relationship between tap dancers and big bands was extremely innovative and lasted until the 1950s. Many purists consider this to be the only true jazz dance form.

Charles Atkins (1913–2003), better known as Cholly Atkins, exemplified his era, reached the top, and then became one of the best perpetuators of the classic black dance style in his later life. His approach to tap was "First you think of a rhythm, then you try to duplicate the rhythm in your feet."[27] Then it could become a "happy marriage" between what the music was saying and what the dancer did. Working with live musicians could also be a challenge. Dancers might find they could come up against some obstinate drummers. In Atkins's words:

We worked with a lot of drummers. I mean big, big drummers, like Cozy Cole, but the one we loved the most was Jo Jones. He has so much respect for dancers and just the right feel for accompanying tap. Jo understood that it was his job to provide musical support for the acts on the bill and he'd stay right up underneath us. Wouldn't try to overplay it. Sonny Payne did the same thing. He found little rhythms in there like a crazy wing I used to do: HIPPYHIPPY-HIPPYHIPPY-SUR, STUR'A'DA'BOP. And every time Sonny would lay on it, he'd do that STUR'A thing with me. . . .

But some of the drummers felt that they should interpret the music. They'd say, "Hey, man, I'm out there playing. I've got to play something for myself." I said, "Yeah, man, but you dropping bombs in the middle of my pretty step. All I want is some time there, HA-CH'BAM, HA-CH'BAM, HA-CH'BAM."[28]

For Atkins, jazz dance not only uses many of the same steps as tap dancing without the sound, but it uses the same rhythms visually by emphasizing the accents in parts of the body. One of the most popular phrases I used to play with as a child was the old "Shave and a haircut—two bits." Inherently this would work out musically with sounds made on the counts of 1, &, a, 2, &, 3&, 4, which syncopates very nicely through the downbeats. One can easily come up with movements that correspond with this phrase audibly or physically, and it is much easier to say the words than to remember the counts. Such is the basic premise behind Atkins's method.

When he teamed up with another tapper, Honi Coles, "Coles & Atkins" became one of the top dance teams on the big band circuit. Most big bands not only played great music, but they carried a boy-and-girl team, a comedy dancing act, and usually a couple of vocalists. There were also popular vocal groups who traveled with bands. Even neighborhood clubs that could hold just a trio of musicians would bring in a singer and a dancing act. Since Coles & Atkins did both singing and dancing, they got a lot of work at the small places as well.

Modern Jazz

The big band era was a very exciting time in America, but nothing remains popular forever. After World War II and especially in the 1950s, jazz music underwent a shift. New taxes on dancing in clubs forced many club owners to cut back on entertainment or, in the case of the famed Savoy, close altogether. Jazz musicians began to play a style more suited for smaller combos—bebop—which, for many dancers, is not that accessible for dance. Bebop is

characterized by complex polyrhythms; steady but light and subtle beats; exciting dissonant harmonies; new tone colors; and irregular phrases. Honi Coles pointed out that to a great extent it was tap dancers who gave birth to bebop—through the work of John Bubbles: 'If you listen to any band before the thirties, the drummer was used just to keep time, then drummers started listening to Bubbles.' Ironically enough, these same Bubbles-inspired drummers helped cut tappers out of jazz shows. In bop's tighter arrangements, the spaces formerly reserved for tappers was gone, and all the percussion was now being done by the drummers.[29]

And with dancers, especially white dancers receiving more training in ballet and modern dance, *modern jazz dance* became a term used during the 1950s and 1960s to denote Afro-American vernacular aesthetics combined with movements from the vocabulary of ballet. This style had its own merits. Several great and memorable choreographers thrived in this era, especially on Broadway. Bob Fosse was born in Chicago in 1927. He took dance classes at the Chicago Academy of Theatre Arts because he was dragged along with his sister, for whom formal dance school was considered essential. The managing director of the school, Frederic Weaver, loved vaudeville and aspired to create child acts for the stage. Fosse was teamed up with another boy from academy, Charles Grass, and together they hit the boards under the name "The Riff Brothers," playing American Legion halls and amateur venues. By the time they were ready to become professional in the late 1930s, the heyday of vaudeville was over. Burlesque, famed for its striptease dancing and comics, was quickly rising in popularity. When they were sixteen, Weaver was booking the Riff Brothers into Minsky's Burlesque. Fosse described this phase as his "strange, schizophrenic childhood . . . a pull between Sunday school and my wicked underground life."[30]

He had a career dancing in Hollywood movies such as *Kiss Me Kate* and *My Sister Eileen* on Broadway, but it was as a choreographer and director that Bob Fosse truly made his mark. *Damn Yankees*, *Pajama Game*, *Bells Are Ringing*, and *Redhead* were a few of the Broadway shows he choreographed. He both directed and choreographed *Chicago*, *Sweet Charity*, *Dancin'*, and the movies *All That Jazz* and *Cabaret*. And he directed straight drama in the movies *Lenny* and *Star 80*. In 1973 he won three directing awards—the Tony Award for *Pippin*, the Academy Award for *Cabaret*, and the Emmy Award for *Liza with a Z*. The Fosse style of jazz dance is one of the sharpest, most understated, sensuous, and coolest, but has also been viewed as blatantly sexual and slightly misogynist. His female dancers have not always been shown in the most flattering light. In his work, Fosse used many aesthetics of African dance such as isolations, polyrhythms, and getting down. He often said, self-depreciatingly, that his style was based on his physical malformities, which he felt had prevented him from making it as major professional dancer. He was bald, his shoulders rounded forward, and he did not have a good turn out so many of his dances incorporate hats and steps that are hunched forward and knock-kneed. Still, Bob Fosse is considered by many to be one of the all time greats whose riveting contributions have been very influential in musical theater history. There is an entire style of jazz dance today known as the Fosse style.

Another great dancer and choreographer both in the ballet and jazz idioms was Jerome Robbins. His most famous shows were *West Side Story*, *Gypsy*, *Peter Pan*, *The King and I*, *Fiddler on the Roof*, *On the Town*, and *A Funny Thing Happened on the Way to the Forum*. He also was a resident choreographer in the golden age of the New York City Ballet, where he created some beautiful, well-crafted ballets. Robbins always felt that his Broadway shows and his ballets were interrelated.[31] And so his 1957 *West Side Story* based on Shakespeare's *Romeo and Juliet* involved young people from different social strata. Unlike most musicals, it actually dared to have a tragic ending. The dancing was very effectively fused with the drama and exquisitely captured the angst of youth by punctuating the choreography with many moves from Afro-American vernacular. Brooks Atkinson in the *New York Times* stated in his review that the show is "profoundly moving . . . As ugly as the city jungles and also pathetic; tender and forgiving."[32] Robbins's choreography was equally succinct in the film version of this show and, much like Gene Kelly, the camera was used to heighten the tension. Robbins's work was indeed a highlight in musical theater history, but it also exemplified the direction jazz was heading in the 1950s.

Other white jazz dance innovators of the time include Jack Cole, Matt Mattox, and Luigi. Jack Cole (1911–1974), originally a Denishawn dancer, took the classical Indian Bharata Natyam, fused it with Harlem's swing and jazz, and then added African and Caribbean steps, creating what he called "urban folk dance." Besides choreographing for film and Broadway, his highly popular dance troupe, Dance Workshop, performed widely in casinos, theaters, and nightclubs. Cole was also a highly sought after teacher and is known as the "Father of Jazz Dance." His advancements in isolation exercises and placement basically codified jazz dance technique, thereby validating jazz dance as an art form. Matt Mattox was a Jack Cole dancer who taught a Cole-based style in New York City. Mattox's classes, accompanied by a single bongo drummer, began with stretches on the floor and then moved to center isolations and improvised combinations. His style incorporated percussion with fluid, liquid-like movements. Luigi, another major jazz teacher, emphasized the line of the body, with arms lifted, chest high, and the head thrown back. Luigi, together with Mattox, dominated the field of jazz dance in New York City in the 1950s and 1960s.

While not authentic jazz dance, George Balanchine, the originator and soul of the New York City Ballet, borrowed very heavily from the Afro-American vernacular in creating his version of neoclassical ballet. Before moving to New York, he worked in Europe and was very impressed with the energy and athleticism of black performers in Paris and London nightclubs. Balanchine liked the rhythm and percussion of jazz music and, with his knowledge of music from his background as a classical musician, he merged ballet's cool aloofness with the African aesthetic of cool, enlivening ballet with a new energy, attack, speed, timing, and off-centeredness. His lines were often angular, with turned-in legs and bent knees. His new, energized, and expansive standard became the norm in contemporary ballet today. He manipulated the ultimate European aristocratic dance form and created a true American version.

The "Rediscovery" of Tap

Afro-American jazz and tap lost much steam in mainstream America to the technically proficient modern jazz dance being performed by trained ballet and modern dancers. With shows such as Robbins's and others such as Cole's 1953 *Kismet* and

Agnes de Mille's[33] 1943 *Oklahoma!*, the post–World War II sentiment in America preferred cathartic dramatic experiences in theater. And for the black tap dancer, remnants of minstrelsy continued to follow him, creating a perception of the black performer as a happy-go-lucky fellow. Then in the 1950s and 1960s, the civil rights movement changed the image of black Americans as they were becoming empowered in their African-American identity. A new image of the American black man was being advocated by the media. "Blaxploitation" movies were very popular in the 1960s and focused on the black hoodlum character or the hardened cop, as exemplified by the movie *Shaft*. Dancers such as Coles & Atkins had a difficult time finding performing work in the 1950s into the 1970s. Atkins bemoaned that

> We were a black *class act*, which in the tap world meant that you were well mannered, well groomed, your attire was excellent, and your material was extremely polished. We refused to play into any of the stereotypes, so a lot of the guys who controlled the swankiest spots thought of us as defiant. Back then many Americans were not ready to see two black men with an act as suave as ours.[34]

So tap went underground for a period of time. Back in 1949 when Bill "Bojangles" Robinson died, a group of the finest black tappers had formed an organization as a tribute to Robinson, calling themselves the "Copasetics" after his favorite saying. Besides Honi Coles and Cholly Atkins, others included Billy Strayhorn, Phace Robert, Milton Larkin, Francis Goldberg, Billy Eckstine, John E. Thomas, Pete Nugent, Ernest Brown, Louise Brown, Peg Leg Bates, Frank Goldberg, Eddie West, Emory Evans, Elmer Waters, Roy Branker, Paul Black, and Chink Collins. The members would put together shows every now and then, and every September they would do a big production. It was as much of a social club as a performance group. In 1962 five members,[35] including Coles and Atkins, performed at the Newport Jazz Festival in an informal production called "A History of the Tap Dance and Its Relationship to Jazz." They were such a hit that they were invited back in 1963. That year they presented "An Afternoon at the Hoofers Club," in which they imitated the old characters who used to hang out there. For the first time, tap dancing was recognized as an art form and not just a form of light entertainment. Another interesting trend worth mentioning began at this time. In the 1960s white American females started making a major contribution to the continuity of tap dance. They studied, apprenticed, and performed with the older generation of black male tap masters and helped to bring attention to this form of pure dance to white concert venues. Tap dance began a slow ascent to a concert dance form.

Motown

Meanwhile, popular music was moving in a new direction. The birth of "rock and roll" has been dated as beginning in 1955, but doo-wop groups had already gained national attention earlier with singing acts such as the Cadillacs in 1953. Although these and other groups had some great songs, many of these young performers did not have a clue as to how to act and move on stage. Cholly Atkins, classy man that he was, was called in to coach them. He taught them stage etiquette, how to bow, and specially tailored movements drawn from the American vernacular—such as trucking, the Charleston, boogie woogie, and the camel walk—that were suitable with the lyrics. In the 1960s Atkins was invited to work at Detroit's Motown Records, which was groundbreaking in concept and material. Motown had been founded by Berry Gordy, whose vision "was to make music with a funk beat and great stories that would be crossover, that would *not* be blues. . . . to try and make melody and words memorable and a dance beat very, very audible."[36] Atkin's vocal choreography was characterized by precise visual polyrhythms. Even when the backup singers were not singing there was continuous movement, with interesting steps from the black chorus line dancing of the 1920s through 1940s. Sometimes the singers were adept enough so that Atkins could give them actual tap steps. He worked with all of the top acts, from Gladys Knight and the Pips to the Temptations to the Supremes.

> The Atkins contribution to American culture has been extraordinarily significant. He not only made polished performers out of rock-and-roll singers who started with a hit single and raw ambition. He taught them to *perform* their music by doing dances that worked their magic not by retelling a song's storyline in predictable pantomime but by punctuating it with rhythmical dance steps, turns, and gestures drawn from the rich bedrock of black vernacular dance. In so doing, he virtually created a new form of expression: vocal choreography. . . . Without knowing it, popular groups of the sixties, seventies, and eighties were performing updated versions of dances of the forties, thirties, and twenties—classic black vernacular dances—and projecting them to a larger audience than ever before.[37]

Tap Really Makes a Comeback

In the 1970s tap came back to Broadway in a very "fluffy" white musical entitled *No, No Nanette*. In 1980 Gower Champion re-created a stage version of 1930s movie *42nd Street*. Suddenly tap was reborn. Black shows such as *Bubblin' Brown Sugar*, *Eubie*, *The Wiz*, *The Tap Dance Kid*, and my favorite, *Sophisticated Ladies*, which featured Gregory Hines dancing to the big band music of the Duke Ellington Orchestra, proved that tap was alive again. And still these shows were not integrated on anywhere near a fifty-fifty basis. They were primarily either white or black. Much like today's music industry, only certain stars have a wide crossover appeal.

More recently, Savion Glover has become the champion of tap dance. When he was twelve he starred in *The Tap Dance Kid*, and he has been the artistic heir of the most revered figures in the history of the dance—Jimmy Slyde, Honi Coles, Harold Nicholas, Bunny Briggs, and Gregory Hines. In 1996 he starred in and choreographed the musical *Bring in 'da Noise, Bring in 'da Funk*, which merged tap and rap, bringing the history of African-American dance up to date. He has since been touring the world with his own young company and is continually trading rhythms with live musicians while advancing the level of today's tap.

Jazz and tap have separated along the way, but some dancers do maintain the improvisational elements that make jazz what it is. Glover does it with his taps. Hip-hop dancers do it with their hard-edged movements—often in a challenge setting, with each soloist trying outdance the opponents. Choreographer Danny Buraczeski did it with old jazz standard tunes. With his company, which only recently disbanded, Buraczeski aspired to create a more intimate, pure style driven by the intricate rhythms of the music. Other choreographers today working in a structured format with moves from the black vernacular create amazing pyrotechnic feats of wizardry for their dancers. Twyla Tharp, originally a modern dancer, choreographed a show on Broadway entitled *Movin' Out* to music by pop musician Billy Joel. Tharp flings her dancers around the stage at breakneck speed, which is reminiscent of the flash dancing of the Nicholas Brothers. Susan Stroman has choreographed several Broadway shows, including *Contact* and *The Producers*, with the same proclivities that were used by Gower Champion. Her steps are designed for audience appeal and she is very adept at inserting very witty morsels in her work.

Jazz dancing is the most accessible of dance forms. Its roots come from ordinary people, street dancers, and club dancing. It is the most visible form of dance for youngsters growing up in the United States via television, the movies, and concerts. For theater-goers, jazz dance continues to be the most common idiom for Broadway and Las Vegas–type shows. The reason for this is still the rhythms. Rhythm is contagious. Just as in African dance, there is something ritualistic in percussion that resonates deep within the soul. Cholly Atkins, in his long life watching the dance world go by, identified movements from the Charleston, Michael Jackson's moonwalk, break dancing, and everything that looks new today as the same steps he saw in National Geographic films of the dances of Africa and the Caribbean islands. He swore that all the "new" dances are

those rhythms. You can go all the way back to primarily just drumbeats. And the dances were just as interesting when you didn't have saxophones, and trumpets and trombones. All of that was just more whipped cream on the Jell-O. That rhythm from those drums was the foundation, the basic beats; and for inspiration in many cases, because when they would increase their volume, it would inspire the dancers to do more energetic things.[38]

References

Atkins, Cholly, and Jacqui Malone. *Class Act: The Jazz Life of Choreographer Cholly Atkins*. New York: Columbia University Press, 2001.

Bond, Chrystelle. "A Chronicle of Dance in Baltimore 1780–1914." *Dance Perspectives*, Summer 1976.

Boross, Bob. "All That's Jazz." *Dance Magazine*, Aug. 1999: 54–58.

Dixon, Brenda. "Introduction." In *Proceedings of the International CORD Conference, July 13–17, 1988: Dance and Culture*, Ed. Sondra Horton. Fraleigh, Toronto, Canada.: 1988.

Emery, Lynne Fauley. *Black Dance from 1619 to Today*. (1988 reprint). New Jersey: Princeton Book Publishers, 1972.

Gottfried, Martin. *All His Jazz: The Life and Death of Bob Fosse*. (1998 reprint). New York: Da Capo Press, 1990.

Gottschild, Brenda Dixon. *Digging the Africanist Presence in American Performance*. Westport, CT: Greenwood Press, 1996.

Hering, Doris. "Jerry's Legacy." *Dance Magazine*, Apr. 1989: 44–51.

Lawrence, Greg. *Dance with Demons: The Life of Jerome Robbins*. New York: Berkley Books, 2001.

Malone, Jacqui. *Steppin' on the Blues: The Visible Rhythms of African American Dance*. Chicago: University of Illinois Press, 1996.

Mazo, Joseph H. "And the Band Played On." *Dance Magazine*, Apr. 1992: SC-20.

Mazo, Joseph H. "The Real Thing." *Dance Magazine*, Mar. 1994: 66.

The New Hampshire Gazette, 20 Aug. 1796, Vol. XL, Iss. 2073. Available online at http://infoweb.newsbank.com.

Payne-Carter, David. *Gower Champion: Dance and the American Musical Theatre*. Eds. Brooks McNamara and Steve Nelson. Connecticut: Greenwood Press, 1999.

Stearns, Marshall, and Jean. *Jazz Dance: The Story of American Vernacular Dance*. (1994 reprint). New York: Da Capo Press, 1968.

Thompson, Robert Farris. *African Art in Motion*. California: University of California Press, 1974.

Valis Hill, Constance. "Tap Dance in America: A Short History." In *The Living Dance*, Ed. Judith Chazin-Bennahum. Iowa: Kendall/Hunt Publishing Company, 2003.

Notes

1. Bob Boross, "All That's Jazz," *Dance Magazine*, Aug. 1999: 54.
2. Joseph H. Mazo, "And the Band Played On," *Dance Magazine*, Apr. 1992: SC–20.
3. Unfortunately "African" has become a general name for the thousands of different cultures with roots on the African continent. Such a reference to African dance is, admittedly, problematic due to the generic appellation of "African." Scholars are just now beginning to identify attributes of specific African cultures and their influences on dances of other continents. More research is still needed on this topic.
4. Brenda Dixon, "Introduction," in Proceedings of the International CORD Conference, July 13–17, 1988: Dance and Culture, ed. Sondra Horton Fraleigh, (Toronto, Canada), 14–15.

5. Robert Farris Thompson, *African Art in Motion* (California: University of California Press, 1974), 43.

6. Lynne Fauley Emery, *Black Dance from 1619 to Today* (New Jersey: Princeton Book Publishers, 1988 [1972]), 91.

7. Marshall Jean Stearns, *Jazz Dance: The Story of American Vernacular Dance* (New York: Da Capo Press, 1994 [1968]), 37.

8. Chrystelle Bond, "A Chronicle of Dance in Baltimore 1780–1914," *Dance Perspectives*, Summer 1976: 13.

9. *The New Hampshire Gazette*, 20 Aug. 1796, Vol. XL, Iss. 2073, available online at http://infoweb.newsbank.com.

10. Lynne Fauley Emery, *Black Dance from 1619 to Today* (New Jersey: Princeton Book Publishers, 1988 [1972]), 184.

11. *Ibid.*, 188.

12. Marshall Jean Stearns, *Jazz Dance: The Story of American Vernacular Dance* (New York: Da Capo Press, 1994 [1968]), 47.

13. Lynne Fauley Emery, *Black Dance from 1619 to Today* (New Jersey: Princeton Book Publishers, 1988 [1972]), 203.

14. Marshall Jean Stearns, *Jazz Dance: The Story of American Vernacular Dance* (New York: Da Capo Press, 1994 [1968]), 89.

15. *Ibid.*, 232.

16. *Ibid.*, 233.

17. *Ibid.*, 236–237.

18. Cholly Atkins and Jacqui Malone, *Class Act: The Jazz Life of Choreographer Cholly Atkins* (New York: Columbia University Press, 2001), 44.

19. *Ibid.*, 222.

20. *Ibid.*, 220.

21. David Payne-Carter, *Gower Champion: Dance and the American Musical Theatre*, eds. Brooks McNamara and Steve Nelson (Connecticut: Greenwood Press, 1999), 73.

22. Jacqui Malone, *Steppin' on the Blues: The Visible Rhythms of African American Dance* (Chicago: University of Illinois Press, 1996), 97.

23. Marshall and Jean Stearns, *Jazz Dance: The Story of American Vernacular Dance* (New York: Da Capo Press, 1994 [1968]), 212.

24. *Ibid.*, 212.

25. *Ibid.*, 282.

26. Constance Valis Hill, "Tap Dance in America: A Short History," *The Living Dance*, ed. Judith Chazin-Bennahum (Iowa: Kendall/Hunt Publishing Company, 2003), 170.

27. Cholly Atkins and Jacqui Malone, *Class Act: The Jazz Life of Choreographer Cholly Atkins* (New York: Columbia University Press, 2001), 19.

28. *Ibid.*, 81.

29. Jacqui Malone, *Steppin' on the Blues: The Visible Rhythms of African American Dance* (Chicago: University of Illinois Press, 1996), 116.
30. Martin Gottfried, *All His Jazz: The Life and Death of Bob Fosse* (New York: Da Capo Press, 1998 [1990]), 28.
31. Doris Hering, "Jerry's Legacy," *Dance Magazine*, Apr. 1989: 50.
32. Greg Lawrence, *Dance with Demons: The Life of Jerome Robbins* (New York: Berkley Books, 2001), 258.
33. Agnes de Mille was listed as the choreographer for the Broadway show *Gentlemen Prefer Blonds*. Coles & Atkins were featured performers. She told them to work something out for their specialty number and then later took full credit for the choreography. Years later when they wanted to perform the piece in another show, they had to get her permission first.
34. Cholly Atkins and Jacqui Malone, *Class Act: The Jazz Life of Choreographer Cholly Atkins* (New York: Columbia University Press, 2001), 114.
35. The roster necessarily changed over time. The five who performed at the 1962 Newport Jazz Festival were Honi Coles, Cholly Atkins, Pete Nugent, Baby Laurence, and Bunny Briggs.
36. Jacqui Malone, *Steppin' on the Blues: The Visible Rhythms of African American Dance* (Chicago: University of Illinois Press, 1996), 120.
37. *Ibid.*, 125.
38. Cholly Atkins and Jacqui Malone, *Class Act: The Jazz Life of Choreographer Cholly Atkins* (New York: Columbia University Press, 2001), 198.

Chapter 7

Dance in India

Dance in India: Where Are We Today?

Ananya Chatterjea

In working with dance histories of nonwestern cultures, one of the most important lessons I have learned is about the inadequacy of existing models of historiography, directly related to the dominance of themes of Western history in selecting and organizing "facts" that make up historical narratives everywhere. This is particularly obvious to me in researching the few historical accounts of Indian dance, all written in current times retrospectively. The lack of historical texts about performance practices from the past is, of course, natural in contexts dominated by direct bodily and oral modes of transmission, which raise questions about the need for documenting developments in cultural practices in the manner of historical texts. It also draws attention to the kind of validation that accrues to embodied practices through textualization and to the logocentric imperative that has come to be our legacy from the West. This, of course, does not mean that there is not evidence about the historicity about performance practices from the past, but rather that such evidence has rarely been narrativized in terms of a linear chronology—a modality that has acquired legitimizing power in conventions of historical narratology. Here of course, knowledge about the distant past is gleaned from various sources: from documents which codify performance techniques and conventions like the ancient *Natyashastra*, written by Bharata-Muni between the second and fifth centuries, a comprehensive scripture of performance, and other such manuals written from time to time; references to dance and dancers in other literary texts; the plethora of sculptures of dancing figures on temple walls and other buildings, etchings on cave walls and paintings, and other visual evidence.

However, the disciplinary institutionalization of history in modern times in accordance with these specific norms of linear chronology and the thematic concerns of European modernity—such as the inevitable march of progress, development, and such ideologies—has meant that those who do not, or perhaps cannot, produce such narratives, often get petrified in some notion of ahistoricity and timelessness. This of course has both fed and been fed by the practice of studying "other" cultures, primarily nonwhite, non-Western cultures from the Third World, through the discipline of anthropology, that unfortunately, has increasingly reified cultural difference in terms of the tradition-innovation binary. Thus it is that the absence of textualized, linear chronologies, standing in for history, has been made to signify that in these "other" cultures, cultural practices originated in an ancient past and have continued as such, as unmoving "tradition," which is the opposite of the constant moving forward of Western performance history, developing and evolving genres of its own and then re-volting against them: baroque, romantic, classical, modern, postmodern.

Of course these genres do not exist in Indian dance, which is organized differently. But the interventions of India's colonial history and the enforcement of English edu-cation among the Indian middle classes by the dictates of Lord Macaulay's famous Minute on Indian Education, have had serious consequences. In this famous docu-ment, Macaulay urged the importance of English education among a group of Indians, who could serve as interpreters for the British, intermediaries between the British rulers, who would be "Indian in blood and color, but English in taste, in opinions, in morals, and in intellect."[1] With the colonial experience and the ensuing struggle for in-dependence, India seemed to be inducted into the modernity that the West had inau-gurated, marked ultimately by its organization into a nation-state in 1947. Huge cultural shifts that were now effected, reflect the inevitability of the implication of the East in the West and vice versa. At any rate, it is largely when we are into the twenti-eth century, that the focus falls on dance as part of the cultural revival movements in-spired by nationalism, the erasures and disruptions caused by colonial rule are brought to light, and efforts to re-stage the existing dance traditions on the contempo-rary concert stage are argued over, leaving us sufficient documentation to construct a history of Indian dance in modern times. This is also the time that terminologies such as classical and folk become part of discussions of dance, and of culture generally. It is largely from the perspective of this body of knowledge that I can, and indeed desire to, speak. For it is largely through looking at the developments in dance at these times that one realizes how vital a cultural-political signifier the dancing body is and how intertwined are the politics of cultural practice and political/governmental policy.

However, to briefly trace the journey to this point. Some of the earliest evidence of dance in India comes from sculptures of dancing women from the cities of Mohenjo-Daro and Harappa, typically described as the pre-historic civilizations of the Dravid-ian settlers in the Indus valley. It is however with the development of Indo-Aryan culture in the Indo-Gangetic belt that marks the time from which performance texts, documenting the existence of a sophisticated movement system, become available to us. One of the founding texts of Indian performance, the *Natyashastra,* was written by the sage Bharata during this period, not later than the third century CE. The *Natyashas-tra,* literally the "scripture of performance," seems to have been written based on a compilation of dominant performance practices of the concert stage, existent across several regions in the country. There are several other texts that are important to take into account when studying Indian dance, but given the limitations of space and the predominant influence this scripture has had on the rearticulation of Indian dance in modern times, I will talk briefly about some of the central emphases of this text.

What immediately becomes clear even from a cursory glance at the *Natyashastra* is that there is little demarcation between theater and dance. Rather, movement, music, and drama are intertwined to create a rich and total theatrical experience. Moreover, there is a clear directive that performance exists as a mode of instruction as well as entertainment for audiences, and that it has immense power in swaying audiences, imbuing them with desirable moral and socio-cultural values. Again, while expressivity is a dominant mode of such performance, it is never realism but rather metaphorical approximations that are used. It is in keeping with this that dance is understood as composed of *nritta*, or pure or non-narrative dance, and *nritya*, expressional dance, where pure dance movements are woven in with *abhinaya*, or expressive intent. In order to chisel the body and achieve finesse in expressivity, whether of an aesthetic in *nritta* or of nonlinear narrative in *nritya*, the body is classified into limbs *(anga)*, subsidiary limbs *(pratyanga)*, and tertiary limbs *(upanga)*. For each limb then is codified a repertoire of movements, the various combinations of which make for different meaning structures.

Thus, for instance, one of the prime repertoires of movements is that of the hand gestures, or *mudras*, or *hastas*. These are further classified as *asamyukta hastas* or *samyukta hastas*. The former, single hand gestures, are gestures that are completed by using one hand, such as the *pataka mudra*, the first *mudra* of the repertoire of hand gestures where the palm is held straight, the fingers held together and the thumb folded into the palm. The latter signifies joint hand gestures, which require both hands in order to complete the formation of the *mudra*. Such, for instance, is the gesture of the fish, *matsya mudra*, where one palm is laid on top of another with the thumbs out on either side, and the thumbs move in a continuous circular motion to convey the sense of swimming through water. In terms of *asamyukta hastas*, each individual hand is formed into the *chandrakala* hand gesture, which is much like the *pataka mudra*, except that the thumb is held out suggesting the curved lines of a sliver of moon. But since both hands in *chandrakala* jointly make the *matsya mudra*, this latter is classified as *samyukta hasta*.

Now the ways of meaning-making here are complex, and particularly with *mudras*, one is always performing layers of metaphor that unravel the many possible interpretations of the emotional landscape being articulated. *Abhinaya* also works with the logic of abstract imagery versus the logic of linear narrative, such that there is no direct and inevitable functionality of meaning attached to a hand gesture or other elements of expressive movement, and the possibility of significance and signification are constantly renewed. This becomes obvious when we look at the *biniyoga*, the applications of the hand gestures in different contexts to signify differently, such as the many possible ways to use the *pataka* hand gesture, which include *natyarambhe* (to begin a dance sequence), *varivahe* (to indicate clouds), *vane* (to suggest a forest), *vastunishedhane* (to point out things), among many other possibilities. Of course, in poetic interpretation, *mudras* blend with eye gestures, body stance, and other elements such that the dancer can make us wonder whether she is talking about the clouds she sees in the sky, or the dark wavy hair of the poet's beloved, or the sadness that cloud over her eyes when she misses her lover. It is this possibility of constant shifts between meaning, resonance, and signification that I would point to as one of the richest and most unique aspects of Indian classical performance.

There are four main modes through which *abhinaya* is worked, and indeed the way the *Natyashastra* specifies these testifies to the immediately correlated existence of theatre and dance, the idea of performance as a richly coordinated theatricalization. All of the above movement categorizations fall into the first of these modes, *Angika*, which refers to the expressivity of movement, embodied techniques; then comes *Vachika*, that which is explored through vocalization, dialogues, singing; *Aharya*, which is the enhancement of thematic concerns, characterizations, and aesthetic framework through costumes, makeup, stagecraft; and last, *Sattvika*, which is the expression of psychic states intimately associated with emotions, such as tears of joy, trembling, fainting, change of color, and such. These different modes, working in concert, allow the performer to communicate with audiences who have become familiar with stage conventions, and can be described as *sahridaya*, close in heart, or *rasika*, one who appreciates. This communication, this resonance of the artistic intention with audience appreciation, makes for and is based on the invocation of *rasa*, or mood, that is at the core of successful performance. This in turn makes for the elaboration of the nine dominant emotional frames or moods of Indian classical performance, once again described as *rasa*; no doubt also suggesting the centrality of such expressivity and communication to performance. These moods, initially codified by Bharata as eight, with the last mood being added later, are now generally referred to as *navarasa* (the nine moods): *sringara* (erotic), *vira* (heroic), *karuna* (tragic), *adbhuta* (wondrous), *raudra* (furious), *hasya* (comic), *bhayanaka* (fearful), *bibhatsa* (disgusting), and *shanta* (peaceful). Of course these are but the dominant moods or *sthayibhava*, and there are variations within them, so that they are qualified by differing *bhavas*, which are composed of determinants or *vibhavas*, consequents or *anubhavas*, and transitory feelings or *vyabhichari bhava*. So, for instance, the articulation of the erotic mood might work through the expression of discouragement, anxiety, indignation, joy, doubt and other such emotions. Moreover, the expression of *sringara* is of one kind, romantic, when the dancer performs longing for her beloved; and of another kind in *vatsalya*, a mother's love for the child, loving even as she scolds him for being naughty. For each different possibility of the same mood, there is a whole repertoire of facial expressions and specific body movements. I have talked about these aspects largely in order to suggest the richness of the classical performance traditions, the detailed techniques that the Indian dancer has access to.

At any rate, what the *Natyashastra* and other texts, such as the *Abhinaya Darpana*, written by Nandikeshwara between the fifth and thirteenth centuries CE, refer to are the conventions of staged performance that evolved early as important cultural practice, ritualized but very much woven from and back into the fabric of life. Applications and manifestations of these codified movement repertoires, however, varied depending on the particular dance style and regional cultural specificities. For instance, the same *mudra* can be performed differently in the different styles, and there is also an additional repertoire of local hand gestures that are specific to each style. These styles were described generally as *margi*, a term which referred to their organization in terms of a specific aesthetic.[2] Other styles developed locally, strung together more as a series of pieces or social dances, and were referred to as *desi*, translating more or less incompletely as vernacular. I have referred earlier to the onslaught of Western modernity and the influence of its categories and themes on the cultural leaders of "modern," i.e., independent, India. The different levels of formality, varying organization and goals of the plethora of cultural practices in India, reflected in loose groupings of these forms as *desi* or *margi*, were reified and hardened with the mistranslation of the above descriptors as "classical" and "folk," with their inevitable implications of high and low art. Inevitably also, these categories remained messy, unable to cover up overlaps, with several forms demanding categorization as at least "semi-classical."

Thus, the recognized classical forms at this time are Bharatanatyam, Kathakali, Kuchipudi, and Mohini Attam from the southern part of India, and Odissi, Kathak, and Manipuri from the northern and northeastern part. The four forms from the south reflect generally the specific preferences of the Carnatic style of musical and rhythmic organization interwoven with local inflections, while Kathak is based more or less completely on Hindustani styles, Odissi works with the confluence of Hindustani, Carnatic, and regional musical and rhythmic styles, and Manipuri with the vernacular forms typical to that region. There are huge and important stylistic and aesthetic differences among these styles, important to maintain in keeping with notions of *angasuddhi* (purity of body/limb, i.e., technique and line), and even among the different schools within those styles. For instance, the history and style of the Jaipur *gharana*, or school of Kathak, which developed from the performative techniques of storytellers, or *kathakars*, and was performed primarily in the temple courtyards of northwestern India, is distinct from those of the Lucknow *gharana* which developed through the performances of the courtesans in courts of Muslim rulers in north India. "Folk" forms are referred to generally through the names of the places where they developed and are practiced, though of course each dance has its own name. For instance, the *Bihu* dance of Assamese folk dance forms from the state of Assam. On the other hand, forms such as the *Chhau* dance style, developed from training in martial movements and the performance of folk mythologies, with three distinct schools of movement developing in Purulia, Seraikella, and Mayurbhanj, fall technically into neither category according to the given specifications, and is generally classified as "semi-classical," as is the Sanskrit dance drama form Kudiyattam, that is aesthetically close to Kathakali, but does not have as strict or elaborate grammatical codes as the latter. As I write, in 2002, there are two movements gathering force, urging the recognition by the highest national cultural organization of the country: the Sangeet Natak Akademi, of the Sattriya dance of Assam and the Guadiya Nritta of Bengal as classical forms.

The notion of the dignity and prestige attendant upon the classical was encouraged through the work of scholars such as Ananda Coomaraswamy who translated and published the *Abhinaya Darpana* as *Mirror of Gesture* in 1917, and familiarized the West with the philosophical underpinnings of Indian cultural practices in his famous book *The Dance of Shiva* published in 1918. The German Orientalist scholars such as

Max Mueller and the notion of the ancient, glorious, and timeless classical traditions of India also influenced him. This foregrounding of the classical traditions found support in the nationalist movement seeking to establish India's cultural heritage, but the ways in which it was done, setting up a binary with Western modern and avant-garde, served, problematically, both to hierarchize the classical and to museumize it, fixating it in the past.

For instance, it was obvious that the dance forms had changed from the time that the above mentioned texts were written, over several centuries, and that there were huge gaps in the continuity of these forms due to the violences effected by colonialism. Yet the attempt during the cultural revivalism movement of the 1940s was to suggest a seamless continuity, or at least a total recovery and recuperation, as if that were possible, instead of a recreation and reorganization. There was little recognition of the fact, for instance, that most of these classical dance forms were performed in the temples, or as in the instance of Kathakali, in the village courtyard, and later in the courts of kings and the royalty, and the dancers, hence, were surrounded by audiences on two or three sides, and specific kinds of audiences at that. This is true even of the three kinds of performance spaces described in the *Natyashastra*. Obviously then, there were many elements to be negotiated when, in the post-independence era, the classical dance forms were reincarnated as concert stage forms, performed on proscenium stages, a concept imported from Western performance traditions, and reformulated as ticketed events. However, many of these issues were left unaddressed, even as the leaders of the cultural movement sought to invoke a continuous tradition from the past, a project aggravated largely by the disruptive story of the *devadasis*, to whom I will turn my attention momentarily.

At any rate, with the cultural revival movement of the late thirties and forties, the vernacular dance from the state of Tamil Nadu known as *sadir nac*, was revived, redesigned in keeping with temple sculptures and other visual and textual evidence and reorganized according to the tenets of the *Natyashastra,* and renamed Bharatanatyam. Apparently the name came from the combination vital to the dance form *(natya): bhava* (mood or emotion), *raga* (music), and *tala* (rhythm), hence *bha-ra-ta*. However, there is no escaping the immediate implications of the reference to sage Bharata, the author of the classic text that was now upheld as legitimizing classical performance. Nor can we ignore that Bharata is also the indigenous name for India, an interpretation that suggests Bharatanatyam is indeed the dance of India, and indeed since it was the first of the forms to be revived and institutionalized, it has acquired the status, both in India and outside, of a near-national dance form, or at least the representative form of Indian dance. This of course has spawned its own kind of political maneuverings, with the other classical styles struggling against what appears to be their marginalization through the implied superiority of Bharatanatyam. Also, because Bharatanatyam was the first to be reorganized according to the scriptured codifications, and to have its repertoire organized in a developmental pathway fit for an evening-length solo dance performance format, and thus establish a model of "classicism," several other dance

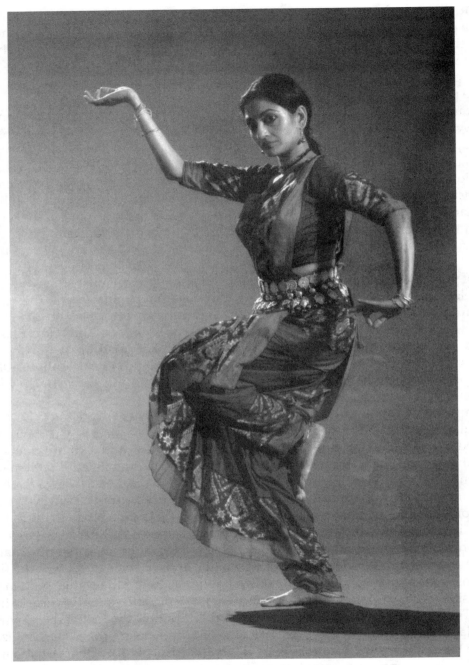

Odissi, Dancer Ananya Chatterjea.
Courtesy of photographer Eric Saulitis.

forms, like Kuchipudi and Odissi followed suit, making this organization formulaic. Along with this, the conventions of the *Natyashastra* came to acquire pan-Indian, prescriptive force, such that, several scholars have argued, the differences among the regional and culturally specific aesthetics that had initially characterized these dance forms came to be minimized. I also feel that currently, there are burgeoning movements urging the recognition of and research on local stylistic elements.

The history of the development of these forms in modern India, which I feel are best described as neo-classical forms, given their history of revival-but-reconceptualization, is inextricably tied up with the history of the dancers, who with embodied knowledge kept these forms alive through time. The practice of *devadasi* dedication was an ancient and widespread one in India. *Devadasis,* literally "servants of the gods," were women dedicated to the service of the gods at a young age, and married to the resident deity of the temple at the time they were initiated into its services. It is their status as brides of the god that earned them a position of importance in society, signs of auspiciousness, since they were forever-brides, un-widowable, *nityasumangali,* for their husband could never die. Hence their presence was required at most important temple services as well as other socio-cultural and religious ceremonies. At the same time, as women married to an immanent deity but often serving their divine lord through earthly representations, engaged in sexual relationships with the king or other royalty, they could only exist at the margins of society. *Devadasis* were organized into groups according to the services they rendered; one of the highest among which was singing and dancing before the idol. Since the dance was an offering to divinity, artistic excellence was obviously a high priority, and a sign of the spiritual dedication of the devotee. But since the *devadasi* was the bride of god, this spiritual expression was in the form of love, primarily erotic love, and there was no denial of the sensual or the sexual. This intertwining of the spiritual-sexual in artistic expression is clearly seen in the plethora of sculptures of dancing figures on temple walls, often highly erotic, which did not obviously interrupt the sacredness of a place of worship. This of course also points to the very different ways in which both spirituality and religiosity were conceptualized and organized prior to colonial rule and the patriarchal agendas of nationalism, which caused major changes.

At any rate, the *devadasis* lived more or less always on or near temple grounds, on land granted to them by the royalty, and their families were organized matrilineally, with the children they had through their liaisons with the royalty. Often they adopted children who followed them in their profession. The daughters become *devadasis* and the sons became accompanying musicians or were inducted into temple services. Even later, when the dance was also clearly developing as a court dance form, with the dancers being regarded more as courtesans, performing elaborate expositions of love and passion, the *devadasis* remained unique women in terms of the general socio-cultural organization, owning property, highly literate, writing poetry and performing it to audiences of connoisseurs. This of course does not take away from the oppressions attendant upon their lifestyle, their enforced sexual availability to particular individuals and groups who stood in positions of power. At any rate, the *devadasi* system, as the temple organization, depended entirely on the financial support of a Hindu king, or benevolent kings of other faiths such as the Mughal emperor Akbar who believed in supporting the religious followings of his diverse subjects. So, while Muslim rulers often dealt severe blows to these systems, these latter continued to resurface and survive till the coming of the British Raj. Not only did the colonial government withdraw all support to temples, it also pronounced moral outrage at the sensuousness of the dance they saw, largely based on their somatophobic reaction to the erotic nature of such spiritual expression. For instance the Bengal District Gazetteers of 1878 reported the words of an indignant British civil servant, William Ward Hunter (1872): "Indecent ceremonies disgraced the ritual, and dancing-girls with rolling eyes put the modest worshipper to the blush . . . The baser features of a worship which aims at a sensuous realization of God appears in a band of prostitutes who sing before the image . . . In the pillared halls, a choir of dancing-girls enliven the idols' repast by their airy gyrations" (quoted in Patnaik, 1990, 71).[3]

The so-called secular colonial government's withdrawal of any support to the temples left the *devadasis* without any income. These women, who could hardly find their way back into a more-or-less strictly regulated social system, were forced to earn their living by accommodating prostitution. The British administrators had already complained bitterly about the indecent and lascivious dancing of the native *"nautch* girls."[4] The officers were seriously disturbed by the increasing sexual encounters between such native women and British officers. Reportedly, red light areas sprung up around British encampments in great numbers. In 1864, the colonial government devised a way of establishing some measure of control over this situation: they passed the Contagious Diseases Act whereby prostitutes were required to be registered and examined medically. Many women committed suicide in frustration at police harassment at this time. However, by this one stroke of pen, the *devadasis* in whose bodies the dance had lived, the *nautch* girls, and courtesans, who had different levels of training in the arts, were all reductively categorized as prostitutes only, supposedly lacking both decency and morals.

From that point on, history usually referred to these dancing women primarily in this negative light, delegitimizing their artistry, without simultaneously theorizing that without any form of support from the state, hounded by daily worries of survival, it was hardly possible for these women to continue to practice their art with the kind of attention and dedication that earlier characterized their practice. The dance gained prominence only years later, during the cultural revivalist movement of the 1940s, when the sculptors of modern India realized that here indeed was a great wealth of cultural practices which should be "revived" and celebrated in the project of reconstructing India's grand culture, a project influenced by the Western Orientalist scholars of the nineteenth century. The influence of Theosophical thought, which can be traced in the philosophical base of the Kalakshetra College of Dance and Music established in Madras in 1936, no doubt entered this arena through the advice given by Annie Besant and Lord Arundale to Rukmini Devi, the architect of modern Bharatnatyam. Dislodged from the practices of the *devadasis*, the dance was reborn when, in 1947, after a long, drawn out anti-*nautch* struggle, it became illegal to dance in the temple. Concomitantly, the secular government of independent India announced its support of the classical dance traditions in their reincarnations as concert stage forms.

There were also other kinds of changes that deeply affected the socio-cultural and economic complex that contexted the dissemination and performative continuity of all of these dance forms. For the classical dance forms, learnt through direct transmission, the primary form of training was the *guru-shishya parampara*. The word *guru* is inaccurately translated as "teacher"; indeed, the entire system of learning, here predicated on the depth of the philosophical-aesthetic base and the notion of the art as education as well as entertainment, is better described as preceptor-disciple system. The notion of continuity is also suggested through the descriptor *parampara*, which means tradition, and suggests continuity across generations. This is not a pedagogic model that encourages students to ask questions right from the beginning, but rather one that demands openness to the process of learning. In fact, once the *shishya* or disciple is initiated into the apprenticeship of the guru, he accepts the guru as a spiritual guide as well, one who will enlighten and dispel ignorance. Thus the disciple spends a lot of time at the guru's household, surrounded by practices that support the art, helping out with household duties, serving the guru and learning the entire context of artistic practice through osmosis.[5] Once training is complete, the disciple is introduced to audiences by the guru in a solo recital. This marks the former's entry into the circuit of professional dancers, and while she/he continues to develop through continued training with the guru, through personal reflection and research, she is now ready to take on her performances. While this system of training was highly effective in evolving a total artist, one who is aware of the multiple facets of the art, it could hardly survive unchallenged in the modern economic system built on Western models. While the *guru-shishya* system continues to exist, the larger modes of proliferation of the dance forms have become smaller training schools, formal and informal, where students are enrolled in classes and take class on specific days of the week. There are also two major universities dedicated to the arts, where renowned gurus often teach. No doubt, however, the most effective mode of training artists has been the guru-shishya system where the individualized relationship between the preceptor and disciple effects, despite the restraints and controls created by the guru, a balance between the continuity of tradition and an individual performer's creativity.

One of the large changes that have affected the folk dance forms has come again with the localization of the nationalist agenda. The central institute for the performing arts established by the government after independence, the Sangeet Natak Akademi and all its local branches in the different states, have continuously encouraged the research and highlighting of folk dance traditions. The government, at both state and national levels, has established forums to support this agenda. As a result, folk dance forms have begun to be staged and as a corollary, to be compositionally altered to make for a more "complex" visual experience. This has also meant that the practice of these forms as a social dance form by village folk, among whom and where they evolved, has been affected. The folk dance forms have also become somewhat more codified and organized in terms of pieces that can be "learned" and thereafter performed. While these have also become part of a larger touring circuit, both national and international, they are also often deployed to feed the growing market for "ethnic chic," once again a result of Western interest in things that create access to the "ethnic other."

For instance, there are the Inter-state Cultural Exchange programs sponsored by state governments, where troupes of performers travel to other states and give concerts in different cities and towns, showcasing the indigenous folk traditions of that particular state. Again, recently the government of the state of West Bengal has sponsored the setting up of a large scale cultural bazaar, Swabhumi (literally translating as "own grounds"), in the city of Kolkata. The typical folk handicrafts from the different states are put on display there through various stalls selling them. Also supporting the national government's policy of unity in diversity, Swabhumi features folk artists of various kinds, Rajasthani folk singers and drummers who perform as they move through the grounds, among the shoppers; a contemporary percussion group on the main stage where performances are held free almost every evening. Once, I watched a Gotipua performance, a theatrical folk form from Orissa, performed exclusively by young boys dressed in drag, as women, where the choreography was marked by some uncharacteristic lunges and themes of ethnic pride. I was interested to know, through talking to the choreographer and master drummer, that all of the choreography was new and created in keeping with some governmental directives to enhance the image of the state and its cultural resources. Obviously, even in fields marked as traditional and folk, the changes necessitated by a "modernizing" society moving surely towards first-world-style capitalism and consumerism, are constantly under negotiation.

At any rate, these are not the only kinds of concert dance that mark the field of contemporary performance. Indeed, while this is still not the norm, there are some choreographers who have produced excellent contemporary choreography based on the existent traditions. Of course there is an important distinction made between such choreography and composition, which describes the work of gurus working within the idiomatic and technical base, and the philosophical and ideological conventions of classical performances, to add to that repertoire, continuing the project of recovery and reconstitution that I talked about before. This is typically the work of contemporary gurus such as Birju Maharaj (Kathak) and Guru Kelucharan Mahapatra (Odissi). Composition also describes better the work of certain artists who again continue to work within the formal boundaries of these forms, but innovate somewhat with the staging, making new group works on themes that may not have been part of the classical base, but do not disrupt it either, such as the work of Kumudini Lakhia. Contemporary choreography, on the other hand, is an entirely different genre, and I would use it to describe the work of choreographers whose work challenges the conventions of classical performance, and extends its ideological and idiomatic base. Such is the work of choreographers like Chandralekha, Daksha Seth, Maya Rao. What to me is valuable about such work is that it is based as much on respect for indigenous forms and cultural practices, as a critique of the hierarchies and prejudices that have come to be immediately associated with them, and on a recognition of the post-colonial experience and contemporary issues.

In this article I have tried to convey a sense of the richness and diversity of Indian dance as the field is today, indicating also some of the problems that it is laboring under today. It is my hope that the reader will get from this article, brief as it is, both a sense of cultural practices that have been handed down through the ages, as well as continuously evolving conventions of staging. Moreover, what I have tried to emphasize is how the dancing body is a vital political signifier and how the history of dance and dancers is completely interwoven with the agendas of governments and policies, economic needs, as much as the desires and hopes of artists. The field of dance in India today is exciting and volatile even as it is frustrating, and while there is no doubt much research to be done, there is always some development that grips my attention and keeps alive my continuous fascination with it.

Notes

1. From *The Speeches of Lord Macaulay with his Minute on Indian Education,* edited and printed by G. M. Young, Oxford: OUP, 1935, and reprinted in *The post-colonial studies reader,* edited by Bill Ashcroft, Gareth Griffins, and Helen Tiffin, London and New York: Routledge, 1995, p. 430.
2. *Marg* means path, so *margi,* the adjective from that, indicates a particular developmental trajectory.
3. Dhirendra Nath Patnaik, (1990) *Odissi dance.* Bhubaneshwar: Orissa Sangeet Natak Akademi.
4. The word *nautch* is a corruption and an Anglicization of the vernacular *naach,* meaning dance. Initially referring to groups of traveling entertainers, the word came to refer to all dancing women, with the implication that they were primarily entertainers, not artists.
5. This traditional mode of learning was prevalent for all education, but while it more or less disappeared with the secularization of general education, it continued to be a strong tradition in the performing arts.

Bibliography

Banerji, Projesh. (1983) *Erotica in Indian dance.* New Delhi: Cosmo Publications.

Bose, Mandakranta. (2001) *Speaking of dance: the Indian critique.* New Delhi: D.K. Printworld.

Bose, Mandakranta. (1991) *Movement and mimesis: the idea of dance in the Sanskritic tradition.* Dordrecht, Boston: Kluwer Academic Publishers.

Bose, Mandakranta. (1970) *Classical Indian dancing: a glossary*. Calcutta: General Printers and Publishers.

Coomaraswamy, Ananda. (1918) *The dance of Siva: fourteen Indian essays*. New York: Sunwise Turn.

Coomaraswamy, Ananda and Gopala Kristnayya Duggirala, transl. into English, with introduction and illustrations. (1917) *The mirror of gesture, being the Abhinaya darpana of Nandike vara*. Cambridge: Harvard University Press.

Ghosh, Manomohan (Ed. with an introduction and various readings.) *The Natyas astra, ascribed to Bharata-Muni*. Calcutta: Manisha Granthalaya.

Kersenboom-Story, Saskia C. (1987) *Nityasumangal: devadasi tradition in South India*. Delhi: Motilal Banarsidass.

Kothari, Sunil. (2001) *K cip di, Indian classical dance art*. New Delhi: Abhinav Publications.

Kothari, Sunil. (1989) *Kathak, Indian classical dance art*. New Delhi: Abhinav Publications.

Kothari, Sunil. (1979) *Bharata natyam, Indian classical dance art*. Bombay: Marg.

Kothari, Sunil and Avinash Pasricha. (1990) *Odissi, Indian classical dance art*. Bombay:Marg.

Marglin, Frédérique Apffel. (1985) *Wives of the god-king: the rituals of the devadasis of Puri*. Delhi and New York: Oxford University Press.

Mukherjee, Bimal & Sunil Kothari (eds.) *Rasa: the Indian performing arts in the last twenty-five years*. Calcutta: Anamika Kala Sangam.

Narayanan, Kalanidhi. (1994) *Aspects of abhinaya*. Madras: Alliance Co.

Singh, Shanta Serbjeet (ed.) (2000) *Indian dance: the ultimate metaphor*. New Delhi: Bookwise India.

Vatsyayan, Kapila (1981). *A study of some traditions of performing arts in eastern India: margi and desi polarities: Banikanta Kakati memorial lectures, 1976*. Gauhati: Dept. of Publication, University of Gauhati.

Vatsyayan, Kapila (1976) *Traditions of Indian folk dance*. New Delhi: Indian Book Co.

Vatsyayan, Kapila. (1974) *Indian classical dance*. New Delhi: Publications Division, Ministry of Information and Broadcasting, Govt. of India.

Vatsyayan, Kapila. (1968) *Classical Indian dance in literature and the arts*. New Delhi: Sangeet Natak Akademi.

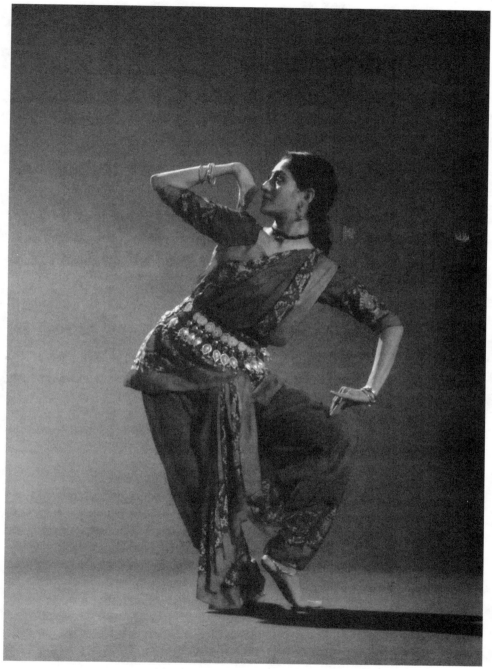

Odissi, Dancer Ananya Chatterjea.
Courtesy of photographer Eric Saulitis.

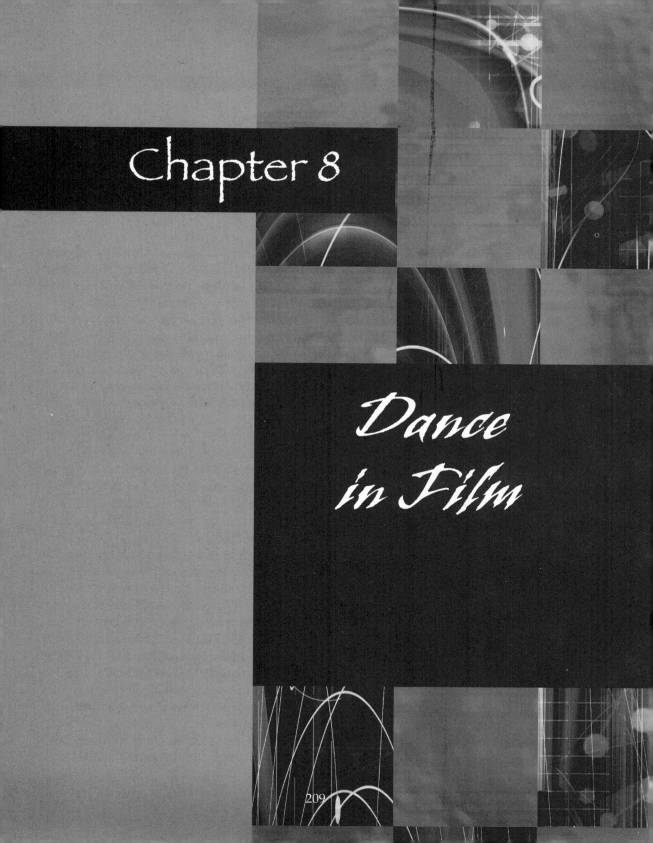

Chapter 8

Dance in Film

Dance in Film

Beth Genné

From the very beginning, dance was a major subject of the new twentieth century art form called cinema, first presented to the public by the Lumière Brothers in Paris in 1895 and soon after by Thomas Edison in New York in 1896. The coming together of the camera and choreography created a new art form: film dance. Film dance, for the first time in history, preserved what had been an ephemeral art form. Like painting and sculpture, film dance can survive the death of the artist. The new medium also offered new visual perspectives on the dancer and the choreography—perhaps the biggest change in Western dance since the invention of the proscenium frame stage. With the moving camera, the dancer and the dance could be seen from any angle and the special effects of editing, lighting, and, in the later years of the twentieth century, digital imagery, would add a new dimension to dance and the dancer on film.

Film also brought dance to new audiences not only in the United States, but all over the world. The vast majority of film dance in the first half of the century was produced in Hollywood, California, as part of the musical films that, with the American Western, were among the most popular film genres between the coming of sound in 1927 and the midfifties when the Hollywood studio system began to slowly fall apart. Movie houses were fixtures of tiny towns as well as big cities and a ticket to the "pictures" was an affordable treat even during the Great Depression in the 1930s. A weekly trip to the movies was a standard part of American social life in the first half of the twentieth century. At the local movie house courtships took place, special occasions were celebrated, and people just got away from it all for a while. In this climate, movie stars became household names and among these stars were dancers: Fred Astaire, Ginger Rogers, Gene Kelly and others. Even those who couldn't see them regularly knew their names and followed their fortunes. The teenage Anne Frank, in hiding during World War II in Amsterdam, had a photo of Ginger Rogers pasted on her bedroom wall, and eagerly awaited delivery of the latest movie news. Artists and intellectuals like Simone de Beauvoir and Jean-Paul Sartre also loved movie dancers like Astaire and Rogers as did people from all classes and callings. They sang their songs, went to ballroom dance class with their images in mind and, outside of the United States, saw them as American icons.

Annabelle Moore may be American film's first choreographer. A follower of Loie Fuller, she manipulated her gossamer skirts to create sinuous and varied patterns in space. Her *Sun Dance* (1896) was an important part of the first press showing of the Edison films in New York City. She and Edison made use of the possibilities offered in the post-production phase of the film—each frame was painstakingly hand tinted to recreate the everchanging flow of light and color created by the swirl of her skirts. In France, George Mélies was fascinated with the movement of dancers and used them in his pioneering films, which explored the possibilities of dance as affected by editing and special effects.

Early modern pioneer Ted Shawn made one of the earliest dance motion pictures, *Dance of the Ages* (with Norma Gould) in 1913. With Ruth St. Denis, whom he married in 1914, he founded the Denishawn School, which would train many film dancers as well as the pioneers of American modern dance, Martha Graham and Doris Humphrey. The great silent film director, D. W. Griffith, insisted that all his leading ladies learn dance at Denishawn. Both Denishawn and their dancers appeared in D. W. Griffith's *Intolerance* (1916) and other silent films.

Dancers, too, joined the ranks of silent film actors. Anna Pavlova, one of the greatest of the Imperial Russian ballerinas, whose tireless touring brought ballet to a worldwide audience, brought her charismatic dancing and acting to the *Dumb Girl of Portici* (1916). The popular ballroom dance team Vernon and Irene Castle brought their theatricalized versions of ballroom dances to *The Whirl of Life* (1915).

The great romantic silent screen idol Rudolph Valentino was an accomplished dancer. In *Four Horsemen of the Apocalypse* (1921), his smoldering tango ignited the enthusiasm of countless fans and his sensuous body language made him one of the most popular screen idols of all time. Silent screen comics could also be seen as "dancers." W.C. Fields famously complimented Charlie Chaplin, describing him as "the greatest ballet dancer that ever lived."[1] He was referring to this comedian's brilliantly choreographed physical comedy. Chaplin did actually *dance* as well—or rather brilliantly satirized various dances in *Tango Tangles* (1914), *Tillie's Punctured Romance* (1914), *The Floorwalker* (1916), *Sunnyside* (1919) and *The Pilgrim* (1922). Perhaps most famously, he hilariously "choreographs" two dinner rolls in *The Gold Rush* (1925). In 1955, his sound film, *Limelight,* would focus on the relationship between a lonely Londoner and an aspiring ballerina. Chaplin, himself, is credited as the choreographer for the film, for which he also wrote the score.

In the final years of silent film, it was a *dance*—the Charleston—that came to symbolize a new generation and its era, The Jazz Age. The Charleston was featured in many movies recording the new and liberated life of the short haired, short skirted twenties "flapper" represented by Joan Crawford in silent films like *Paris* (1926) and *Pretty Ladies* (1927) and continuing in sound films like *Our Dancing Daughters* (1928) and *Our Modern Maidens* (1929).

The musical accompaniment of silent film dances like the Charleston depended on the talents of the local movie house pianist or organist, except in big cities where on special occasions symphony orchestras played specially commissioned scores for major releases. With the coming of sound to films around 1927, choreographers suddenly gained some control over the music that accompanied their dances. Suddenly composers and musicians were added to the staff of film studios to specialize in creating music especially for soundtracks. One of the first sound films in England featured a short dance by three of the centuries most famous dancers, Alexandra Danilova, Anton Dolin and George Balanchine, who would go on to make important contributions not only to the history of dance, but to the history of dance on film.

In Hollywood, the coming of sound resulted in a newfound popularity for the film musical, copying one of the great American art forms then burgeoning on the stage in New York. Song and dance formed the core of the film musical and a number of choreographers who had first appeared on Broadway were brought to Hollywood to work in the new medium. Among them was Busby Berkeley (1895–1976), who eagerly seized the opportunities for innovation provided by the new medium of sound film. His extended dance sequences, featured in films such as *Forty-Second Street* (1933) and *The Gold Diggers* Series (1933–38), used the moving camera to add another layer of excitement to the movement of dance itself. He choreographed the camera as well as his dancers. He placed his cameras on wheels or suspended them, like monorails, from the sound stage ceiling and exploited the new freedom of perspective thus offered on his dancers as his cameras glided high above them, swooped around them, and tracked through their legs. In doing so he, in Gene Kelly's words, "tore down" the proscenium arch frame of the stage as his dancers moved through seemingly unlimited space.[2]

Berkeley also created special effects achievable only in the controlled and spacious environment of the movie studio; he used dramatically lit, large masses of dancers, moving stages and props and creative editing devices that added yet more "movement" to the dance. As Berkeley explored the possibilities of the camera, he relied less and less on his dancers actually *dancing,* moving through space. They remained in relatively stable positions, moving parts of their bodies to form decorative patterns while the camera became increasingly more active than the dancers.

As Berkeley explains: "It wasn't because I didn't know how to create (dance) and do it, but I wanted to do something new and different. Something that has never been seen before. Had they ever seen seventy or a hundred pianos waltzing? Had they ever seen lighted violins before? The same goes for all my various formations. It isn't particularly the steps but what you do with them."[3]

Not to say that there were no solo dancers in Berkeley's films. His most famous star was Ruby Keeler (1909–1993). She helped popularize the jazz tap dance which had been developed by the melding of African American and Irish step dancers (see Constance Valis Hill article). Keeler, like most dancers in musical films, needed to be multi-talented: to sing as well as dance, for most dance numbers in films, as on Broadway, began with a song—and many of the dancers who performed in musical films came to be known as singers as well as dancers.

This was true of the next great star of the 1930s, Fred Astaire, who, like Berkeley, would bring his own innovations to film dance and whose dances to the songs written for him by the great American composers George Gershwin, Jerome Kern, Irving Berlin and Cole Porter would create some of the greatest dances of the twentieth century—or indeed in the history of dance. Born in Omaha, Nebraska, Astaire (1899–1987) began in vaudeville, teamed with his sister Adele, and moved on to star with her in musical comedy on Broadway and in London. Astaire's style drew on the Broadway dance styles of his teacher Ned Wayburn and absorbed influences from the great African American jazz dancers Buddy Bradley as well as John Bubbles and Bill "Bojangles" Robinson who Astaire knew and admired. (Astaire's tribute to Bojangles can be seen in his 1937 film *Swing Time*). In his films, Astaire performed his own distinctive form of jazz tap dance modified and transformed by influences from other dance forms like ballet and, most importantly, the theatricalized ballroom dances of Vernon and Irene Castle.

In most of his dances for films and in contrast to his African American jazz tap dance colleagues, Astaire was interested in the narrative and emotional aspect of the dance and its relationship to the plot of the film musical stories of which they were a vital part. Whatever else film musicals were about, courtship was always a major theme and Astaire's dances with his partner Ginger Rogers explored in movement the trajectory of growing affection between a man and woman in a form of expanded and theatricalized ballroom dance, combined, on occasion, with jazz tap.

Ginger Rogers (1911–1995), born in Texas, appeared first on Broadway and then went to Hollywood to work in the movies as both a dancer and dramatic actor. Rogers was an adept Broadway dancer but did not specialize in it. Working with Astaire, however, she became one of the foremost female dancers in films: her elegance, brilliant timing and comedic wit were displayed in both her solo work and with Astaire. Rogers and Astaire became among the top box office draws in Hollywood and around the world, consistently attracting large audiences to their movies, and enhancing and promoting the popularity of social dancing in the United States and abroad. They made ten films together—*Flying Down to Rio*, 1933, *The Gay Divorcee*, 1934, *Roberta* and *Top Hat*, 1935, *Follow the Fleet* and *Swing Time*, 1936, *Shall We Dance* in 1937, *Carefree*, 1938, and *The Story of Vernon* and *Irene Castle* in *The Barkleys of Broadway*, 1949. In these films, choreographed for the most part by Astaire and his colleague Hermes Pan, dance became the vehicle for the expression of a full range of emotions between a man and woman displayed in inventive and formally fascinating pas de deux which followed the ups and downs of what came to be seen as an iconic American romance. Their couple dances were both serious (e.g., "Cheek to Cheek" in *Top Hat*, "Never Gonna Dance" in *Swing Time*) and light hearted (e.g., "Isn't it a Lovely Day" in *Top Hat*, "They all Laughed" in *Shall We Dance*).

Along with these couple dances, Astaire also choreographed solos often artfully incorporating everyday inanimate objects into his dances: from his hat and cane to increasingly interesting "found" objects—golf clubs, chairs, tables, sofas, coat racks, and, in the "Slap That Bass" number in *Shall We Dance,* the working engine of an ocean liner. Astaire's dances, both with Rogers and his later screen partners, stand among the greatest of American dance of the period and became major influences on dancers and choreographers working in every genre, throughout the twentieth century, from

George Balanchine to Michael Jackson. They continue to exert their influence on new generations through DVD and video.

Unlike Berkeley, Astaire and his colleague Hermes Pan were interested in making the *dancer*, the human body shaping space, the focus of the viewer's experience. In doing so, they set new standards in dance filming. To this end Astaire (who had control over the filming of his dance sequences) kept camera movement to a minimum. He insisted on framing the whole of the dancer's body at all times with no close ups or cutting away to breakup the unified image of the dancer in space. Most of his dances were filmed in one take, so as not to break the coherency and flow of the choreography. But it is important to understand that Astaire's dances are not merely documents of stage performances. He took advantage of the greater latitude and space offered by the sound stage and, on occasion, the special effects offered in postproduction. The camera was placed and moved along with the dancers, so as to allow each audience member an ideal view of the dance, no matter the position of their seat in a movie theater—an effect impossible to create on stage.

When Astaire and his directors experimented with special cinematic effects they had a great impact on film dance. In the Bojangles number in *Swing Time*, Astaire used multiple image devices such as three giant silhouettes of himself. He also used slow motion effects in the dream dance in *Carefree* and incorporated distorted mirrors in the Fun House sequence in *Damsel in Distress*. These devices all had an impact on the future of dance. In addition, Astaire and his directors used outdoor locations and a moving camera in the "Things are looking up sequence" in *Damsel in Distress* in which Astaire danced through a wooded landscape with Joan Fontaine.

Another pioneer of film dance in the first decade of sound films was George Balanchine (1904–1983). Trained at the Russian Imperial Ballet School in St. Petersburg, Balanchine would leave his mark on dance in film between 1938 and 1942. Although he was not the first to present ballet dancers on film, Balanchine made Hollywood sit up and take notice of the art form that he eventually transformed into a modern American classical ballet style. The dancers, from his newly formed American Ballet whom he brought to Hollywood, were, with exception of Anna Pavlova, perhaps the most rigorously trained to appear in sound films until that point. The two ballets he choreographed for the *Goldwyn Follies* (1938), both featuring Vera Zorina and with specially written scores by Vernon Duke, set a model for film ballet. Balanchine demonstrated conclusively that an extended segment of modern ballet, without song or dialogue or overwhelming spectacle, could hold an audience's attention and effectively convey an emotional mood or narrative.

Balanchine admired both Astaire *and* Berkeley. He understood that film offered all sorts of new possibilities for dance. Like Berkeley and Astaire, Balanchine directed as well as choreographed his segments—and his approach to film dance fell somewhere in between the two. Like Astaire, he focused on the human body in motion shaping space, but like Berkeley, he took advantage of the variety of perspectives offered by the moving camera and editing. He was the first major director-choreographer, before

Gene Kelly and Vincente Minnelli, to create the illusion of a seamless, full body centered performance, while moving the camera both to enhance the formal impact of the dance and at the same time convey a dance drama—a story in dance—using a variety of perspectives integrating close-ups, medium shots, low and high angled shots, and the editing required to integrate them without losing the flow and coherency of the dancer's movement or the drama. Balanchine worked with Vera Zorina (b. 1917), whom he married, in all his Hollywood films; in *On Your Toes* (a film version of the stage musical which Balanchine had also choreographed) Balanchine, as he had on Broadway, used the climactic "Slaughter on 10th Avenue" ballet to provide the denouement of the film narrative largely in dance terms reconceiving the dance for cinema and taking advantage of multiple camera set ups. In "That Old Black Magic" segment of *Star Spangled Rhythm,* he captured Zorina's dance with a swiftly moving camera and incorporated a special effect in which Zorina seems to jump from a photograph frame onto the bedside table of the lonely soldier who sings the song yearningly to her picture.

The interest in film musicals led to demand for good teachers in Hollywood. These teachers taught dance skills to Hollywood stars and chorus members, alike, as well as choreographing for many films. They included the Russian trained, former *Diaghilev's Ballets Russes* dancer Theodore Kosloff (1882–1956) and London trained Ernest Belcher (1882–1973), both of whom opened important dance schools in Los Angeles. Viennese ballerina Albertina Rasch (1896–1967), like Kosloff and Belcher, introduced classical ballet technique to Hollywood and its dancers. The great Russian choreographer Bronislava Nijinska (1891–1972) became an important teacher in Hollywood as well, training future dancers not only for the ballet stage (like Maria Tallchief) but film dancers, like Cyd Charisse who would become one of the most prominent dancers of the 1940s and '50s. Nijinska, herself, choreographed one film, *A Midsummer Night's Dream* (1935), directed by Max Reinhardt.

The brilliant African American jazz tap dancers of the first half of the century, whose creations were so vital to the development of jazz dance, were largely barred by race prejudice from film stardom. They did appear in feature motion pictures— but too often in short, easily cut cameo appearances. These all-to-brief appearances have immortalized their artistry, providing some of the most exciting moments of dance on film: John Bubbles in *Cabin in the Sky,* Harold and Fayard Nicholas in *Stormy Weather* and *Down Argentine Way* and Bill "Bojangles" Robinson dancing alone and with Shirley Temple in the *Little Colonel.* A number of film shorts also featured their dancing.

Race prejudice also affected the film career of the African American choreographer, Katherine Dunham (b. 1912), who made several films, but like her male colleagues, was often relegated to short segments. Dunham revolutionized modern dance with her use of dance sources from the Caribbean and West Indies culled, in part, from her research as a student of anthropology at the University of Chicago. She choreographed and appeared as a dancer in both feature length and short films including *Carnival of*

Rhythm (1941), *Star Spangled Rhythm* (1942), *Stormy Weather* (1943), *Casbah* (1948) and in the Italian film *Mambo* (1955).

In the forties a new generation of dancers and choreographers, like Dunham, brought new innovations to dance on film at the same time that they built on the advances of their predecessors. The most important worked at Metro Goldwyn Mayer (MGM) studios, which would become famous for its dance musicals of the forties and fifties.[4]

The forties saw the turn from black and white to color film. Director Vincente Minnelli explored the potential of dance and color film. Working with a roster of distinguished cinematographers, including Charles Rosher, Harry Stradling, Joseph Ruttenberg and John Seitz as well as costume designer Irene Sharaff, Minnelli incorporated brilliant light and color effects into his dance sequences with Fred Astaire and Lucille Bremer in *The Ziegfeld Follies* (1946) and *Yolanda and the Thief* (1945). These works set a new standard for the film "ballet," or dance drama sequences, that became an increasingly regular part of film musicals as well as their stage counterparts in the forties and fifties. Minnelli followed Balanchine, in his dancer centered ballets, seamlessly editing together a variety of camera angles to convey a coherent dance drama or mood without sacrificing the formal coherency of the dance. Minnelli, like Berkeley, especially delighted in the use of the moving boom camera (a camera mounted on wheels and attached to a crane, which moved in height, as well as on the ground) but he eschewed Berkeley's emphasis on spectacle for spectacle's sake. Minnelli went on to direct some of the landmark dance film musicals of the century, working further with Fred Astaire in *The Bandwagon* (1953) and in *The Pirate* (1947), *An American in Paris* (1951), and *Brigadoon* (1954) with Gene Kelly with whom he would create one of the most productive partner ships in film dance. Together and separately the two would revolutionize dance in film in the 1940s and '50s.

Gene Kelly (1912–1996), born in Pittsburgh, Pennsylvania, joined Fred Astaire as the major male dancer in films in the first half of the century. He spent much time on the streets, and the rough and tumble sports he learned there, as well as gymnastics, strongly influenced his choreography. He also grew up with the movies—idolizing silent film actors like comic Charlie Chaplin and romantic swashbuckler Douglas Fairbanks, who could create drama and comedy with their choreographed body language and virtuoso physical prowess. African American jazz dancers Dancing Dotson, who combined tap and acrobatics, and Frank Harrington, were also heroes. Other powerful influences included Russian ballet taught by his teacher, Berenice Holmes, a pupil and sometime partner of Adolph Bolm, and his contemporaries, the American modern dancers, Charles Weidman, Doris Humphrey, and Martha Graham. Kelly also learned Spanish dance forms and folk dance from his own Irish tradition. He blended these into a style that combined the emphasis on line and attention to upper body carriage of the ballet dancer, with the force and gravity of modern dance, the vernacular gestures of the street and the syncopated swing of jazz tap dance.

Like so many of his contemporaries in the world of stage dance, Kelly was interested in finding a uniquely American style, but unlike them, Kelly shaped his style within the new medium of cinema. A political progressive taught by the Great Depression and aware of the social issues of his time, Kelly deliberately made the choice to go to Hollywood. He wanted to present his work to people who could not otherwise afford to see dance. The working class dance persona he projected differed from Astaire's casual, elegant, Anglo-American image. Kelly's forceful, athletic dances fit with his stockier and clearly muscled body—the body of an athlete or physical laborer. His most famous dances, like *Singin' in the Rain* in the film of the same name, used gestures with which every American could identify—rhythmic walking, running, skipping, splashing, balancing on the curb and stomping, but transformed them into something extraordinary.

Kelly became an important director in his own right: the first dancer to extend his prowess as a director of the whole film. He collaborated with another young dancer and film maker, Stanley Donen (b. 1934), and together the two created some of the most innovative films of the 1940s and '50s beginning with sequences in *Cover Girl* (1944), *Anchors Aweigh* (1945) and *Take Me Out to the Ball Game* (1949). Kelly and Donen fully co-directed *On the Town* (1949), *Singin' in the Rain* (1952), and *It's Always Fair Weather* (1955). Together, they experimented with new sites for dance; the on-location opening for the opening number of *On the Town* was a landmark in film musicals. As in his *Singin' in the Rain* dance, Kelly often chose the long and extensive area of a city street as a dance site using the moving camera to photograph the dancer from a variety of angles thus eschewing Astaire's pavilions, ballrooms and nightclub floors. Kelly and Donen also experimented with new special effects in film dance combining the dancer and animated figures in *Anchors Aweigh*, when Kelly dances within an animated landscape with Jerry the Mouse ("The Worry Song") and multiple image effects in the "Alter Ego" dance in *Cover Girl* in which Kelly dances with a transparent image of himself to demonstrate the psychological conflict of a jealous lover. Donen later went on as a solo director to make several important dance musicals: most famously, *Seven Brides for Seven Brothers* (1954), choreographed by Michael Kidd, and *Funny Face* (1957) with Fred Astaire and Audrey Hepburn.

Kelly was also an important force, as Balanchine had been, in inviting classically trained dancers to the screen. He was responsible for bringing the young Leslie Caron, whom he first saw in Paris working with Roland Petit, and the *Ballets des Champs Elysées* to Hollywood to star in *An American in Paris*. In his ambitious all-dance film *Invitation to the Dance* (1956), he choreographed three ballets for dancers including Claude Bessy, Claire Sombert, Diana Adams, Igor Youskevitch, Tamara Toumonova and jazz dancer Tommy Rall. He was aided in this by the immense success of *The Red Shoes* (1948), a film directed by the English directors Michael Powell and Emeric Pressburger, which starred the young British ballet dancer, Moira Shearer, and also featured performances by Leonide Massine and Robert Helpmann. *The Red Shoes* concluded with a seventeen-minute ballet, which furthered the acceptance of pure dance sequences in films. *The Red Shoes'* impact on the development of film history was felt outside the world of dance and dance films as well. Martin Scorsese has cited it as one of his favorite films. Powell and Pressburger also asked the British choreographer Sir Frederick Ashton to create dance sequences for *The Tales of Hoffman* (1951), also featuring Moira Shearer.

Donald O'Connor (b. 1925) was also a major dancing star at Metro Goldwyn Mayer appearing in numerous musicals including *Call Me Madam, There's No Business Like Show Business* and *Anything Goes*. His virtuoso tap-dancing, acrobatic and comedic skills helped to make *Singin' in the Rain* a classic dance musical. His "Make 'Em Laugh" number, choreographed and improvised by himself, is probably one of the most famous dance comedy routines in movies.

Metro Goldwyn Mayer and other Hollywood studios also presented brilliant female dancers to movie audiences. Eleanor Powell, like many American dancers, studied a variety of dance forms: ballet, tap, social dance and what was then called "interpretive" dance. Her forceful and intricate tapping and cheerful up front American girl presence made her one of the most popular female dancing stars of the late 30s and '40s. Her many films include *The Broadway Melody of 1940* in which her tap duet with Fred Astaire to Cole Porter's "Begin the Beguine" is one of the most stunning of such displays in the history of film. Her choreographers often exploited her ability to perform in multiple styles blending acrobatics, tap and ballet in her dances and in films like *Honolulu*, the Hula. The forceful and enthusiastic Ann Miller (b. 1919) also combined jazz tap, acrobatics and social dance in numerous musicals including landmark films: *Easter Parade* (1948), *On the Town* (1949), and *Kiss Me Kate* (1953). Miller's hilarious interpretation of an inept but enthusiastic would-be American ballerina, instructed by a Russian ballet master in Frank Capra's *You Can't Take It with You* gives insight into the popular American perception of expatriate Russian ballet masters in the 1930s and '40s. Rita Hayworth (born Margarita Carmen Cansino in 1918) came from a family of Spanish dancers and became one of the most elegant and virtuosic dancers in the movies. Hayworth's brilliant and varied dances with Astaire in *You'll Never Get Rich* (1941) and *You Were Never Lovelier* (1942) and with Kelly in *Cover Girl* (1944) are landmarks.

Cyd Charisse (b. 1923), perhaps the dominant female dancer in American musical films in the late '40s and '50s, was paired with both Gene Kelly and Fred Astaire in MGM films. A long legged and sensual sculptor of space with an impeccable sense of timing and phrasing and a beautiful line, her work in *Singin' in the Rain, The Bandwagon, Brigadoon* and *It's Always Fair Weather* displayed her skills in both jazz dance and a modern lyrical style which combined ballet and modern dance. In Rouben Mamoulian's film *Silk Stockings* (1956), a musical remake of Lubitsch's film for Greta Garbo, *Ninotchka*, Charisse was also a wonderful comedic actress. Playing a Russian commissar who falls in love with an American producer (Fred Astaire) during the Cold War, she ranges from playful and sensuous duets to lyrical and jazz dance solos.

Vera Ellen made several important films in the 1940s and '50s. She starred as "Miss Turnstiles" in *On the Town*, dancing with Gene Kelly to Leonard Bernstein's music "Day in New York Ballet" and with Fred Astaire in *Three Little Words* (1950) and *The Belle of New York* (1952). Leslie Caron, who first appeared in *An American in Paris*, continued on in musical films made to especially exploit her gamine charm as dancer and actress and her ballet background. They include *Lili* (1953), *The Glass Slipper* (1955), and *Daddy Long Legs* (1955), in which the ballet sequence was choreographed by her mentor, Roland Petit. Marge Champion (b. 1919) was another major presence in the forties and fifties films. She met her husband Gower Champion (1919–1980) when they were both pupils of her father, Ernest Belcher, and they became one of the most successful of dance partnerships in films of the fifties appearing together in films like *Give a Girl a Break* (1953), *Jupiter's Darling* (1955) and *Showboat* (1951). As a teenager, Marge Champion was the live action model for the Walt Disney animators: as Snow White in *Snow White and the Seven Dwarfs*, the Blue Fairy in *Pinocchio*, and even the dancing hippos in *Fantasia* (1940) which she helped to choreograph. Both Marge and Gower Champion would go on to work—both together and separately—as choreographers and dance directors in television and on Broadway.

The second half of the century saw the demise of the film musical as a popular form. From the 1960s, dancers, so easily employable in the first part of the century, now had to look elsewhere and the studio system that had housed and employed the numerous creative artists and technicians necessary to the creation of film dance, gradually fell apart. There were, however, some very important exceptions. Jerome Robbins (born Jerome Rabinowitz in New York in 1918) brought the dances from some of his most successful Broadway shows to film. They included *The King and I* (1956), *Fiddler on the Roof* (1971) and *West Side Story* (1961). Like Kelly and Astaire, Robbins demanded control over how his dances were filmed. His opening dance for *West Side Story* with its brilliant choreographed camera movement and rhythmic editing takes off from and develops innovations first brought to the screen by Kelly and Donen in *On the Town*. Robbins' painstaking, perfectionist approach to film dance slowed *West Side Story* filming and ultimately only Robbins was responsible for the direction of the opening number. The rest of the film was choreographed by Robbins but directed by Robert Wise. However, Robbins received a special Academy award "for his brilliant achievements in the art of choreography on film."

In *West Side Story*, Robbins took the Astaire-Kelly notion of the street dance and developed it further as his gang members, the Jets and the Sharks, did battle in dance along the streets of New York City. Robbins' style in *West Side Story* combined jazz dance, ballet and athletics and drew, like Gene Kelly's, on the close observation of American male behavior that he had been developing on Broadway and in ballets like *Fancy Free* and *Interplay*.

Agnes De Mille (1905–1993) also recreated and reconceived some of her Broadway dance sequences for film—most famously her dream ballet for the 1943 *Oklahoma* (film, 1955) in which Bambi Lynn and James Mitchell re-created the roles of the dream Laurey and Curley. Jacques d'Amboise enlivened de Mille's ballet sequence in *Carousel* (1956) playing the carnival barker who thrills the young daughter of Julie and Billy Bigelow. Working in the 1950s, De Mille, like Robbins, Kelly and Astaire, had to contend with the new wide screen processes of film (Cinemascope, Vista Vision and others). The wider than high format meant that choreographers again had to readjust their notion of the relationship of dancer to camera.

Robbins and De Mille, however, made their careers on the stage. The choreographer who followed Berkeley, Astaire and Kelly to become the next major force in film dance was Bob Fosse (1927–1987). Fosse began his career at MGM, appearing as a dancer in *Kiss Me Kate* (1953) and *Give a Girl a Break* (1953) and *My Sister Eileen* (1955), which he also had a hand in choreographing. His early dance persona and choreography drew heavily on the jazz ballet dance style developed by Gene Kelly. He was also strongly influenced by Astaire. However, Fosse quickly evolved a distinctive new choreographic voice, which he developed on both Broadway and in the movies. His dances for *Pajama Game* (1957) and *Damn Yankees!* (1958) reveal his off beat, witty, sexy style—concerned with isolations of limbs and torso often working in counterpoint to one another. *Sweet Charity* (1969) demonstrates the mature Fosse, both as choreographer and film director. The most radical step in a new kind of choreography for dance and the camera came in his award winning film *Cabaret* (1972) that used dance and music to examine the decadent political and artistic atmosphere of pre-World War II Berlin. In *Cabaret* Fosse expanded the jump cut editing of his predecessors—brilliantly juxtaposing dance with dramatic images to create an ironic commentary on both the choreography and the film's social context. He also increasingly moved away from the full body framing that had been the rule in films since Astaire, instead moving quickly and abruptly from close to medium to long shot in his later dance sequences thus giving the editing a new, more vigorous, pace. Fosse's *All That Jazz* (1979), winner of the *Palme d'Or* at the Cannes Film Festival, was openly autobiographical, interweaving episodes from a choreographer's personal and professional life and tackling psychological issues rarely seen in film musicals. Like Kelly and Donen, Fosse went on to apply his knowledge of choreography to the creation of movies not directly concerned with film dance, including *Star 80.*

Fosse and Robbins were interested in socially relevant themes that reflected the new political and social awareness and upheavals of the '60s and '70s and led to other such dance musicals. In the anti-Vietnam war musical *Hair* (1977), Twyla Tharp and her dancers explored the joys and fears of the pacifist counterculture in dance, chronicling the tale of a young draftee who is befriended by a group of hippies. *Saturday Night Fever* (1977) examined the anomie and restlessness of a young Brooklyn man who tries to see beyond the narrow world of his low-level job and teenage buddies. *Saturday Night Fever* both reflected and promoted the disco dance craze that swept the country in the 1970s and '80s in New York, becoming one of the most popular films of the second half of the twentieth century. *Saturday Night Fever* also created a new star. John Travolta was the first screen idol since Astaire and Kelly to be identified as a dancer. *Saturday Night Fever* was followed by sequels and a spate of disco dancing films. Emile Ardolino's film *Dirty Dancing* (1987), set at the beginning of the sixties, used dance to trace an upper middle class young woman's (Jennifer Grey) coming of age. Her worldview is challenged and forever changed by her relationship with a working class dancer. *Dirty Dancing* made a star of dancer Patrick Swayze who recreated the social, rock, jazz and Latin American dances of the fifties and sixties. *Flashdance* (1983) examined the difficult life of a single working class welder (Jennifer Beals) trying to make it as a dancer. *Flashdance* introduced another popular dance craze to a wider public: break dancing.

Herbert Ross (b. Brooklyn, New York, 1927), was another dominant presence in film dance in the second half of the century. Trained in both ballet and modern dance and also as an actor and dancer on Broadway, Ross was briefly resident choreographer of American Ballet Theatre. From 1959, he collaborated with his wife, American ballerina Nora Kaye, to bring dance subjects to film, including the story of the great *Ballets Russes* dancer, Nijinsky, and a portrait of life in a fictionalized American Ballet Theatre in *The Turning Point* (1977), featuring dancers Mikhail Baryshnikov, Leslie Brown and Shirley MacLaine. Ross also addressed the clash of dance and fundamentalist religion in small town America in the film *Footloose* (1984), starring Kevin Bacon.

Despite the relative unpopularity of the film musical form in the second half of the century, the explosion of interest in classical dance of the 1970s and '80s resulted in a number of films focusing on the world of ballet and exploiting the talents and sensational notoriety of the dancers who had defected from the Soviet Union (then cut off from the United States by the Cold War). Rudolph Nureyev appeared in and, as choreographer, made several movies including *Romeo and Juliet* (directed by Paul Zimmer, choreographed by British Sir Kenneth MacMillan) and his own productions for the Australian ballet, *Don Quixote* 1973, (after the nineteenth century choreographer, Marius Petipa). Mikhail Baryshnikov appeared not only in Ross's *Turning Point* but also with jazz tap dancer Gregory Hines in the cold war thriller *White Nights* (1985). George Balanchine's ballets *A Midsummer Night's Dream* (1967) and *The Nutcracker* (1993) were released as feature films. And British choreographer Frederick Ashton choreographed *Peter Rabbit and The Tales of Beatrix Potter* (1971), starring members of the Royal Ballet in the beloved characters of Peter Rabbit and other of Potter's characters.

Set in Australia, Baz Luhrmann's *Strictly Ballroom* (1992) drew on the immensely popular culture of competition ballroom dancing which had spread from the West all over the world. So too, did the Japanese film, *Shall we Dansu?* (1997) in which a Japanese businessman learns to dance (and to live) in his off-hours; it drew for its title on the *Shall We Dance* sequence of Robbins's *The King and I*. More recently, ballroom dance films including American remakes in 2004 of *Shall We Dance* and *Dirty Dancing (Dirty Dancing: Havana Nights*) as well as *Take the Lead* (2006) and the documentary *Mad Hot Ballroom* (2005) have introduced new audiences to dance as means of self-discovery and revitalization. In the world of ballet, *Billy Elliot* and *Center Stage* (both 2000) traced the professional journeys of aspiring young ballet dancers, while the 2005 documentary, *Ballets Russes*, introduced audiences to their progenitors in the great tradition of Russian ballet. *Moulin Rouge* (2001) and *Chicago* (2002) and most recently *Idlewild* (2006) drew inspiration from the film and stage musical dance forms developed in the first part of the century. *Chicago* was originally conceived by Bob Fosse for Broadway and the editing and camera movement techniques of both *Chicago, Moulin Rouge* and *Idlewild* owe much to him and to the MTV generation of directors who have brought their own digital-age devices to expand and enhance screen dance.

It is too soon to know whether or not *Moulin Rouge, Chicago* and *Idlewild* herald a new age of dance film musicals. Film dance has not thus far regained the popularity it enjoyed in the first half of the last century in the West. However, dance remains a vital part of film in the so-called "Bollywood" films of South Asia. The huge film industry based in Mumbai (formerly Bombay) turns out more films every year than Hollywood in its heyday, and regularly produces films with extensive dance sequences that combine South Asian dance influences with the popular dance styles of the West. Whether drama or comedy, most Bollywood films contain dances and their most popular stars—both male and female—must be skillful dancers as well as actors. Dance numbers in movies such as *Kaho Naa . . . Pyaar Hai* (Say . . . . You Love Me) (2000) starring Hrithik Roshan and Amisha Patel show influences from the courtship dances of Astaire, the street and location dances of Kelly, the spectacles of Busby Berkeley and the dances of MTV stars like Michael and Janet Jackson. These are blended with movements from classical, folk and popular Indian dance forms as well as Western popular dance from swing and disco to break dancing. Indian directors also employ and are expanding the repertory of color and lighting effects, camera movement and musical editing developed in Hollywood to add to the drama and excitement of film dance. Bollywood musicals draw huge and devoted audiences not only on the Indian subcontinent, but also throughout Southeast Asia, Japan, and Africa. They are also becoming increasingly popular in Great Britain and United States—countries where the Indian population is substantial and continues to grow, and where second generation directors like Gurinder Chada offer audiences their own distinctive take on the blend of East and West as in Chada's *Bride and Prejudice* (2004).

In the West however, film dance has moved for the most part to television, where the MTV culture has popularized dance. Michael Jackson (b. 1958), perhaps the most popular and influential male dancer since Kelly and Astaire—and influenced by them both—brought the dancing star back firmly into mainstream popular culture with his dance videos. Choreographed by Michael Peters (1948–1994), Jackson, himself, and others and directed by luminaries such as Martin Scorsese (*Beat It)* and John Landis (*Thriller 1983)*, Jackson's "mini-musicals" have evolved directly from the tradition of Hollywood film dance, but expanded with digital imagery made possible by the computer age. In *Black or White*, for example, Jackson seamlessly morphs from dancer to leopard and back again and moves through a surreal, digitally enhanced landscape. Madonna (who was a modern dance major at the University of Michigan) and her choreographers also draw on the Hollywood film dance tradition as well as modern and social dance in her videos, as does Michael's sister Janet Jackson. Influential choreographers for film videos include Paula Abdul (b. 1963) and Vincent Paterson (b.1950).

African American street dance culture has been the other major influence on dance music videos—most notably those dances arising from hip hop culture—and including forms such as break dancing, popping, locking and other moves drawn directly from those created on the streets of New York, Philadelphia, Los Angles and Chicago by groups such as Rock Steady Crew (now called GhettOriginal). Although *Flashdance* (1983) brought break dancing into mainstream films, the form was more thoroughly documented in the films *Wild Style* (1982) and *Beat Street* (1984). Latin and Caribbean dance forms are also part of the rich multi-cultural dance video scene which incorporates Reggae, Salsa and other Latin American forms. This rich melting pot of dances is foundation and inspiration for the new millenium's first generation of dancers, choreographers and directors who are now making their mark on screen dance in the twenty first century.

Experimental Dance Film

Outside the mainstream Hollywood studio films with their populist tradition and mass audience base, a group of independent filmmakers combined choreography and camera work to create experimental dance films. These filmmakers allied themselves with the tradition of the European and American avant-garde and their relatively smaller and selfselected audience of artists, intellectuals and academics. Working within limited budgets but without the often-strict restrictions of length and censorship of subject imposed on Hollywood dance filmmakers, they produced innovative short film dance. Perhaps the most famous of early experimental dance films was the French painter Fernand Léger's *Ballet Mécanique* (1924) described by Arthur Knight as a "dance created out of the movement of levers, gears, pendulums, egg beaters, pots and pans—and incidentally people."[5] Like Leger, and later in Hollywood Busby Berkeley, experimental filmmakers used the moving camera and creative editing to make both bodies and inanimate objects "dance." But unlike Berkeley, experimental filmmakers were increasingly interested in suggesting nonnarrative, nonlinear imagery, thus evoking an emotional and aesthetic response rather than conveying a story in dance. Maya Deren's films beginning with *Meshes of the Afternoon* (1943) experimented with creative editing and printing techniques, the dancer's body and evocative lighting to create a dream-like, almost surrealist film dance vision. In her 1958 film, *The Eye of Night,* she collaborated with choreographer Anthony Tudor to give the illusion of dancers moving through horizonless space. Deren's other films include *At Land* (1944), *Choreography for the Camera* (1945) and *Ritual in Transfigured Time* (1946). Inspired by Deren, Shirley Clarke went on to create her own highly evocative film dances including *Bullfight* (1955) and *A Moment in Love* (1957). Canadian Norman MacClaren's *Pas de Deux* (1967) ingeniously traced the trajectory of the dancers' images as slowed by the camera; they moved, frame by frame, through space and time. MacLaren continued experimenting with variable camera speeds and other special effects in *Ballet Adagio* (1972) and *Narcissus* (1983).

Film was an important part of the post modern dance world in the 1960s and continues to be so today. Yvonne Rainer, Trisha Brown and their contemporaries at the Judson Theatre either created film dances or incorporated film into their live performances and that tradition has continued. Meredith Monk has created a number of challenging and evocative films including *Ellis Island* (1983) and *Book of Days* (1988). Choreographerdancer Amy Greenfield has focused primarily on film dance since 1970, creating numerous short films and a feature length dance film, *Antigone/Rites of Passion* (1991). Visual artist and choreographer Pooh Kaye has experimented with the integration of live action and animation, and also uses brilliant evocative color in her films, including *The Painted Princess* (1993). And "old master" Merce Cunningham's collaborations with film and video makers Charles Atlas and Elliot Caplan have resulted in a number of important dance films including *Atlas-Cunningham's Locale* (1979–80), *Channels/Inserts* (1981–1982) and *Coast Zone* (1983) and Caplan-Cunningham's *Points in Space* (1986) and *Changing Steps* (1989).

With the advent of the computer age and the increasing incorporation of digital imagery into the world of experimental dance films, as well as popular dance films and music videos, young choreographers and film makers continue to be attracted to the mediums of dance film and video—not only in the United States and Canada, but in Great Britain and Europe where an especially rich and varied dance film culture continues to grow and be nourished and enriched by the continually evolving new techniques in digital and other imagery and the enthusiastic collaboration of young choreographers and film makers. At the beginning of the twentieth century, dance is everywhere on television as well as easily obtainable at stores on DVD and video. The ability to buy and show DVDs and videos on computers and home television systems means that it is now possible for audiences to see and "re-see" professional dance in a way never before available in the history of the art of dance. Like books and recordings, dance performances will be preserved for the ages—people hundreds and (hopefully) thousands of years from now will be able to see what we saw and how we danced.

Notes

1. Fields quoted in Larry Billman, *Film Choreographers and Dance Directors: An Illustrated Biographical Encyclopedia with a History and Filmographies* (North Carolina and London: MacFarland & Co, 1995), 262.
2. Kelly quoted in ibid.
3. Larry Billman, *Film choreographers and Dance Directors* (Jefferson, North Carolina and London: McFarland and company, 1997), 35: Berkeley quoted from Bob Pike and Dave Martin, *The Genius of Busby Berkeley* in L. Billman, ibid.
4. These included Vincente Minnelli, Gene Kelly, Stanley Donen, Eleanor Powell, Cyd Charisse, Vera Ellen, Marge Champion, Lucille Bremer, Leslie Caron and choreographer-dancers and sometimes directors Charles Walters, Robert Alton, Jack Cole, Eugene Loring, Gower Champion, Nick Castle, Michael Kidd, Russ Tamblyn, Tommy Rall, Carol Haney, Jeanne Coyne and the designer Irene

Sharaff. Fred Astaire and his colleague Hermes Pan would continue their careers at MGM—as would, briefly, Busby Berkeley.
5. Knight quoted in Nancy Becker Schwarz and Jody Sperling, "Film and Video: Choreography for the Camera" in Selma Jeanne Cohen, ed. *International Encyclopedia of Dance* (London and New York: Oxford University Press, 2000), 603.

Bibliography

Altman, Rick. *The American Film Musical.* Bloomington: Indiana University Press, 1989.

Billman, Larry. *Film Choreographers and Dance Directors: An Illustrated Biographical Encyclopedia with a History and Filmographies,* North Carolina and London: MacFarland & Co, 1995.

Croce, Arlene. *The Fred Astaire and Ginger Rogers Book.* New York: Galahad, 1972.

Dodds, Sherill. *Dance on Screen: Genres and Media from Hollywood to Experimental Art.* London: Palgrave, 2001.

Delamter, Jerome. *Dance in the Hollywood Musical,* Ann Arbor: UMI Research Press, 1981.

Genné, Beth. "Dancin' in the Rain: Gene Kelly's Musical Films" in *Envisioning Dance on Film and Video.* ed. Judy Mitoma. London and New York: Routledge, 2002.

Hirschhorn, Clive. *The Hollywood Musical.* New York: Crown, 1981.

Jordan, Stephanie and D. Allen, ed. *Parallel Lines: Media Representations of Dance.* London: Libbey, 1993.

Mitoma, Judy, ed. *Envisioning Dance on Film and Video.* London and New York: Routledge, 2002.

Mueller, John. *Astaire Dancing.* New York: Knopf, 1985.

Prevots, Naima. *Dancing in the Sun: Hollywood Choreographers 1915–1937.* Ann Arbor: UMI Research Press, 1987.

Stearns, Marshall and Jean Stearns. *Jazz Dance: The Story of Amercian Vernacular Dance.* New York: Da Capo Press, 1973.

Thomas, Tony and Jim Terry with Busby Berkeley. *The Busby Berkeley Book.* New York: New York Graphic Society, 1973.

Chapter 9

Dance and Video Technology

Who's Dancing the Dance?

Jennifer Predock-Linnell

Interface: The theatre lights dim, the performance begins. Off to the side of the stage in the wings stand a man, a table and a laptop. The man's hands are poised on the computer, his eyes focused on the female solo dancer. Miniature, mobile, robotic video cameras traverse back and forth at the front edge of the stage on tracks. The dancer, dressed in a 'wired' body suit with hidden transmitters, is wearing pressure sensitive switches that activate sound and music bites and movement from the screen through the laptop computer. The screen at the back of the stage remains blank, waiting for an image from the movements of the dancer to then be projected onto the screen in "photo-realism" images. The computer becomes the tool for the nondancer, (the man) to organize and choreograph digital movements elicited from the wired dancer's body. With its industrial robot-like arms and legs, the dancer's movements are limited to flailing and thrashing, actions that induce images of a trapped animal.

Moving out of the twentieth century and grounding ourselves in the twenty-first century, the media culture has come to inhabit and influence every facet of our lives. Technology is a part of our daily lives. We wear technology inside and outside of our bodies and although we revel and indulge in their use, we also carry fears of their perceived control over our lives. Babies are lulled to sleep to the electronically simulated sounds of their mother's heartbeat. Animals talk in movies. We walk, work, cook, run, sit plugged into pre-recorded sounds or transmitted voices. Global and universal images are broadcast into private and public spaces connecting us immediately to foreign galaxies or the horrors of hate and destruction. A quick daily fix of TV is just as common in our morning routine as a sip of caffeine. A flip of the television channel and we instantly become mimetic dancers in our own living rooms.

From the early part of the twentieth century, and progressing rapidly into the twenty-first century, dance and technology have had a close, reciprocal relationship with each other. Have dance and technology created a new visual vocabulary? If so, what are the elements?

Some of the digital media tools applied to dance practice today are motion capture and choreographic animation, interactive and real-time performance software that manipulates image and sound for dance performance. Dance in digital and telematic spaces refers to web-dances, dancing on line, and remote performance collaborations. Some dance technologies include motion-sensing systems, which connect movement with sound, video and text. Contemporary dance has had an intimate relationship to the shifting, evolving fabric of technology and pop culture. In the past few decades, dance has become rooted within the visual world of media technology and digital art. Yet dance and technology may appear to be strange bedfellows, co-existing yet conceptually colliding.

Dance—the art of movement in time and space—is all about humanness. It is about live, visceral bodies, physical display, breath, sweat, muscles and skin. Dancing and dances are ephemeral, moving bodies charged with emotional and psychological meaning that momentarily electrify a prescribed performance space. Movements vanish as quickly as they appear. Real dance bodies make mistakes; mistakes in turn can then become a resource for problematizing a creative dance idea. Dancers forget steps, dance out of sync with other dancers, perform an improvisation, and make conscious choices to re-interpret a choreographic sequence. A dance performance is never repeated or embodied exactly the same way by the same dancer. A dance experience embodies training, rehearsal, creative process, performance and reception. Expression, form, content, meaning, organic or embodied dance techniques and memories that intersect with culture and consciousness are contextually located in the dance and the dancing body. Dance is a process-oriented live art with an insistence on presence and on the sensory materiality of the body. Dance focuses on the corporeality of the body. "[Live] bodies have dimensions, orientations, inclinations, weights, stances, and postural alignments," they *live in space*.[1] Technology's most complex form ultimately is of course the human body.

Technology is all about pixels, chips, wires, cameras, sensors, transmitters, tapes, film, CD-ROMs, animation, computers, cyberspace, projections, etc. A digitized or animated dance is performed flawlessly each time it is viewed yet the virtual or "motion capture" body we witness reveals no flesh, no muscular delineation, only a ghost of an outline of an image; there is the lost pleasure of admiring a well trained, sculptured dancing body. Moving bodies can be choreographed inside a flat frame on a computer then projected onto a larger screen(s); movement can be interfaced with living bodies or transmitted across continents. Illusions and suspension of time and space are manipulated. Motion capture technology has moved dance beyond flesh and breath to phantom-like, skeletal figures and "dots in space" that primarily exist in cyberspace. Bodies become transparent. Yet despite their differences, the complex, historically evolving dialectic of live dance, screened dance and now digitized dance continues. Choreographers, video artists, filmmakers, techno/computer scientists and sound and lighting designers are collaborating together continuing an experiment that mirrors the rise of technology itself.

Who, historically, has been responsible for the introduction of these elements? Dance moved from gaslight in the nineteenth century to electricity. Loie Fuller, The

Futurists and Oscar Schlemmer were some of the early dance artists who experimented with the beginning of the technological world. During these periods of experimentation artists broke away from humanizing the body to a more mechanical view of the dancing. Suddenly the body was able to dismiss all the Romantic notion of presenting the body on stage. The early use of technology allowed us to almost x-ray the body to display its physical life.

How did this visual vocabulary become recognized? In the 1890s Loie Fuller was the first dancer to exploit electricity. Appearing to escape the human, Fuller created lighting effects, along with enormous amounts of draperies, to transform her body into a variety of flowers, butterflies, etc.

Early influence of technology on contemporary dance came from photography, recorded sound, and film. Photography froze, contained and framed spatial images contextualizing the evolutionary history of contemporary dance through dance styles, costumes, and body representation. These images tell us who was doing what, where, how and why. Photographs of dancers taken at unguarded moments reveal performative nuances, the flow or truncated energy of the body in space. The mechanical reproduction of photography recorporealizes the body and locks it in time forever. Recorded sound liberated dance making and dancing from the financial burdens and the limitations of live musical performance. Records, tapes and now discs influenced the creative process of dance making through various forms of sound design-recording and inventing sound, re-mixing, looping and designing sound collages. Multiple track recording and digital engineering has transformed our sense of musical time and space through fragmentation and dispersion, which in turn has influenced current dance styles and movement invention. From us, recorded sound elicits emotional, psychological, intellectual, and physical responses through dance films and videos, as an audience member or performer at a dance/theatre concert, in a studio rehearsal, or at a rave club. How does this new visual vocabulary become established?

The evolving technology of film began in the early part of the twentieth century with the end of the 'silent era,' and again in the 1930s with the creation of Hollywood's film musicals. Video appeared in the late 1960s, when Sony gave us portable video. Once liberated from the still frame of photography the genre of Dance For the Camera has been practiced with considerable vigor over the course of the last 100 years. "Currently, given the availability and increased awareness of new media in the form of web sites, cd-rom and digital technology, dance again finds itself the object of much [attention] within the frame . . . [One] of the most recognizable features of dance for the camera is the attempt to fix ephemeral moments written by dancing bodies and render them in the medium of film or video." What is seen on the screen is less momentary. The image lives in the realm of timelessness and imagination. "From the earliest days of photography, the body has been a constant source of subject matter . . . we (have come to) see in film and later video the changing morals and attitudes toward the body."[2] As a documentary vehicle, film created a "moving" history of dance that became an educational and ethnographic resource for dance studies. Videos, computers and CDs are now used in abundance in dance education, performances, workshops, and and have replaced film.[3] Photography, recorded sound and film became part of a developing visual vocabulary that was forming in the dance culture because of technology. The development of this language—light, sound and film/video—created a new environment in which to explore dance performance, new layers of a new visual language in the making. How are these new layers going to be integrated with the dance and the performer?

The current waves of contemporary dance include physical theatre/dance, new dance, hyper dance, video dance and digital dance. Dance companies like Merce Cunningham, Bill T. Jones, Lloyd Newson's DV8 Physical Theatre, Wim Vandekeybus's Ultima Vez, Edoudard Lock's LaLaLa Human Steps, Meredith Monk, Trisha Brown and Lucinda Childs have been exploring and integrating film, video and computer generated images into their creative process and performance theatre since as early as the 1960s. The counterculture of the 1960s brought us an era of self-examination. The age of video art overlaps the coming out of post modern dance and the Judson Church. In 1963 the presentation of film *as* dance became a choreographic concept that was explored in Concert 1 by a number of artists associated with the Judson Dance Theatre. Trisha Brown, a fledgling member of JDT, performed a solo, *Homemade,* with a film projector strapped to her back. "As Brown moved, the projector haphazardly cast an image of her doing the same dance, with the projector, around the space . . . [resulting in] a playful duet between choreographer in the flesh and celluloid alter ego."[4]

The major visual vocabulary was put in place the later part of this century. Dance artists and technologists began to come together for the purpose of forging a new dance art form creating a new environment for dance. Choreographer Lucinda Childs created a multidimensional dance/film work, *Dance* (1979) with music by Philip Glass and film/setting by Sol LeWitt at the Brooklyn Academy of Music, during the time large-scale intermedia productions were being promoted. Contemporary Critic Susan Sontag gives this work a rather metaphysical, early modernist reading:

> The synchronized ongoing of film and dance creates a double space: flat (the scrim/screen) and three-dimensional (the stage); provides a double reality, both dance and its shadow (documentation, projection), both intimacy and distance. Recording the dancers from different angles, in long shot and close-up, LeWitt's film tracks the dancer sometimes on the same level, sometimes above—using split screen and multiple images. Or it immobilizes them, in a freeze-frame (or series of still shots) which the live dancer passes through.[5]

As choreographers and filmmakers began to work together with more frequency, they had to find new ways to relate dance and camera. The difference between performance space and film space was heightened by movement capabilities of the camera itself and new conceptual issues concerning the relationship between

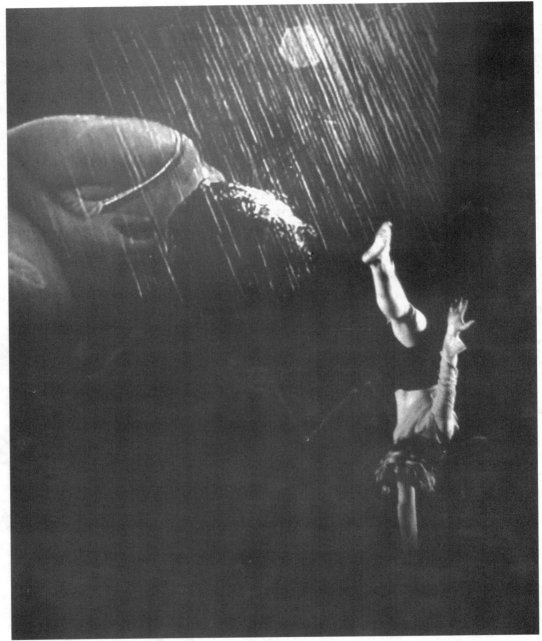

"No Visible Trace," 1999. Dancer Rebecca Blackwell Hafner.
Choreagraphy by Jennifer Predock-Linnell.
Courtesy of photographer John Bauer.

the filming process and postproduction process (editing and manipulation of the filmed images).[6]

Coming from the Futurist drive, the next 'anti-romantics' choreographer Merce Cunnigham and designer/director/choreographer/conceptual artist Robert Wilson massaged time, repetition, and abstraction and layered their productions with projections and film. Now there is a new dance/visual language that Cunningham and Wilson have created since Fuller, the Futurists and Schlemmer. These two artists began to integrate the dance performer into this new expressive art form; the dance is a partner in a bigger vocabulary.

Cunningham's interest was bringing technology into the dance performance. He didn't do anything in particular to alter his dancer's bodies with the use of technology. Instead there was a coalescing of technology and dance in his works. Cunningham began to add layers of complex sound scores, complex visual scores in combination with what the dancers were performing live. Cunningham may perhaps be considered the supreme dance/techno maker who has routinely utilized computer technology as an essential component of his choreographic process. He was also one of the first to raise questions "about issues of creativity, representation, mechanization in their exploration of the possibilities of using computer technology for dance."[7]

> One can wonder about the accuracy of expression which will be possible. Can the soul of a dance be animated? Or is it too much to ask . . . Can the effort of a movement be computerized? . . . we must always remember that dancing is for people.[8]

By the mid-seventies, Cunningham began to show an interest in figure/character animation and visual space composition. Cunningham began to videotape his performances and choreograph videodances in collaboration with film and videomaker Charles Atlas. Their collaborative projects for television, their experimental films and video dances were challenged by the problem of filming dancers effectively [and convincingly] within film and video space.[9] Also, different technologies produce different illusions of movement. Film has a temporal character based on its production and re-assemblage process while the electronic image transmission has a more spatial character with its flatness and lack of depth. The transition from dance to video image or digitized/manipulated image is not fluid; whatever dynamic movement video and computer can simulate in "real time," they cannot capture the full spatial context, nor can they adequately compensate for body heat, sweat, breath and visceral and tactile feedback.[10]

Cunningham's nonfrontal use of space in his dance works influenced his affinity for screen choreography. His collaboration with film/video maker, painter Elliot Caplan began in the 1980s. Together they exploited the camera's ability to show dance from a variety of vantage points, creating memorable video dances such as: *Points in Space* (1986), *Changing Steps* (1989), *Beach Birds for Camera* (1991–92), and *CRWDSPCR* (pronounced "crowd spacer") (1993).[11] As a painter and filmmaker,

Caplan was trained to "see" and to work with the film screen as a canvas. Caplan explains:

> One of the ways I apply the notion of process in filmmaking is by taking advantage of details that occur behind the main action both in picture and in sound . . . In film [small] details of movement are perceptible to the viewer. The details can be a dancer's hand moving or the twitch of an eye which conveys their own rhythms and when seen become part of of the overall experience. I look for these events and accent them as a way to exaggerate movement and convey choreographic ideas.[12]

Robert Wilson was influenced by Cunningham's aesthetic. In 1976 Wilson wrote and directed *Einstein on the Beach* and forever changed the image of opera with advanced technology. Wilson and his collaborator, composer Philip Glass, emerged from the New York art world from the 1960s and began collaborating when musical theatre was at the center of experimentation in the arts. *Einstein* was an opera where dancers were the featured performers. Wilson challenged our ways of seeing and hearing. He asked the spectator to re-think the definition of opera. He thought about gesture, lights, movements, sound and stage environments as separate objects and took these scenes of visual images along with slide projections and billboard-like light walls and layered them against each other. There was no obvious link between words, music, image or movement. According to Wilson, there was no narrative, the opera did not tell a story. Instead it gave a poetic interpretation of Einstein.[13]

Lucinda Childs, a founding member of the Judson Church Dance Group, was the main choreographer. Her choreography produced a whole mechanization of the performing body that made the dancer appear as a mechanical robot-like moving image. Cunningham and Wilson's productions showed us how this period broke away from humanizing the body in favor of a more mechanical view of the body. Cunningham and Wilson didn't do anything particular to the dancer's body. They didn't change the body with or through technology. In the later part of the 20th century, there was a coalescing of technology and dance in the works of Cunningham and Wilson. It gave us a different way of looking at the dance in the performance environment of the stage by adding to the dancer's movement a layering of complex sound scores, or visual scores in combination with what the dancer was doing physically and emotionally.

Now we have completely accepted this triangle of dance, technology and culture. We have seen how this partnership has developed over the past century and how we have come to acknowledge this marriage of dance and technology as a natural performance presentation.

How can we continue to look at the dance in the performance environment of the stage? By videoing a particular movement sequence or groupings of dancers, the movement viewed frontally or the group viewed from the side creates new interpretations of the movements within a prescribed space. New points in space will be created; the dynamic timing will become re-interpreted, viewed from an unfamiliar angle. When there is an interrelationship of live dance (real bodies moving in space) and the projected image of video or film, the performance space becomes even more visually complex. Projecting from behind, from above, from side angles, onto multiple projection surfaces, moving surfaces, or moving bodies begin to distort the traditional rectangular image space in ways that disturb the geometries in the space and in our visual perspective. What is then seen on the screen will become more dream-like; the image(s) lives in the realm of timelessness and imagination.

If a dance video work is created for particular dancers and the projected video images are replications of those dancers and the re-recorded images mimic the real dancers, the work cannot exist outside of those specific dancers. If by chance they are recreated or restructured for other dancers, the dance/video work becomes an interpretation of the original. The dancers who reconstruct the original piece are "filling in" and providing a "copy" of a particular creative process that the original dancers developed. At the same time, the imaged copy of the original dancers creates a "ghosting"—bodily memory juxtaposed or layered against the mimeticized body which now dances the dances of the "other's" memories and techniques.

One particular problem with video, sound, film and movement interlinking in a performance is that the mediated images and/or the sound could become stronger than the dance, especially since we are culturally conditioned now to be drawn to the mediated image, to the "big" screen image. The dance could then become a weakly illustrated movement language that failed to speak on its own terms in a reflective relationship to the content of the video or film. Or the video or film projection could end up looking decorative, disconnected, or overwhelming to the live dancers and the choreography if the choreographic mark is stronger than the mediated images.

Canadian director/writer Robert LePage[14] conceived one of the most convincing uses of video and live body interaction in his theatre/dance/video production, *The Far Side of the Moon* (2001). What made this production so successful is what lies at the heart of dance and theatre—transformation and connections. LePage transcended a body in space through the reflected illusion created by mirrors and chairs. Full-length mirrors[15] were suspended at the back of the stage and tilted on a 45° angle towards the audience. A row of straight back chairs were placed in front of the angled mirrors, only they were lying on their backs on the floor, facing the mirrors above. A man lay on the floor, sitting in one of the chairs looking up. What we saw from the viewer's perspective was the normal position of a man sitting in a chair upright, facing us. As the man gradually and progressively moved off the chair and onto the floor he moved in very slow motion, floundering across the floor away from the row of chairs. But what we saw from the mirrored reflection was the illusion of a man floating in space as if he had freed himself from gravity.

As more contemporary dance artists utilized dance and video in their productions, Cunningham had already moved on to newer, riskier, provocative dance technology. In 1989, Cunningham stepped into the world of computer technology and created new dances with computer-assisted choreographic software LifeForms™. *Trackers* (1991), *Beach Birds for Camera* (1991–92), and *CRWDSPCR* (1993)[16] were three of his early works that were conceived on Lifeforms, Cunningham's "living sketchbook" computer. The computer choreographic software LifeForms™, a 3D human figure animation software, was developed in1986 through a joint adventure between the Dance and Science Departments at Simon Fraser University in British Columbia.[17] Lifeforms™ functions as a compositional tool for the artist/choreographer to create realistic and accurate movement sequences in time and space and provides the artist with a mechanism for visualizing dance. Some of the digitized figures are drawn in concentric circles. The computer program allows artists to go beyond restrictive assumptions about movement. A choreographer could conceivably create, with the onscreen figure, individual chunks of movement for the torso, the arms and the legs (the legs, arms and torso do not correspond to anything each other are doing). The "live" dancers learn these individual and separate movements and then glue them together so they are all being performed on the dancing body at the same time. In other words, you are more or less "colliding" dissimilar parts of the body to create a whole moving body in time and space.

Lifeforms™ also acts as a memory device and as a method of preserving dances. If used in a studio class, a dance teacher or choreographer may put into the memory of the computer exercises that were given in class that then could be viewed later by the students forclarification of movement phrases.[18]

In conjunction with a group of computer artists, American born director and choreographer William Forsythe developed a very important educational tool that can be used by dance educators in choreography classes. He developed a CD-Rom, *Improvisation Technologies* for his Frankfurt Ballet Company, which documents and preserves his creative process in dance making. Fleeting, ephemeral moments of improvisational exploration become the seeds of a new dance, which are immediately captured and archived. A body-movement library can be accessed at any moment from the CD-ROM and further explored by the choreographer and/or dancers or revisited and remembered. These new forms of dance technology liberate the artist from trying to remember and recall movements s/he just created in a rehearsal.

Motion-capture is the most recent of the technological advances in this new world order of living bodies and digitized "sketches" of dancers moving across space and time. Several such collaborative creations were Cunningham's "Hand Drawn Spaces (1998), "Biped" (1999) and Bill T. Jones's "Ghostcatching" (1999). These three dances in collaboration with multi-media computer artists Paul Kaiser and Shelly Eshkar used this newer and more radical digital technology to fashion a dance minus the dancer. But these transparent dancing forms are stripped of all human life—no cells, blood, breath, skin, muscle, memory, impulse, intellect or psyche. They are simply representations of movements dancers created and performed. Lifeforms™ employed computer animated figures to generate new movement possibilities and to choreograph movement dancers would eventually learn to perform. Motion capture begins with living, breathing, three-dimensional bodies moving in three-dimensional space in a studio.[19] [Dancers perform] in front of a digital/video camera while wearing light

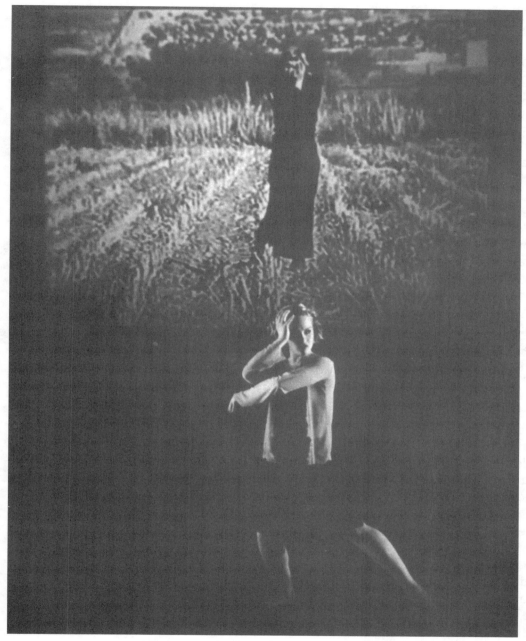

"No Visible Trace," 1999. Dancer Rebecca Blackwell Hafner.
Choreography by Jennifer Predock-Linnell.
Courtesy of photographer John Bauer.

sensitive disks called "motion capture sensors". . . . The movements of these sensors [were] optically recorded as "points in space" and then converted into digital 3D files . . . [which captured] the position and rotation of the body-in-motion without preserving its mass or musculature. Movement is thereby [captured] from the performer's body.[20] Hence the label, "motion-capture." The "real" body is now and forever plugged into virtual reality; it has become the temporal body in space devoid of any internal impulse that motivates the movement.[21]

Dance is traditionally a live performance form, in and of a space, and not visible externally to the performers. In the new world order of media culture, areas of dance/technology have become a digital package; you can make a piece of dance art, experience it yourself as intended at any stage in the future, and maybe even sell thousands of copies to the public either online, or in shops. Are we saying then that digital dance as a package can be sampled, recorded, edited, manipulated, reorganized, and that any movement image (dance) from any source/environment could thus be utililzed, produced on CD-ROM and subsequently distributed, implying the total portability, transportability, transmutability of the dance environment, just like music?[22]

These few examples of dance and technology are only the tip of the iceberg. Before the next word is printed, new technology will inhabit our lives. What was an innovative idea today has become a disposable item by tomorrow. Technology for dance has become a useful device in dance education. Through the use of the Internet, new artforms for expressing and sharing movement concepts can materialize and expand globally, creating new bridges of communication with cultures all over the world. It is now possible for choreographers from three or four different local or global locations to use collaborative online methods to share and respond to a variety of choreographic ideas as they collectively create a dance. One choreographer may create a virtual dance on a computer, send it to multiple choreographers asking or allowing them to add on, manipulate, subtract or re-arrange the initial dance structure. Although two minds might be better than one sensing and feeling through images and actions sent by others, this practice also signals concerns of directorship, ownership and appropriation, which will forge future debates between artists and viewers.

With these new forms—such as MIDI, motion capture, Digital—of technological dance making and dance performance, does there need to be a re-thinking of our current notions of what dance, performance, and interactivity are or should be? There are fundamental questions of whether sensor-base interactive technology really has any place within traditional choreographed dance performance. If it does, what would this place be and what forms would these works take? Are we, in fact, creating a new dance vocabulary, e.g., *cyberography* instead of choreography?

Technology in dance raises endless philosophical issues about performance and the value of the human body and human movement. In the virtual world of dance and technology how do we incorporate digital tools of composition into our creative

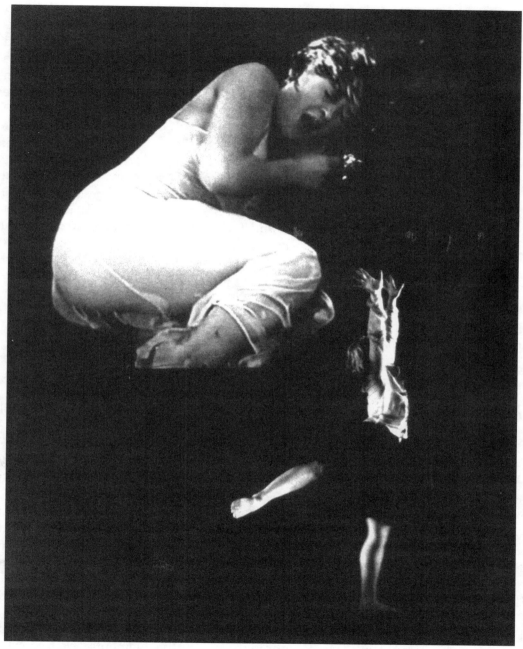

"No Visible Trace," 1999. Dancer Rebecca Blackwell Hafner.
Choreography by Jennifer Predock-Linnell.
Courtesy of photographer John Bauer.

process? How will projected computer-generated temporality and space (digitized form, content, movement, image, sound) affect the kinesthetic and psychological experience in our lived bodies? Have our creative work habits been permanently altered by this evolving partnership of dance and technology? What does all this mean for the future of dance, dance making, dance viewing and dance writing? The (re)definition of the phenomenon of dance and dance making, even ideas about space and time, have forged new meaning and intent.

Notes

1. Birringer, Johannes. *Media and Performance: along the border* (Baltimore and London: The John Hopkins University Press, 1998), 38.
2. Rosenberg, Douglas. "Opening Remarks and Manifesto," Dance for Camera Panel. International Dance and Technology Conference, Arizona State University, 1999.
3. For a comprehensive discourse on film and video for dance, see the section of "Choreography for Camera" under Film and Dance in the *International Encyclopedia of Dance*. Cohen, S.J. Ed. Vol. 2 (New York/Oxford: Oxford University Press, 1998), 603–612.
4. Ibid., p. 605.
5. Sontag, Susan. "For Available Light: A Brief Lexicon," *Art in America* 71 (December 1983) 102, quoted from Birringer, Johannes. *Media and Performance: along the border* (Baltimore and London: The John Hopkins University Press, 1998), 72.
6. Birringer, Johannes. *Media and Performance: along the border* (Baltimore and London: The John Hopkins University Press, 1998), 69.
7. Schipshorst, Thecla "Merce Cunningham: Making Dances with the Computer" Vaughan, David. ed. "Merce Cunningham: Creative Elements," *choreography and dance: an international journal* Vol. 4(3) (harwood academic publishers: 1997), 81.
8. Ibid., "From Notation to Video," *The Dancer and the Dance*. Marion Boyers Inc.: 1980) pp. 188–89. Quoted in Vaughan's *Merce Cunningham: Creative Elements*, 81.
9. "Choreography for Camera" in the *International Dictionary of Dance*. Vol. 6 (New York/Oxford: Oxford University Press, 1998), 607. One attempt to document dance on film is to convey a *feeling* of the stage event.
10. Birringer, Johannes, *Media and Performance: along the border*. (Baltimore and London: The John Hopkins University Press, 1998), 82.
11. Caplan, Elliot. "Dance on Film: Notes on the making of CRWDSPCR," quoted in Vaughan, David. ed. "Merce Cunningham: Creative Elements," *choreography and dance: an international journal* Vol. 4(3) (harwood adacemic publishers: 1997), 100.
12. Ibid., 102.

13. For a comprehensive examination of the making of "Einstein On the Beach" look at the VHS video of *Einstein On The Beach: The Changing Image of Opera*. The video presents interviews with Glass and Wilson plus clips of rehearsals and the restaging of the 1976 performance at the Brooklyn Academy of Music in New York City in 1984. Director and Photographer, Mark Obenhaus. An Obenhaus Film.

14. For further insight into Lepage's creative process see: Charest, R. *Robert Lepage, Connecting Flights*. (New York: Theatre Communications Group, 1998).

15. In Kent De Spain's footnotes from his article, *Dance and Technology: a Pas de Deux for Post-humans*, De Spain suggests "that mirrors were the first imaging technology to pull us out of our somatic experience, toward seeing aspects of the dancing as separate from ourselves." *Dance Research Journal* 32/1 (Summer 2000), 17.

16. Caplan, Elliot. "Dance on Film: Notes on the making of CRWDSPCR," quoted in Vaughan, David. ed. "Merce Cunningham: Creative Elements," *choreography and dance: an international journal* Vol. 4(3) (harwood adacemic publishers: 1997), 100.

17. See Calvert, T., Welman, C., Gaudet, S., Shiphorst, T., Lee, C., "Compostition of Multiple Figure Sequences for Dance and Animation," Visual Computer (1991), 7:114–121

18. Schiphorst, Thecla. "Merce Cunningham: Making Dance with the Computer." In Vaughan, David. ed. "Merce Cunningham: Creative Elements," *choreography and dance: an international journal* Vol. 4(3) (harwood adacemic publishers: 1997) 79–98. Also find information on Lifeforms™ at: www/wired.com/wired archives/ 4.10/ Schiphorst.html; www/mercelorg:80/technology/html; //hotwired./ ycos.com/kino/95/29/feature.

19. Copeland, Roger. "Dancing For the Digital Age: Merce Cunningham's Biped." *Proceedings of the Society of Dance History Scholars Twenty-Fourth Annual Conference*. Goucher College, Baltimore, Maryland, June 2001. (Fall 2001), 23–28.

20. Ibid.

21. For a lively discussion of Bill T. Jones's *Ghostcatching*, see Ann Dils' critical essay, "Absent/Presence" in Dils, A. and Cooper Albright. *moving history/dancing cultures: A Dance History Reader*. (Connecticut: Wesleyan University Press. 2001), 462–471.

22. Birringher, Johannes. *http://www.dance-techlists.acs.ohio-state.edu*. 4/8/99.

Bibliography

Auslander, P. *Liveness*. London and New York. Routledge Press. 1999.

Birringer, J. *Media and Performance: along the border*. Baltimore and London: The John Hopkins University Press, 1998.

_____. *http://www.dance-tech @lists.acs.ohio-state.edu*.

_____. A Report," NDA website: *http//www.aahperd.org/nda/ dance_mouse.html* _____.

"Environments: Dancing with Technologies," *Dance Magazine*, *http://www.dance magazine.com/sterns/bodytech_frame.html*.

Birringer, J. ed., "Connected Dance: Distributed Performance across Time Zones," hypertext essay with Ellen Bromberg, Naomi Jackson, John Mitchell, Lisa Naugle, and Doug Rosenberg, in "Transmigatory Moves/Dance in Global Circulation," *Congress on Research in Dance Conference Proceedings*, New York University, October 2001. 51–77.

Bolter, J.D. and Grusin, R. *Remediation: Understanding New Media*. Cambridge. MIT Press. 1999.

Caplan, E. "Dance on Film: Notes on the making of CRWDSPCR." David Vaughan, ed. "Merce Cunningham: Creative Elements," *choreography and dance: an international journal* Vol. 4(3) harwood adacemic publishers: 1997.

Calvert, T., Welman, C., Gaudet, S., Shiphorst, T., Lee, C., "Composition of Multiple Figure Sequences for Dance and Animation," Visual Computer. 1991.

Charest, R. *Robert Lepage, Connecting Flights*. New York: Theatre Communications Group, 1998.

Copeland, R. "Dancing For the Digital Age: Merce Cunningham's Biped." *Proceedings of the Society of Dance History Scholars Twenty-Fourth Annual Conference*. Goucher College, Baltimore, Maryland, June 2001.

DeSpain, K. "Dance and Technology: a Pas de Deux for Post-humans." *Dance Research Journal* 32/1. Summer 2000.

Dils, A. "Absent/Presence" in Dils, A. and Cooper Albright. *moving history/dancing cultures: A Dance History Reader*. Connecticut: Wesleyan University Press. 2001.

Gladstone, V. "Sereendance." *The Nation*. March 22, 1999. 31–34.

Feliciano, R. "Steady Souls." *http://www.dancemagazine.com/sterns/bodytech_frame.html*.

International Encyclopedia of Dance. Cohen, S.J. ed. Vol. 2. New York/Oxford: Oxford University Press, 1998.

_____. Vol. 6. New York/Oxford: Oxford University Press, 1998.

Kahlich, L. "Dance Technology—Moving into the Future." *Dance Research Journal*, 24(2):63–64, Fall 1992.

Keith, C. "Image After Image, the Video Art of Bill Viola." *Performance Art Journal*, H59. Vol. 44. no. 2. May 1998.

Lemmon, R. "Mirror and Smoke" *http://www.dancemagazine.com/sterns/bodytech_frame.html*

McKenzie, J. *Perform or Else: From discipline to Performance*. London and New York: Routledge Press. 2001.

Popat, S. Interactive Awakenings: Heightening Consciousness of the Dance Artwork for Artist and Audience Member. *Consciousness Reframed III: Art and Consciousness in the Post Biological Era*, Proceedings of the Third International Research Conference at the Centre for Advanced Inquiry in the Interactive Arts. Newport: University of Wales College. August 2000.

Popat, S. and Smith-Autard, J. "Dance-Making on the Internet: Can On-Line Choreographic Projects Foster Creativity in the User Participant?" *Leonardo*, 35(1):31–36. 2002.

Schipshorst, T., "Merce Cunningham: Making Dances with the Computer." David Vaughan, ed. "Merce Cunningham: Creative Elements," *choreography and dance: an international journal* Vol. 4(3) harwood academic publishers, 1997.

Sontag, Susan. "For Available Light: A Brief Lexicon," *Art in America* 71 December 1983, 102, quoted from Birringer, Johannes. *Media and Performance Along the Border.* Baltimore and London: The John Hopkins University Press, 1998.

Chapter 10

A Critical Appreciation of Dances

The Critical Appreciation of Dances

Larry Lavender

I want to tell you something about the work of appreciating dances and how I think it should be done. I use the term "work" because appreciating dances goes beyond merely enjoying them. It involves a kind of specialized attention to the specific character of each dance seen. To begin I must explain the difference between ordinary *looking* and the specialized *seeing* that is the trademark of the astute dance critic. By "ordinary looking" I mean the general human capacity to make sense of the visual environment. Critical seeing, on the other hand, is more focused and precise than this, and in fact, is a kind of overdevelopment of our general capacity for vision. Indeed, it is a luxury that is enjoyed only by those with few other pressing concerns or responsibilities.

The extra effort required for seeing a dance and other kinds of art is reserved (in Western culture, anyway) for those extraordinary occasions when one is presented specifically with *something to see,* or something *for* seeing. These occasions typically occur inside theatres, concert halls, and galleries. Such "art spaces" isolate from the general environment that which is to be seen, or attended to, and provide the physical conditions under which the specific form of attention that is required may most readily be obtained. Seats are usually comfortable and arranged to make ideal seeing possible. Lighting systems and stage masking direct vision just where it is intended to go. Acoustical systems amplify and transmit those sounds that are supposed to enter our ears and minimize or eliminate the rest. In galleries the walls are usually painted white to permit the art to stand alone in claiming attention. All of these spaces act as a kind of frame for the performance or work of art.

To engage in *informed* and *appreciative* talk, or writing, about works of art requires one to start with *focused and open-minded seeing.* Your task as a dance appreciator, then, is to attend to the work—*see* it—in a concentrated, contemplative way. Afterward, you must engage reflectively with your experience of the work, and describe its visible features. The next step will be to articulate on the basis of your experience of the work an interpretation of its meaning or significance, and perhaps to formulate a judgment of its value—i.e., the *way* in which it rewards attention and the *kind* of reward it offers.

Taken as a whole, the process is a way of showing respect to dances. Underlying this sense of respect is the knowledge that each work is what it is *by design;* it is no accident. Even when an artist uses "accidental" or "chance" procedures, the work that is made is the result of an intelligent activity of making that usually includes experimentation, decisionmaking, skilled crafting, revision, and almost always a bit of luck.

The creative making process through which works of art are made is, for many, a sacred human activity. Others consider it as nothing more or less than the application of tried and true techniques for the manipulation of specific materials. Either way, the work that stands (or moves) before our eyes is composed of details that must be perceived both individually and in relation to one another.

It is often assumed that the appreciative viewer will approach art with a set of questions in mind, or a list of "things to look for" in the work. For example, some have suggested that the perception of art should be motivated by such questions as "What is the artist trying to say here?" or, "How does this work express the character and values of its society?" While these are interesting questions, they exert too much influence on *how* the work is seen, and even on *what* is seen (and not seen) in it. For example, to approach every work armed with the question, "What is the artist saying?" is to assume that art is a kind of semantic activity, akin to speaking, through which artists "tell" the world things. But this is not the case. Many artists (in every medium) work without these kinds of intentions. Their works "say" very little, if anything, in the familiar sense of "saying something" that we link with words.

Appreciative seeing is best accomplished with a mind unburdened by preconceptions about what art is or should be, what artists are or should be up to, and what art works ultimately "mean." Those notions are certainly important, but not during the first encounter with a work. At the start, we should simply enter the world created by the work, just be with it, experience its contours, ride its currents, sense the pulse of its rhythms, allow it the opportunity to exist in perception as nothing else ever has. This attitude of openness— what some call the "aesthetic attitude"—permits the fullest experience of the work to be obtained, and puts us in a strong position later to deal with its complexities, ambiguities, and subtleties.

At this point you may ask, "Am I just supposed to *forget* everything I know about art, or *ignore* my standards of art?" The answer is "Yes and No." In the initial encounter with a work you should "forget" in the sense of suspending or putting aside for the moment your knowledge and beliefs about art and artistic assessment. Such temporary "forgetting" gives the work a chance to be seen for what it is—to exist on its own terms, so to speak— before being subjected to tests, comparisons, and interpretive or evaluative analysis. But of course you should not *literally* forget anything—you should be ready to apply to the work whatever analytical tools you have, but not during the period devoted to the *seeing*. Later, in *reflection* on the work, is when substantive analysis of it appropriately takes place. Reflective analysis may include such things as questioning the "message" of the work, or of the artist, comparing the work, to historical and/or contemporary standards of excellence, categorizing it in terms of period, style, or social function, and a host of other similar kinds of activities.

Following open-minded seeing, you must describe the work's visible features—i.e., gather the evidence and organize the impressions that comprise the basis of informed and appreciative talk about the work. Making written notes is the best way to do this. Writing permits subtle details about the work to be recalled that would be forgotten otherwise; you recollect more, and what you recollect is clearer when you write than when you just "think" or "remember."

Describing a dance sets the wheels in motion for such other operations as *interpreting* and *evaluating,* and *explaining* dances. Think of a basic description as a straightforward account of the perceptible features of the work as you experienced it; what took place, what happened, what are the basic components that make this work the particular work that it is? In writing a reflective description of a dance you state what anyone who watches it ought to be able to see. There were three dancers, for example, all wearing red, except that one had a black scarf tied around her waist. The dancers danced in unison, in a quasiballetic style that was lyrical, expansive, and featured rather quick footwork, a series of leaps, and sudden transitions to slow and sustained adagio passages. Then, the dancer with the black scarf split off and performed an introspective solo downstage while the others repeated earlier movements together upstage . . . and so on.

In providing such a descriptive account of the dance you do not *interpret* its meaning or significance; you do not, for example, assert that the black scarf symbolizes Death, or that the three dancers are creatures from another world. Nor do you *evaluate* the merit of the dance. Nor do you *explain* the dance by giving a history of the choreographer, the artistic period from which her movement is derived, or anything else that might touch on how the dance came to be. You just tell what you saw.

And yet there are complex operations going on in description. For example, the remark that the soloist came downstage as the others danced behind her was a *formal analysis* of the spatial relationship between two moving elements of the dance. And when I said that the movement style was "expansive" and "lyrical," and that the solo was "introspective," I departed from basic description to *characterize* the dance in terms of its *aesthetic qualities.*

The critical activity that I call "description," then, is composed of three things. Think of these as three dimensions of description, and practice doing each one separately, and looking for them in criticisms that you read. The three dimensions of description are: (1) *Basic information statements* about what is there to be seen, such as "three dancers in red, one with a black scarf tied around her waist." (2) *Formal analysis* statements that describe time/space relationships between and among parts of the dance. (3) *Characterizing statements* that give the mood, feeling tone, ambiance, or qualitative sense of something in the dance, or the dance as a whole.

It might seem to you that category (3) does not really fit because a characterizing statement seems more a matter of opinion, more "subjective," and less informative than basic descriptions and formal analysis statements. It is true that the same movement, or phrase, or section of a dance—indeed, an entire dance—can and probably will be characterized differently by different viewers even when their basic descriptions are compatible. Where one characterizes the slow raising of a dancer's arm as *melancholy,* another may see it as *selfabsorbed,* and a third may consider it merely a design element with no emotional importance whatsoever. But it does not follow from this that such claims are mere opinion and thus have no place in descriptive accounts.

In characterizing a dance, what you describe is not just the work as a series of physical activities, but *as you experienced it as art.* I am talking here about the difference between a dance as it occupies a particular space and time within the public world, on the one hand, and a dance as it enters into and merges with your private sensory world, on the other hand. One should write both about the dance "itself" and the dance as experienced by you, the public *and* the private dance. Characterizing statements bridge the apparent gap between these "two dances" by describing the aesthetic qualities expressed by the dance in your experience of it.

As one watches dances, one typically notices such things as lifted arms, footwork passages, black scarves, and so on. These are the plain physical properties of the dance. In reflection, one describes these things and the ways in which they relate in the dance. But in experiencing a dance *as art,* one experiences its physical properties as possessing some aesthetic quality or another, and these need also to be described. Characterizing language does this work. In my sample description I used the aesthetic quality term "introspection" to characterize the dancer's solo. Presumably I would be able to provide a *basic description* of the solo to explain my use of that aesthetic quality term. I might say, "I see the solo as introspective because the dancer's visual focus is inward, toward herself, and her movements are mostly in the near space, with gestures of wrapping around and enveloping herself. She does not relate to or engage with the space outside her kinesphere." Insofar as they are *grounded* in basic descriptions, then, characterizing statements belong in descriptive accounts. While characterizing statements do have a place in reflective description, it is nonetheless true that they point us in the direction of interpretation and evaluation.

The first thing to say about interpretation and evaluation is that they are fundamentally different from description. When I say "description" I mean the three distinct operations we just finished discussing (basic informative statements, formal analysis, and characterization). All of those, and the focused seeing on which they are based, comprise "exploratory criticism." This term refers to all the work we do in the interest of *coming to know* the dance as it exists in perception.

In contrast to exploratory criticism, "argumentative criticism" is composed of the operations of interpretation and evaluation. Through these operations we make *arguments* that the work is most appropriately understood in one way or another, that its *value* is of such and such a kind, and that this value may be found in, or obtained from, the work to this or that degree. Whereas exploratory criticism does not try to *convince* anyone of anything, but merely to *report* on what is there to be experienced in the work and how it was experienced, argumentative criticism does seek to convince others to understand and to value the work in one way rather than another.

Exploratory and *argumentative* criticism work hand in hand; we have the best chance of being convincing in our arguments if we have done good exploratory work and are thus able to employ descriptive information to support our conclusions. Without descriptive support, interpretations and evaluations are just *unsubstantiated* claims, rather like idle speculations.

A critical interpretation makes a *claim* about the meaning of the dance. Specifically, it claims that the dance is best seen as having one particular meaning or another. The term "meaning" itself has multiple meanings. For our purposes the meaning of the dance is what it is seen as "being about," or "expressing," or "communicating." All those terms are as philosophically slippery as "meaning," of course, but they have ordinary uses with which you are familiar. Generally, the "meaning" of a work of art is what one "gets from it," or finds it to "be about."

Interpretation is thus a matter of describing how and why a work is best, or at least reasonably, seen in terms of meaning. For example, the introspective solo I described, and the work in which it appears, can be interpreted as signifying the virtue of following one's personal path despite its departure from the norm. To make this interpretation strong I will need to gather descriptive evidence to support it such that others may reflect on their experience of the dance and say, "Yes, I see what you mean."

Often the same work will give rise to two or more reasonable interpretations. It is possible, for example, that another viewer will see the introspective solo and the dance as a whole, not as a validation of individualism but as a warning against it; a cautionary tale of the loneliness and loss that can befall the rebel who departs from custom. It is neither a weakness in art nor a flaw in criticism when multiple interpretations of the same work arise, it just happens. When we meet rival interpretations of the same work we must return attention to the work itself, and to whatever information about it that an interpreter might have drawn from other sources, and evaluate the soundness of each interpretation. The point is not to find the "true" interpretation, for there is none. But there are complete and satisfying ones, interpretations that afford a good match with the work as we experience it.

The idea of interpretation I am advancing decentralizes what artists say about their works, putting them in the same position as others in terms of making an interpretation. A work cannot be said to mean something because the artist *says* that is what it means. The artist may certainly be sincere in having intended or hoped that the work would mean one thing or another, but that sincerity and those hopes do not necessarily mean the artist has done what she intended. Thus an artist no less than other viewers must draw upon descriptive evidence to persuade others of the reasonableness of her interpretations. The same holds for *evaluative* claims that seek to convince us of the merit or value of a work.

I want to say one more thing about interpretation as it fits into my general theory of dance criticism. The theory described in this chapter is a theory of *aesthetic* criticism because it concerns itself first and foremost with the visible features of the work of art—in our case, dances. Thus the theory prioritizes descriptions, analyses, and characterizations of what we see when watching the dance, and these form the primary basis of subsequent interpretations and evaluations.

Yet there are other dimensions of art besides the aesthetic, and other ways to investigate and talk about works of art. For example, one could focus on the *biographical* details and personal idiosyncrasies of artists, and research how they live, how they come to do what they do, and what they think about their lives and work. Or, one could concentrate on the *psychology* of responses to art, the reactions people have to works of different kinds, and the sorts of things people say about them. In a more academic vein, one could devote energy to grouping and classifying works of art in terms of period, style, genre, and the like. Such *art-historical* inquiry helps us to make sense of art across the ages and to recognize our place in the broader histories of art. Separate from these modes of inquiry, or perhaps together with them, one might investigate the social and cultural roles that artworks, or things like artworks, play in different societies. *Cultural/anthropological* inquiry prevails in many quarters today as members of various cultural groups feel an urgency to understand one another.

I admire all of these modes of inquiry—the biographical, psychological, art-historical, and cultural/anthropological—for the richness of the various dimensions of art each mode permits us to discover. Yet I place the direct encounter with the work as an aesthetic entity at the heart of my critical method. The reason is that it is only on the basis of the work of art as an aesthetic entity that the other modes of inquiry may even emerge. Without the *aesthetic facts* of art works—their *intrinsic* features—there is no further inquiry into art, for there is no art in the first place. Thus, my method of criticism is one in which the proper place to begin is with the work itself. I argue further that those who are sufficiently disciplined to come to know and understand art works aesthetically will make the most meaningful contributions to the discussions going on in the other modes of inquiry.

I turn now to the often-controversial topic of evaluation, or judgment. There are many who think that art should not be judged because judgment is really just an expression of personal opinion. Behind this claim is often found the notion that there is an insurmountable barrier between "objectivity" and "subjectivity." All criticism, on this view, is subjective and so critical judgments—if they even exist—are a folly because they just pretend to possess objectivity they can never actually have.

I disagree with the above line of thinking for several reasons. First, whether critical judgments are objective, subjective, or something else, the dance world is built upon and sustained by them; judgments keep the engines of the dance world running. Dance historians judge which works best exemplify an artist's style. Critics are widely expected to judge the works they review, and choreography teachers must evaluate students' works if the notion of "teaching choreography" is to retain any semblance of meaning. For dance professionals in these and other domains to abandon judgments would be absurd, and probably not possible.

As for the suspicion that judgments are merely "subjective opinion" and thus of no use, the accusation itself is false and the conclusion incorrect. Criticism in general, and judgments in particular, are *both* objective and subjective. Judgments are objective (rational, reasonable, intelligible) insofar as they direct attention to aspects of works of art that are there plainly to be seen, and provide comprehensible readings of those aspects, and thus of the works whose aspects they are. At the same time criticism is unashamedly subjective in the sense that the evaluative conclusions a critic reaches about art, and the ways she organizes and presents evidence in support of them, are *her* ways of doing these things; her critical perspectives are *uniquely* hers. If we find them to be clearly and persuasively presented and our appreciation of the work under review is enhanced, we might adopt her perspectives as our own. This is an important *function* of judgments in criticism: they invite us to understand, and perhaps to embrace perspectives that we might not otherwise have gained.

Critical judgments are objective also in dealing with facts and ideas drawn from the work, as well as from the history and philosophy of art, and from the skills and knowledge that compose a particular art discipline. But since criticism deals equally well with the emotional, feeling "sides" of life, and of art, judgments are also subjective. Critics regularly include in judgment references to their emotional states and feelings as well as to feelings and emotions they find expressed in the work. But like a good critic, you need to make such references clear by grounding them in description. If you do this, the alleged contradiction between "objective" and "subjective" falls away as a threat to judgment.

The important thing to ask is how well a particular judgment incorporates and deals with what we can see in the work, and how relevant to the work are the *reasons* provided in support of the judgment? Judgments are not always directly stated, but are found embedded within or implied by descriptive passages. But all judgments boil down to the basic form: "the work is good (or poor) because . . ." and then a reason is provided. A good evaluative reason forges a link between visible features of the work and standards of value appropriate to the work.

It is not always clear what sorts of standards are appropriate to the evaluation of works of art, and no one can provide a definitive list of standards. I can say this: there are *aesthetic* standards that appear to hold across the fine arts, and there are *artistic* standards that arise out of specific art disciplines. In classical ballet, for example, standards of judgment have evolved in tandem with ideas about what composes good ballet *dancing:* pointed feet, clear body lines, grace and lightness of motion, etc. Related standards stipulate the qualities of good ballet *choreography:* architecturally clear formations, qualitative adherence to the music, intricately designed steps, and the like. Critical standards like these grow up around all artistic disciplines; it is part of what makes a certain body of knowledge and skills a "discipline" in the first place.

It is important to note that some art disciplines—modern dance, for example—traditionally have valued "breaking the rules." We might say that breaking the rules is itself one of the "rules" of modern dance. For this reason, the tradition of modern dance is one of those that philosophers of art call a "transgressive tradition." (To transgress means to go beyond a boundary or limit.)

As concerns *aesthetic* standards, I will explain three of those historically used within the Western fine arts tradition and which remain in wide use today. Works of art are often evaluated in terms of *unity,* the ways in which their elements or parts fit together to form a coherent whole. Exhibiting unity is generally considered to be a good thing in art, but obviously this is not always the case. Many works of art, particularly within the last century or so, have been deliberately chaotic, disorganized, and lacking in unity. Thus the evaluative question is not whether a work has unity, or how much unity it has, but *in what ways* whatever unity, or disunity the work exhibits functions within the work. Many dances in which the performers face front, dance in unison, stay in precise rhythmic relation with the music, and remain in the same spatial configuration are judged as weak because the unity of elements undermines visual and/or emotional/intellectual interest. On the other hand, cluttered and busy dances often collapse into messes because too much is going on that does not relate to anything else.

Another traditional category of value is *complexity.* As in the case of unity, what matters is *how* complexity is made to function within a work, what kind of necessity it is seen as having. In many dances, for example, the dance idea is relatively simple and can be expressed without much complication among choreographic elements. In these cases, the work is valued in part because it has just the complexity needed to express its idea, and no more than that. Other dances are found insufficiently complex (or overly simple). In these cases perhaps the dance idea demands for its expression more or different kinds of complexity than the choreographer recognizes or is able to deliver.

A third traditional and widely used criterion of value in art is that of *intensity of quality.* I discussed aesthetic qualities earlier in relation to characterizing statements having to do with the mood, or ambiance, of the work.

In dance, the term "aesthetic quality" refers to aspects of movement that critics describe with such words as "agitated," "billowy," "calm," "convulsive," "delicate," "effusive," and the like. There are hundreds of such words. It is recognized that we discern such qualities through our perception of the basic *physical properties* of a work. We may, for example, see a dancer running across the stage and glancing back over her shoulder. But in seeing this we may also see expressed in it the quality of *frightened anxiety,* or perhaps of *playful teasing.* The movements of running and glancing back over the shoulder will produce entirely different aesthetic qualities depending on *how* the dancer performs those movements, her *manner* of doing so.

A dancer in rehearsal may be asked to perform the running/glancing sequence in several ways to generate different aesthetic qualities that the choreographer wants to try out. "Do it as though you were being pursued," the choreographer might say. Or, "try it as though you were teasing your lover." Similarly, a dancer may be asked to perform a sequence first as if she were a rag doll, then as a princess, and finally as an angry child. If the choreographer has a specific aesthetic quality in mind, the dancer may be prompted to produce that quality. "Improvise something *pulsating* and *jubilant*," the choreographer might say, or "do that sequence again in a *rowdy* and *raucous* manner." Each of these prompts will change the quality expressed in the movement. Through such prompts, accomplished dancers can deliver a broad range of clear qualitative "statements" in movement. Indeed, this is partly what it means to be an accomplished dancer. The richness of dancers' capacity to make fine-grained qualitative adjustments to movement provides for a richness of expression in dance. Similarly, language gives you all you need to characterize danced expression. You must work as diligently at your part of the bargain as dancers work at theirs.

In making judgments, critical viewers often remark on the richness, or *intensity*, of the aesthetic qualities they discern in dances, and discuss how these qualities contribute to the meaning and value of the work. Again, the important thing is not how intensely a quality is exhibited, or even what quality it is, but the appropriateness of *that* degree of intensity of *that* particular quality, or set of qualities, in *this* work.

It is important here to note that the evaluative standards related to unity, complexity, and intensity of quality are central to the Western fine arts tradition. Briefly, the main purpose of art within that tradition is to capture and reward aesthetic attention rather than, say, to summon or control forces of nature, to ward off or attract spiritual entities, or to mark the significant occasions within a social group. While there is ample evidence that artistic activities in all cultures have developed around some notion of visual and/or aesthetic appearances, it is not safe to assume that aesthetic standards particular to one culture are relevant to the art of others. Certainly it is a mistake to think that Western fine arts standards are superior to those by which the art of other cultures may be understood and evaluated. As concerns such art, the critical operations of interpretation and evaluation must be undertaken with caution. For each cultural tradition generates its arts (whether or not that term is used) out of its own necessities and in its own ways, and these may elude the understanding of outsiders. Thus the artistic and cultural practices of one culture may not be assimilated to those of another. This means that the art of cultures less technically advanced than those in the West may not legitimately be seen either as on the same developmental curve as the Western fine arts tradition, or as part of a developmental curve inferior to that one. In fact there is no hierarchy of artistic traditions such that one or another is superior to, or farther along the "true path of art" than the others. Each viewer, when faced with the art of another culture, should try to learn as much as can be learned by an "outsider" about its inherent values. Attempts to evaluate the art of other cultures strictly in terms of the values of one's own are misguided and ultimately shed little light.

On the other hand, it is perfectly all right to mention the fact that art from another culture satisfies aesthetic attention in some or all of the same ways as art from within one's culture. It is commonplace to discover that Chinese art, for example, exhibits some or all of the aesthetic qualities that members of other cultures value in "their" art. There is no reason to shy away from this, and there is no reason to imagine of any culture that "their concept of art" is all that different from yours; while "their" art might be quite different, the reasons people everywhere draw, paint, carve, dance, compose music, literature, and verse have more in common than they have differences.

I hope it is clear that while there are no definitive standards of value for art, there are in wide use *artistic* standards derived from specific art disciplines, and *aesthetic* standards derived from the Western fine arts tradition. It is important to develop your own stance with regard to these standards, as well as to maintain a mind open to stances adopted by other artists and viewers. Your standards for evaluating art will ideally arise through a merging of your perceptual attention and your capacity for open engagement with works of art, on the one hand, and the values and qualities found alone and in relation with one another within each work, on the other hand. Critical evaluation is a complex transaction whose success depends less on what standards you employ and more on how clear, complete, articulate, passionate, and reasonable you are in connecting those standards—i.e., showing their relevance—to *each particular* work. With practice you will find that engaging in the activities of critical appreciation will enhance your own and others' experiences of dances, and other works of art.

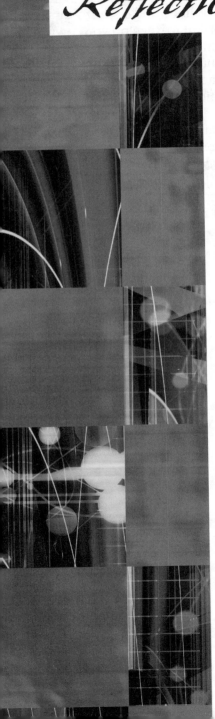

Reflection Journal

Chapter 1:
Native American Dances of
New Mexico

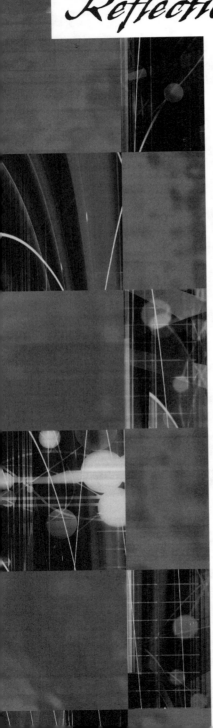

Reflection Journal

Chapter 2:
Mexican and New Mexican
Dances

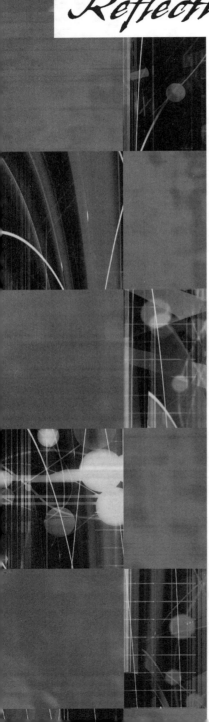

Reflection Journal

Chapter 3:
Flamenco Dance

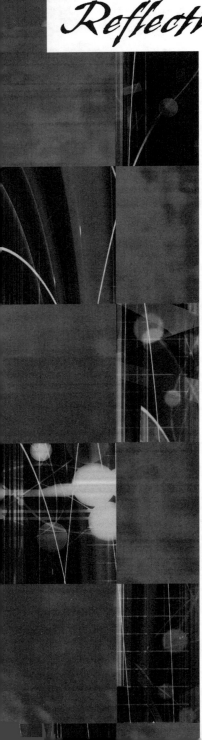

Reflection Journal

Chapter 4:
Modern Dance

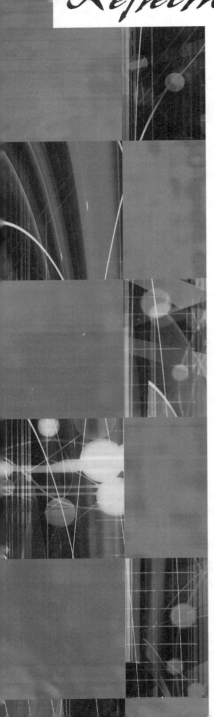

Reflection Journal

Chapter 5:
Ballet

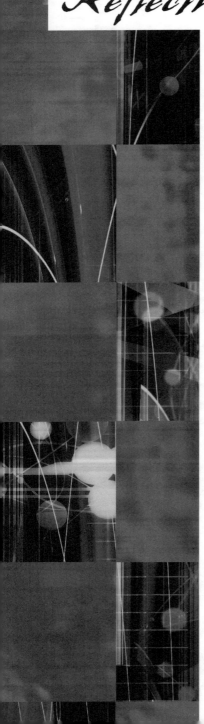

Reflection Journal

Chapter 6:
African American
Influences on Dance

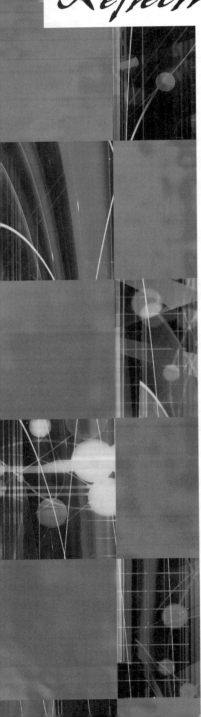

Reflection Journal

Chapter 7:
Dance in India

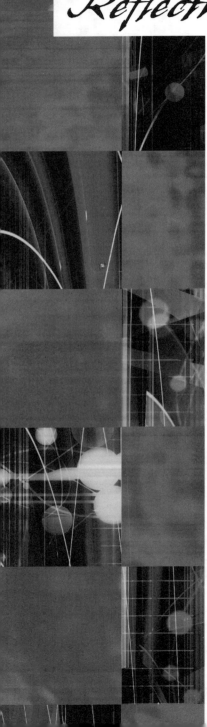

Reflection Journal

Chapter 8:
Dance in Film

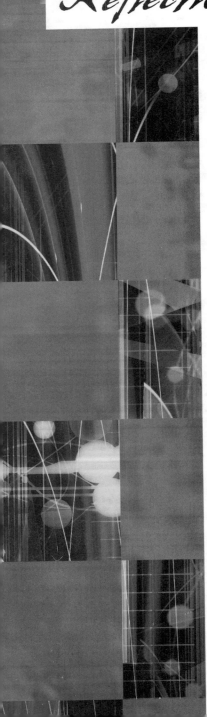

Reflection Journal

Chapter 9:
Dance and Video
Technology

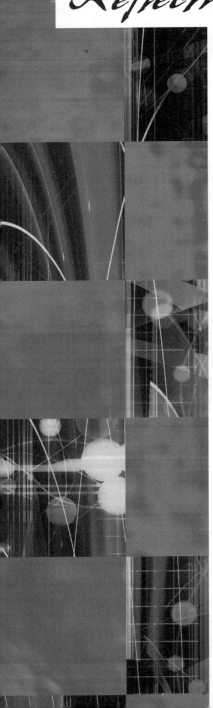

Reflection Journal

Chapter 10:
A Critical Appreciation
of Dances

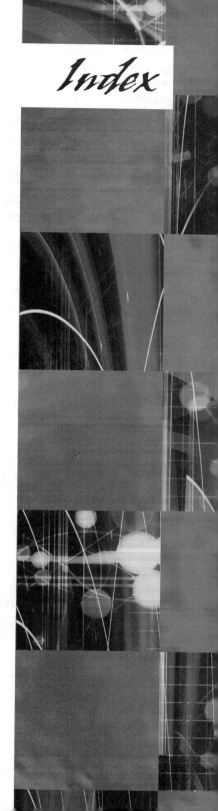

Index